The Nuts and Bolts
of Implantable
Device Therapy
Pacemakers

The Nuts and Bolts of Implantable Device Therapy Pacemakers

Tom Kenny, FHRS, CCDS

Director of Education, PrepMD, Braintree, MA, USA

WILEY Blackwell

Library of Congress Cataloging-in-Publication Data

Kenny, Tom, 1954– , author.
   The nuts and bolts of implantable device therapy pacemakers / Tom Kenny.
      p. ; cm.
   Includes index.
   ISBN 978-1-118-67067-5 (pbk.)
   I. Title.
   [DNLM: 1. Cardiac Pacing, Artificial–methods.   2. Pacemaker, Artificial.   WG 168]
   RC684.P3
   617.4′120645–dc23

                          2014027299

A catalogue record for this book is available from the British Library.

Cover images: © iStock.com/angelhel; © iStock.com/RASimon

Wiley also publishes its books in a variety of electronic formats. Some content that appears in print may not be available in electronic books.

Set in 9.5/12pt Minion by SPi Publisher Services, Pondicherry, India

1   2015

Contents

Preface

Cardiac pacing has changed dramatically in the past decades, and yet certain things have not changed at all. While technology has advanced cardiac pacing to provide benefits to more and more patients while streamlining device function and downsizing the pulse generators, cardiac pacing is still a field that can be difficult to learn and slow to master. Those who become cardiac pacing specialists are those who take the time to learn the concepts, work systematically through follow-up, and listen carefully to their patients. It has been more than three decades since I entered the cardiac rhythm management field and two decades since I wrote my first workbook on pacing to assist those trying to learn the field—and while everyone talks about how much cardiac pacing has changed in the past decades, it strikes me how much has stayed the same.

After all, it is still about a battery, a wire in the heart, and timing tiny electrical pulses to fire at precisely the right split-second. It is still about knowing rate and mode and being able to find a pacing spike on an ECG. And it is still about restoring as near-to-normal a cardiac rhythm as possible to our patients.

For those embarking on a career in cardiac pacing or clinicians who just need to know more about device-based cardiac rhythm management therapy, it is my hope that this book will help break down some of the complexities of this cardiac pacing. Cardiac pacing can seem overwhelmingly complex because it involves the simultaneous interplay of many different factors. Somebody once told me that there are more than a million possible device parameter combinations available in today's most advanced pacemakers. So how does a busy clinician find that one-in-a-million pacing prescription? The number of options may have changed, but it is still about the basics. You find the right mode. The right rate. You program an AV delay. You just work through the programming one simple step at a time. For those willing to learn the concepts and approach things systematically, cardiac pacing can be mastered.

It has always been about the patient and how that patient interacts with the pacemaker. Our patients come to the clinic—often nervous about their new "battery-powered" status—and expect to find in us clinicians both expertise and reassurance. I hope this book conveys my sentiment that the greatest expert is one who not only knows what to do but also knows how to talk warmly, frankly, and helpfully to each and every patient.

Tom Kenny
November 2014

Acknowledgments

Nobody writes a book alone, even if there is just one name on the front cover. First, I must acknowledge with deep gratitude my students, past and present, over the years. From these men and women I have learned a great deal about the kind of person who seeks a career in device-based therapy and how to break down difficult concepts to make them not just understandable but logical. I think every time one of my students had an "ah-ha!" moment, I had one too! I hope that my instruction, my explanations, my anecdotes, and my method of teaching serve you well in your future clinical work. I would also like to thank my mentors that have taught me so much over the years. I know much of what I know because of people like Orlando Maytin, Michael Chizner, Kathy King, Barbara Perra, and Eliot Ostrow. Thank you for sharing your clinical expertise and sparking my interest in cardiology.

Second, I want to thank my friends and family who supported me in the writing of this book.

I owe a great debt to my publishers, who not only believed in this project but who went the extra mile to make it a reality.

Third, I must thank my editor, Jo Ann LeQuang, who assisted in all of the work that goes into turning a course into a manuscript. She worked with me on my very first workbook when I worked in industry and she was a key contributor to this project as well. I want to thank Matt O'Neal, Bob Matioli, and all of the folks at PrepMD, where I work today, for their support and encouragement with this project.

Finally, I want to thank the many people who encouraged me to write about cardiac pacing. No matter how much I teach this subject, lecture on it, or write about it—I still have a lot to say! That shows the depth of this subject and also my passion for it. It is my wish that this book not just informs future pacing experts but inspires them as well.

CHAPTER 1

Cardiovascular anatomy and physiology

Learning objectives

- Point out the key landmarks in the human heart relevant to cardiac rhythm management.
- Name the four chambers of the heart, the four valves, and the major vessels.
- Describe the flow of blood through the heart.
- Define AV synchrony and explain why it is important.
- State the difference between the body's arterial versus venous systems.

Introduction

An encyclopedia could be written on the anatomy and physiology of the human heart, and that is not our purpose. Device clinicians must understand the cardiovascular system to understand arrhythmias and device therapy. This chapter will introduce the important concepts of cardiac anatomy and physiology necessary for an understanding of cardiac rhythm management. To that end, this chapter will describe the chambers, valves, and major vessels of the heart and how these control the flow of blood in the body. Although we think of the heart—rightly—as a pump, it also possesses a complex electrical system. The cells of the human heart are unique in many ways, and how they produce, conduct, and dissipate electrical energy is very important, particularly to pacing. Our goal here is to describe the anatomy and physiology of the healthy heart and cardiovascular system in terms of what device clinicians need to know.

The healthy heart

The human heart is a double pump (right and left) that sits in the middle of the chest, slightly to the left, and rotated so that the right side is more anterior than the left. An average adult human heart is relatively large, about 13 by 9 by 6 cm and weighing about 300 g. The heart is protected by the rib cage and sits directly behind one of the body's thickest bones, the sternum. The bottom of the heart rests on the diaphragm muscle. The heart is encased in this protected but somewhat crowded area—it also contains the lungs (three lobes on the right, two on the left), the stomach, and the intestines.

The bottom tip of the heart (called the apex) taps up against the chest when the heart contracts. By placing his hands on the chest, a physician can feel the place where the apex of the heart makes contact with the chest; this place is called the point of maximal impulse (PMI). Knowing the precise location of the PMI can be very useful in treating cardiology patients, because the PMI of a healthy heart occurs slightly to the left, while the PMI of a person with an enlarged heart is going to occur much farther to the left, even off to the side. A healthy heart is roughly the size of the fist, but when hearts enlarge, such as occurs with disease progression, the enlargement occurs toward the left. Thus, PMI can

The Nuts and Bolts of Implantable Device Therapy Pacemakers, First Edition. Tom Kenny.
© 2015 John Wiley & Sons, Ltd. Published 2015 by John Wiley & Sons, Ltd.

provide a fast, noninvasive way of determining if and to what degree the heart has enlarged.

The left ventricle composes most of the mass of the heart, being by far the largest of the four pumping chambers. A healthy heart circulates about 4–6 l of blood a minute—which is the entire blood volume of the body! That means the entire circulating volume of blood in the body moves around every minute or once per beat.

The heart consists of four chambers: two upper chambers called atria (singular atrium) and two lower and larger chambers called ventricles. To understand the healthy heart, it is useful to think of the heart in terms of right side (right atrium and right ventricle) and left side (left atrium and left ventricle). The right side of the heart circulates deoxygenated blood to the lungs (where it can be oxygenated). The left side of the heart pumps oxygenated blood out to the rest of the body (see **Figure 1.1**).

The heart is a muscle and consists of four distinct layers. The endocardium is the innermost layer and composes a lining for the interior of the heart. The epicardium is the outer layer of the heart. Between the endocardium and epicardium lies the myocardium—the thickest layer—which is muscle. The entire heart is encased in a

liquid-filled sac called the pericardium, which acts like a shock absorber for the heart. The pericardial sac contains about 15–20 cc of pericardial fluid in a healthy individual. In the event that fluid builds up to abnormally high levels in the pericardial sac (such as might occur when a lead or catheter inside the heart perforates the endocardium, myocardium, and epicardium and goes exterior to the heart), this fluid can place pressure on the heart in a condition known as cardiac tamponade. Since the heart is contained in a relatively small space, this pressure can compromise the heart's ability to fill with blood and pump efficiently. During device implantation, perforation is an important concern because it can lead to cardiac tamponade. In the event that perforation results in cardiac tamponade, a needle is inserted into the pericardial sac (through the chest wall) to drain the blood. Lead perforation does not always result in cardiac tamponade, but it is a serious concern.

Blood flow through the heart

The heart is a pump and it is located amid a network of vessels that carry deoxygenated blood into the right side of the heart and reoxygenated blood into the left side of the heart. The flow is actually

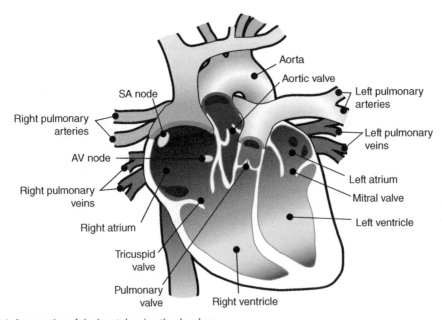

Figure 1.1 Cross section of the heart showing the chambers.

fairly simple. Deoxygenated blood enters the right side of the heart and is pumped over to the lungs via the pulmonary arteries and is returned back (as oxygen-rich blood) to the left side of the heart by way of the pulmonary veins (PV). While both right and left sides of the heart contract at the same time as a single unit, the right side is busy pumping deoxygenated blood to the lungs, while the left side is pumping reoxygenated blood out to the rest of the body.

Deoxygenated blood enters the right side of the heart via the superior vena cava (SVC), but once it has become oxygenated again, blood is pumped back out from the left side of the heart into the aorta. The aorta is the largest vessel in the body, and it forms a U shape at the top of the heart. These portions of the aorta are called the *ascending*, the *descending*, and the *arch*. Coming off the aortic arch are three main arteries: the left subclavian artery, the left common carotid artery, and the brachiocephalic trunk.

To better understand the blood flow through the heart, it is important to review the structure of the heart. The atria or upper chambers of the heart are smaller, have thinner walls, and are smoother on the inside than the ventricles. Within the ventricles is a network of fibrous strands known as trabeculae. These structural differences become important in lead implantation within the heart; it is much easier to affix or lodge a lead in the trabeculae of the ventricles than to try to anchor the lead to a smooth atrial wall. Historically, atrial leads have almost always been active-fixation screw-in-type leads, while ventricular leads were almost always passive-fixation leads (fins or tines that lodge in the trabeculae). Today, active-fixation leads are often used in both chambers since they facilitate lead removal (**Figure 1.2**).

Overall, blood flow to the heart is discussed, *right* and *left* sides, although it is important to recognize that what happens in the heart, that is, systole (contraction) and diastole (relaxation), are happening on both sides at the same time. The right atrium of the heart receives blood from the SVC, the inferior vena cava (IVC), and the coronary sinus (CS). The CS is technically a vein and it has an opening or ostium (sometimes just called *os*) at the base of the right atrium, slightly posterior. The CS delivers oxygen-depleted blood

to the right atrium from the coronary arteries that encircle the exterior of the heart. The CS is of interest in cardiac resynchronization therapy (CRT) because the left ventricular lead is passed through the CS (counter to the flow of blood) in order to be placed into the coronary vessels to pace the left ventricle. CRT is used in patients with heart failure, whose hearts have remodeled, that is, enlarged and changed shape. (It may be said that with heart failure, the heart changes from the shape of a football to the shape of a basketball!) The CS may be relocated in this remodeling, which can be challenging in implanting a CRT lead because the physician must first locate the os of the CS and then navigate through it in order to implant the left ventricular lead.

Anatomically, the heart is dominated by the large muscle mass of the left ventricle, which makes up about two-thirds of the heart in terms of weight and volume. This greater size is typically ascribed to the fact that the left ventricle must pump blood throughout the whole body, whereas the right ventricle only has to pump blood to the lungs. The left and right ventricles pump blood to different destinations, but the left ventricle is larger and more muscular for a reason—pressure. It is important to review the pressures against which the heart must work to understand cardiac blood flow (**Figure 1.3**).

Deoxygenated blood in the right side of the heart must travel over the lungs to pick up oxygen. This means that blood in the right ventricle travels across the pulmonary valve into the pulmonary artery and then out toward the lungs. The pulmonary valve opens automatically when pressure from the contracting right ventricle forces it open. This occurs *when the pressure in the right ventricle exceeds the pressure in the pulmonary artery.* Pressure gradients are key concepts in understanding blood flow. Valves are like gates that open and close in response to pressure. In general, the pressure in the PV is fairly low, around 12 mmHg. Thus, the right ventricle does not need to create a lot of force to open the pulmonary valve.

Meanwhile, as the left ventricle contracts, it creates pressure on the aortic valve, leading to the aorta. In order to open the aortic valve and pump blood out into the aorta, the heart must overcome the pressure in the aortic valve. Pressure in the

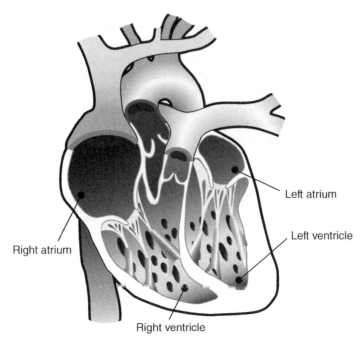

Figure 1.2 Note that the atria are smooth walled, while the ventricles contain a spongelike fibrous network of trabeculae.

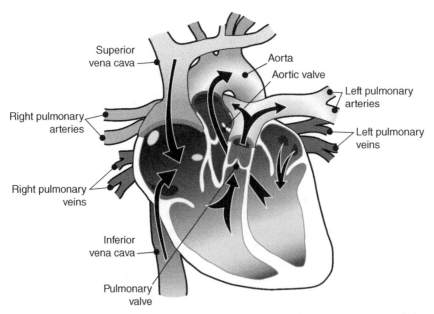

Figure 1.3 The blood flow within the heart takes oxygen-depleted blood from the body into the right atrium, where it flows to the right ventricle and is pumped out over the lungs; the reoxygenated blood from the lungs is pumped into the left atrium where it flows to the left ventricle and is pumped out via the aorta to the body.

aorta is high, around 120 mmHg or *ten times higher* than the pressure in the PV. The left ventricle must therefore work much harder to pump blood than the right ventricle. This requires the left ventricle to be larger and more muscular than the right ventricle (see **Figure 1.4**).

On the right side of the heart, blood travels from the right atrium into the right ventricle via the tricuspid valve. The tricuspid valve gets its name from its characteristic shape involving three leaves or cusps. Attached to these cusps are cords that anchor into the base of the ventricle; known as chordae tendineae, they look almost like little parachutes. The strands of the chordae tendineae attach to tiny papillary muscles. These chords attach to the valve leaves at one end and a papillary muscle at the other end. On the right side of the heart, the tricuspid valve is associated with three papillary muscles. The purpose of these chords and muscles is to assure that the valve is

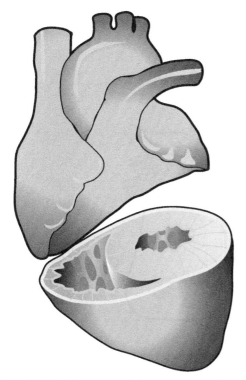

Figure 1.4 The left ventricular is far more muscular than the right ventricle because it must overcome 10 times the pressure of the right ventricle in order to pump blood out via the aortic valve and into the aorta.

effectively closed and opened at the proper times (**Figure 1.5**).

The heart can rightly be thought of as a pump, but it must be remembered that the heart is also a muscle and all muscles need a steady supply of oxygen-rich blood. The heart muscle is supplied with blood through a network of coronary arteries that surround the outside of the heart. Blockage in a coronary artery results in ischemia, which can lead to death of cardiac muscle, including the chordae tendineae and papillary muscles. While the patient may survive such an ischemic event, the damage to the heart may lead to an incompetent valve, that is, a valve that is no longer able to function effectively.

In tracing the blood flow from the right ventricle to the pulmonary artery, it should be clear that the blood has to go from *down* in the right ventricle to *up* through the pulmonary valve and into the pulmonary artery. The blood is able to make this journey because of the pumping pressure of the heart. The route the blood takes as it exits the right ventricle and journeys up toward the pulmonary valve is known as the right ventricular outflow tract (RVOT). On the other side of the heart, there is also a corresponding left ventricular outflow tract (LVOT) of approximately the same size. Cardiac leads are sometimes fixated in the RVOT (see **Figure 1.6**).

Blood pumped out of the right ventricle crosses the pulmonary valve and enters the pulmonary artery, which splits into two branches: right and left. The right pulmonary artery takes blood to the right lung, while the left pulmonary artery takes blood to the left lung. In this respect, the pulmonary artery is unique in the body in that it is an artery but it carries deoxygenated blood! Blood travels through the lung to the alveoli where it gains oxygen and loses carbon dioxide. Once it is reoxygenated, the blood gathers into the PV (which are also unique being the only veins to carry oxygenated blood). There are four PV in total; the two right-sided PV take oxygenated blood from the right lung, while the two left-sided PV take oxygenated blood from the left lung, and they all bring this reoxygenated blood to the left atrium.

The left atrium is smooth walled, like the right atrium, and although the left atrium is much

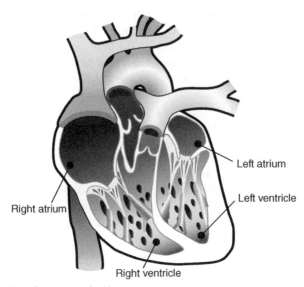

Right atrium

Left atrium

Left ventricle

Right ventricle

Figure 1.5 The leaflets of the valves are attached by chordae tendineae at one end and papillary muscles on the other, which assure the effective opening and closing of the valves.

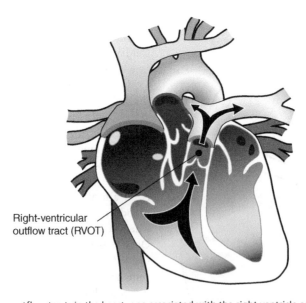

Right-ventricular
outflow tract (RVOT)

Figure 1.6 There are two outflow tracts in the heart, one associated with the right ventricle and the other the left ventricle. These outflow tracts are roughly the same size. The illustration shows the right ventricular outflow tract (RVOT), a preferred location for right ventricular lead fixation. The left ventricular outflow tract (LVOT) cannot be seen in this illustration, as it is posterior.

smaller than the left ventricle, it is larger than the right atrium. The blood will travel from the left atrium into the left ventricle by way of the mitral valve. The mitral valve gets its name from the miter, a bishop's hat. The mitral valve has two cusps and papillary muscles connected by chordae tendineae. Once blood is in the left ventricle, a contraction will force it toward the aorta by way of the LVOT. In persons with hypertrophic obstructive cardiomyopathy (HOCM), the septum or wall in the heart can become thick and enlarged, effectively narrowing the LVOT. In the healthy heart, the blood flows up the LVOT, across the aortic valve, and into the aorta. From the aorta, blood will be directed upward toward the head, downward toward the legs and feet, and some blood will be redirected back to the coronary arteries of the heart.

The blood flow from the left ventricle to the aorta and back to the coronary arteries is unique in the body in that *most of that flow occurs during diastole rather than systole.* Think of it this way: as blood is pumped by the left ventricle during systole upward and downward, to the brain and the rest of the body, some of that blood flows back during diastole and drains into the coronary arteries. Although it may seem counterintuitive, it is important to remember that coronary artery perfusion occurs primarily during diastole.

Volume, valves, and pressure

While it is tempting to think of the heart as simply a pump with an electrical system, it is more accurate to say that the heart moves blood because of variations in volume and pressure.

The heart has four valves: two are atrioventricular (AV) valves because they connect the atrium to the ventricle and two are semilunar valves, connecting the heart with pulmonary arteries or the aorta. The right AV valve is the tricuspid, while the left AV valve is the mitral valve. The flow or movement of blood is guided and controlled by the heart's muscular action in the form of systole (contraction) or diastole (relaxation).

When blood pours into the right atrium, it distends and expands the right atrium. When this volume of blood creates sufficient pressure, it forces the tricuspid valve open. Think of it as volume creating pressure and pressure opening valves. When the tricuspid valve opens, the blood dumps into the right ventricle. During this period of diastole, blood pours into the right ventricle, creating volume and expanding it. As blood pours in and ventricular diastole nears the end, the atria contract while the AV valves are still open in something nicknamed *atrial kick. Atrial systole occurs at the end of ventricular diastole.* Atrial kick forces the maximum amount of blood from the atria into the ventricles. It is estimated that atrial kick delivers 20–30% of cardiac output.

The atrial contribution to ventricular filling (atrial kick) is of enormous clinical significance. Patients with certain atrial arrhythmias, such as atrial fibrillation (AF), lose atrial kick. Even milder forms of atrial tachyarrhythmias may compromise atrial kick. Moreover, patients who do not have AV synchrony (one atrial beat corresponding to one ventricular beat) will lose atrial kick. The loss of atrial kick can reduce cardiac output by 20–30%.

Once the atria have contracted and the ventricles are filled with blood, the AV valves snap closed. The ventricles now start to contract and push open the semilunar valves. For example, as the right ventricle contracts (systole), it opens the PV. (The PV is sometimes called the pulmonic valve; it's the same thing.) The whole process works on volume, pressure, and contraction/relaxation.

Of the four valves in the heart, the tricuspid valve is of most interest to device specialists, because at least one lead will be placed into the right ventricle. This means that pacing and defibrillation leads typically cross the tricuspid valve. These leads may interfere with the proper closing of the tricuspid valve, particularly if the lead is large diameter or several leads are passed over the tricuspid valve. A single lead through the tricuspid valve is likely to cause minimal to no dysfunction. However, it is not unusual to see patients with three or more leads in the right ventricle, and these leads may hamper the tricuspid valve in its closing, leading to tricuspid regurgitation or backflow of blood. Patients with multiple leads (such as children who grow up with pacemakers) may need to have some of them removed to avoid tricuspid regurgitation.

Right ventricular leads are typically fixated at the right ventricular apex or in the RVOT and may be

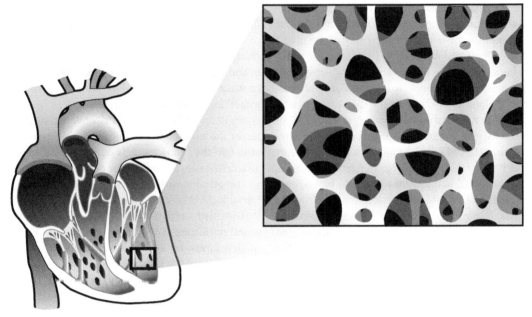

Figure 1.7 Trabeculae form a fibrous network within the ventricles. Passive-fixation ventricular leads are held in place by lodging their tines or fins in the trabeculae.

lodged in the trabeculae. Trabeculae are a fibrous network that could be described as similar to the pores of a sponge (see **Figure 1.7**).

On the left side of the heart, the blood flow pattern is similar. Blood flows into the left atrium, over the open mitral valve, and into the left atrium. At the end of ventricular diastole, as the ventricle is distended and stretched, atrial kick delivers more blood into left ventricle. The volume of blood creates pressure. The mitral valve closes. As the left ventricle contracts, the growing pressure overcomes the resistance on the aortic valve and it opens, allowing blood to flow out into the aorta and beyond.

While any valve can become diseased or dysfunctional, valvular disease more commonly affects the mitral and the aortic valves (left-sided valves) than the right-sided valves (tricuspid and pulmonary). These left valves are more likely to suffer damage or disease because of the high-pressure environment in which they function, exposing them to more potential damage. Other damage can occur when plaque builds up in the coronary arteries and the aorta. The aorta can become

diseased, typically in the case of an aortic aneurysm or dissection. Carotid arteries in the neck are also frequently a site for atherosclerotic disease.

The right atrial appendage

The right atrial appendage (RAA) is an area near the right atrium, which is a preferred site for attaching active-fixation atrial leads (see **Figure 1.8**). The RAA serves no obvious purpose and may be sacrificed in certain heart surgeries, such as a coronary artery bypass graft (CABG) procedure. CABG or *bypass* surgery involves stopping the heart and running the blood through a machine to reoxygenate it during the course of the procedure. This is done by attaching a large-diameter hose to the RAA; when surgery concludes and this hose is removed, it can damage the RAA to the point that it is completely or partially surgically removed. In patients who have had a CABG procedure, the RAA may not be available for right atrial lead placement. For such patients, the right atrial lead is often placed against the lateral wall of the right atrium. It is sometimes possible to fixate a right atrial lead in the remnants of the RAA, if a portion of it is preserved.

Arteries and veins

Any discussion about the heart necessarily involves the vasculature, which is why we commonly refer to our circulatory system as the *cardiovascular* system. As most of us remember from anatomy classes, arteries carry blood away from the heart, while veins transport blood back to the heart. (The exceptions are the PV and arteries described earlier.) Arteries carry oxygen-rich blood, while veins carry deoxygenated blood. What is of importance to device clinicians is that arteries are *high-pressure* vessels, while veins are *low-pressure* vessels. Arteries tend to be more muscular in structure and muscular contractions of the arteries help to move blood outward into the body. Veins tend to be less muscular than arteries, but unlike arteries, they contain a system of tiny interior valves. The purpose of these little valves is to maintain a unidirectional flow of blood (see **Figure 1.9**).

Some of the most important veins in the body are the SVC and its counterpart, the IVC. The SVC takes blood from the upper part of the body and delivers it into the right atrium, with the IVC doing the same for blood from the lower part of the body. The coronary veins, networked around the outside of the heart, carry blood from the heart tissue and deliver it back to the right atrium; they are closely linked to the coronary arteries, which carry reoxygenated blood from the left ventricle back to the heart muscle. The CS is the site where

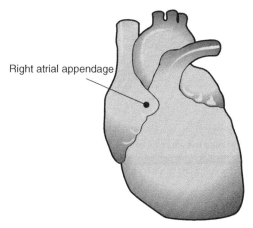

Figure 1.8 The right atrial appendage serves no obvious hemodynamic purpose, but is often the site of fixation of atrial leads.

Right atrial appendage

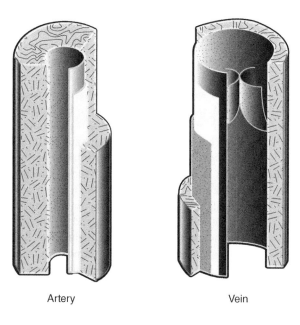

Artery   Vein

Figure 1.9 Veins and arteries have different purposes, different anatomical structure, and different pressures. Overall, veins are low-pressure systems that move blood by a series of little valves that keep blood flowing in the same direction. Arteries are high-pressure systems and are more *muscular*, so that they force blood forward by squeezing.

the great, middle, and small cardiac veins all drain; the CS takes this blood and delivers it back to the right atrium.

The PV carry reoxygenated blood from the lungs and deliver it to the left atrium so that it can be pumped back out to the body by the left ventricle.

The most important artery in the body is by far the aorta. The aorta is connected to the left ventricle, and it is the first and main conduit that takes reoxygenated blood from the left ventricle and sends it out to the body. As this reoxygenated blood makes its way out into the body, its first two stops are the head (brain) and the heart muscle. Inadequate oxygenated blood to the brain can very quickly provoke symptoms. This is the reason that depressed cardiac output is associated with symptoms like dizziness, light headedness, feeling woozy, and fatigue. Severe symptoms might include syncope.

The coronary arteries arise from the root of the aorta, just above the cusps of the aortic valve. Coronary arteries receive most blood during diastole, so blood is more or less *pouring back into these vessels*. The coronary artery system is a network—almost a mesh—of middle-sized to very small vessels that cover the exterior surface of the heart (see **Figure 1.10**).

Coronary arteries get their name from the Latin word for *crown* (such as in our word *coronation*) because this network of vessels sits like a crown atop the heart and encircles it. The heart gets blood *from outside in* as oxygen-rich blood in these coronary arteries is delivered to the exterior of the heart muscle. Coronary arteries are not within the heart; they are epicardial structures. The two main coronary arteries are the right coronary artery (RCA) and the left coronary artery (LCA). The RCA and LCA come off the aorta and are located in the AV groove, an exterior structure below the atria and above the ventricles. The RCA runs from the aorta in the right AV groove, while the LCA comes off the aorta and quickly branches to the left main. The left main is a very short artery (about the size of a thumbnail), which branches quickly into the left anterior descending artery (LAD) and the circumflex artery. The LAD travels down the front of the

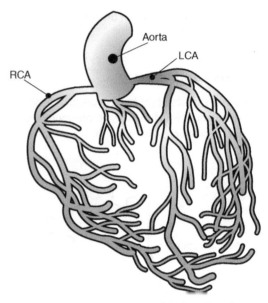

Figure 1.10 The coronary arteries of the heart branch out to surround the entire heart muscle. The two most prominent coronary arteries are the right coronary artery (RCA) and the left coronary artery (LCA).

left side of the heart. The circumflex artery can be found in the left AV groove.

The RCA bifurcates to the posterior descending artery. The right atrium and right ventricle get their supply of oxygen-rich blood from the RCA. Much of the cardiac conduction system is right sided, that is, it commences with the sinoatrial (SA) node in the high right atrium and travels down to the AV node on the right side of the septum. These important electrical structures get their oxygen-rich blood supply from the RCA. The electrical system travels down the ventricles to the inferior wall of the left ventricle (located at the bottom of the heart but belonging to the left ventricle); the inferior wall is also fed oxygen-rich blood by the RCA. An occlusion of the RCA, such as might occur in a myocardial infarction (MI), may result in death of the heart muscle it feeds, which includes the right atrium, the right ventricle, and the inferior wall of the left ventricle, and it might affect the conduction system, including the SA node and the AV node. An inferior wall MI is typically the result of a clogged RCA.

For an MI, the more distal the occlusion (that is, further from the aorta), the less potential damage the heart attack will have. In other words, the worst occlusions are proximal. Whether or not a patient survives an MI comes down to the numbers. The loss of over 40% of the left ventricular muscle mass results in death. However, that 40% is cumulative. For example, a person can survive an MI that costs him 30% of left ventricular muscle mass, but if that heart attack is followed by another that kills 15% of the left ventricular muscle mass, the second (milder) heart attack will prove fatal. This is the reason many people survive a first heart attack but die of a second or third attack, even though their fatal MI may be relatively mild.

The LCA branches quickly to the left main, which branches almost at once to the LAD. The LAD runs on the outside of the heart along the front of the heart along the septum. The left main supplies the left atrium and the majority of the left ventricle, in other words, the major pumping portion of the heart. An occlusion in the left main can be particularly disastrous because it is so far upstream and affects the heart's left ventricular muscle mass. No wonder they call the left main the *widow maker*!

The coronary arteries do not run in straight lines; they twist and turn and sometimes make very sharp bends. People with coronary artery disease (CAD) typically have plaque buildup in the areas where the coronary arteries bend at sharp angles. These are areas where the blood flow creates a lot of turbulence and plaque and other substances can collect and build up. It is typically to find blockage and occlusions at these places.

The LAD supplies the anterior wall of the left ventricle and the septum with oxygen-rich blood. Since part of the heart's conduction system runs through the septum (the right and left bundle branches), an LAD occlusion can damage the heart's ability to conduct electricity properly.

The circumflex artery runs along the AV groove laterally and thus supplies oxygen-rich blood to the lateral wall of the left ventricle along with the left atrium. The circumflex runs along the AV groove to the left, heading toward the back of the heart, where it meets with the RCA, which travels along the AV groove to the left toward the back of the heart. Both the circumflex and the RCA are responsible for providing oxygenated blood to the posterior wall of the ventricle. But which is the more important provider? That depends on *crux* and whether the heart is right or left dominant.

The *crux* refers to an imaginary line drawn exactly down the middle of the ventricular posterior wall without any regard to anatomical landmarks. If the RCA crosses the crux, then the heart is said to be *right dominant*, and the RCA is the greater supplier of oxygenated blood to the ventricular posterior wall. On the other hand, if the circumflex crosses the crux, then the heart is said to be *left dominant*, and the circumflex is the more significant provider. Roughly 60% of the population is right dominant.

While this information about the vasculature is important, it is even more important for clinicians to recognize that there is tremendous interpatient variability in terms of venous anatomy. While we can describe major structures and typical venous formations, anomalies are very common. These anomalies may be minor variations or they can be very pronounced, such as missing veins and arteries. Clinicians who deal with the cardiovascular system must be prepared for large and small differences in vascular anatomy. The cardiovascular system is incredibly resilient and can adapt to some anomalies by building up collateral circulation. For example, a person with a missing or incompetent vessel may over time build up a network of smaller collateral vessels that compensates by doing the same job. It is not unusual to see vessels grow larger or branch out to compensate. Sometimes, when an artery is blocked, collateral circulation will build up and compensate by delivering oxygen-rich blood to the heart muscle.

Every artery in the body has a matching or corresponding vein, usually located in close proximity. This applies to the coronary system as well. Note that there are great differences in coronary venous anatomy among patients, which becomes important when implanting left ventricular leads for CRT devices (see **Figure 1.11**).

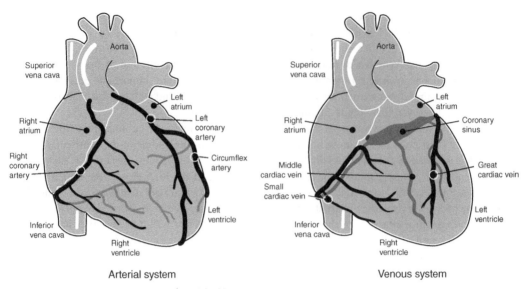

Arterial system   Venous system

Figure 1.11 The coronary artery system is matched by a coronary venous system.

The nuts and bolts of cardiovascular anatomy and physiology

- The heart consists of four chambers, which may be considered the upper chambers (right atrium and left atrium) and lower chambers (right ventricle and left ventricle) or may be thought of as the right heart (right atrium and right ventricle) and left heart (left atrium and left ventricle).
- Deoxygenated blood enters the right atrium, flows to the right ventricle, and is pumped out via the pulmonary valve to the lungs. The blood is reoxygenated in the lungs and then enters the left atrium and flows to the left atrium and out of the aortic valve into the aorta and the rest of the body.
- The heart has two outflow tracts: a right ventricular outflow tract (RVOT) and a left ventricular outflow tract (LVOT).
- The largest chamber of the heart is the left ventricle, making up about 2/3 of the cardiac mass. The left ventricle is muscular and massive because it must pump against approximately 10 times the pressure against which the right ventricle pumps (120 vs. 12 mmHg).
- The two cardiac valves most susceptible to dysfunction and disease are the mitral and aortic valve because they function in a high-pressure environment.

- The chordae tendineae connect the leaflets of the valves to the papillary muscles and look like little parachutes. These help the valves open and close properly.
- In general, arteries transport blood away from the heart, are muscular and contract to help move the blood on its way, and have thicker walls than veins. Veins have thinner, less muscular walls and carry oxygen-depleted blood back to the heart using tiny interior valves to keep the blood flow moving forward. Arteries transport oxygenated blood and can be considered high-pressure systems, while veins transported deoxygenated blood in a low-pressure system.
- Cardiac contraction is systole; cardiac relaxation is diastole. Atrial systole occurs at the very end of ventricular diastole in something nicknamed *atrial kick*. In a healthy individual, about 20–30% of cardiac output comes from atrial kick.
- The heart is a muscle that is fed with oxygenated blood through a network of coronary arteries. Coronary arteries get oxygen-rich blood from the aorta, and they perfuse the heart muscle during diastole as blood drains back.
- Although arteries and veins generally take blood away from or to the heart, respectively,

the pulmonary vessels are the exception. The pulmonary artery transports deoxygenated blood, while the pulmonary veins carry oxygenated blood. This is because of their special location and the fact that their work is taking blood from the right side to the left side of the heart.
- The main coronary arteries are the right coronary artery and the left coronary artery. The left coronary artery branches quickly to a short vessel known as the left main (the *widow maker*) and the circumflex artery.

- A myocardial infarction can kill the heart muscle. The clogged arteries determine the location of the affected muscle. A right coronary artery occlusion will affect the right atrium and ventricle and the inferior wall of the left ventricle, while a left coronary artery occlusion will affect the left atrium and most of the left ventricle. By far the most dangerous occlusion is in the left main because it feeds the majority of the heart muscle with oxygen-rich blood.

Test your knowledge

Fill in these anatomical landmarks of the heart. They include the four chambers, the four valves, and the body's main artery.

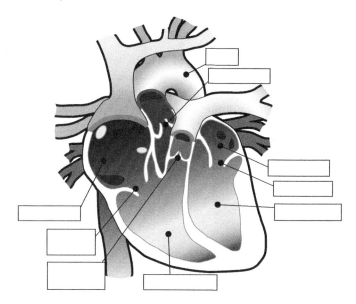

Answer the following questions

1 What are the names of the two atrioventricular valves of the heart?
   A Atrial and ventricular
   B Tricuspid and mitral
   C Pulmonary and pulmonic
   D Aortic and superior vena cava

2 Which chambers of the heart contain trabeculae?
   A Atria
   B Ventricles
   C Right-sided chambers only
   D Left-sided chambers only

3 Why can trabeculae be important to device clinicians?
   A They are good places to secure a passive-fixation lead
   B They help regulate blood pressure
   C They prevent atherosclerosis
   D All of the above

4 Which of the following is *not* true about the aorta?
   A It is an artery.
   B It consists of an ascending portion, a descending portion, and an arch.
   C It carries only oxygenated blood.
   D It is the largest vein in the body.

5 From which artery does blood enter the right atrium?
   A Superior vena cava
   B Inferior vena cava
   C Coronary sinus
   D All of the above

6 What is *atrial* kick?
   A Ventricular pressure on the tricuspid valve, forcing it shut
   B Electrical impulses originating in the atrium to cause the heart to beat faster
   C Atrial systole that forces the most blood possible into the already-full and diastolic ventricles
   D A type of arrhythmia

7 Why would a person with chronic AF likely have decreased cardiac output?
   A AF is associated with low blood volume.
   B AF causes the heart to beat very slowly.
   C AF may cause the heart to experience frequent pauses.
   D AF reduces or eliminates atrial kick—and atrial kick contributes to cardiac output.

8 Which of the following is often a preferred location for affixing a cardiac pacing lead?
   A The right ventricular outflow tract (RVOT)
   B The left ventricular outflow tract (LVOT)
   C The excised right atrial appendage
   D The tricuspid valve

9 What connects the valve leaflets to the papillary muscles?
   A Trabeculae
   B Arteries
   C Chordae tendineae
   D Tiny valves

10 Which coronary artery is nicknamed the *widow maker* because an occlusion in this vessel will deprive the majority of the heart's muscle mass of oxygen-rich blood?
   A Left main
   B Circumflex
   C Right coronary artery
   D Inferior vena cava

CHAPTER 2

Cardiac conduction system

Learning objectives

- Describe the electrical conduction system of the healthy heart.
- List the main anatomical landmarks of normal cardiac conduction.
- Name the anatomical location of the heart's *natural pacemaker*.
- Explain depolarization and repolarization in electrical terms and how it relates to the cardiac contraction.
- Define the term automaticity and how it relates to cardiac conduction.

Introduction

The sinoatrial (SA) node is the heart's *natural pacemaker*. In the healthy heart, the SA node fires and the electrical stimulus conducts along special pathways through the heart that cause cells in specific areas to depolarize. After the stimulus passes the area, the cells repolarize. Myocardial cell depolarization and repolarization govern the heart's contraction and relaxation sequence—in other words, the heart rhythm. Rhythm disorders occur when this healthy conduction system is in some way disrupted or impaired.

The conduction pathways

When the SA node *fires* and sends out electrical energy, the stimulus travels from the SA node in the high right atrium out over the atria via pathways known as internodal tracts. Most of these internodal tracts are located in the right atrium; the main tract over to the left atrium is called Bachmann's bundle. It is because of Bachmann's bundle, linking the right atrium to the left atrium, that the atria can contract simultaneously, that is, as these two upper chambers contract as one coherent unit. After traversing the atria, the impulse comes down through conduction tracts to the atrioventricular (AV) node.

The AV node is an area of highly specialized tissue located below the atria and above the ventricles on the right side of the septum. Anatomically, the AV node rests in the AV groove. The tissue in the healthy AV node has the ability to change the speed of the electrical impulse; specifically, it slows the stimulus down. The slowdown serves two important purposes. First, slowing the impulse allows the atria time to contract and provide the very valuable *atrial kick* to ventricular filling. Second, the slowed impulse protects the ventricles from being forced to beat too quickly, that is, to beat before they have been adequately filled with blood.

Once the impulse crosses the AV node, it travels down into the ventricles and accelerates its speed. The impulse travels through the bundle of His (pronounced hiss), to the bundle branches (right and left), and then out to the network of Purkinje fibers. This allows both ventricles to depolarize and contract simultaneously (**Figure 2.1**).

Polarization, depolarization, and repolarization

Cardiac conduction is driven by the ability of myocardial cells to be depolarized and repolarized. Depolarization occurs at the cellular level and is,

The Nuts and Bolts of Implantable Device Therapy Pacemakers, First Edition. Tom Kenny.
© 2015 John Wiley & Sons, Ltd. Published 2015 by John Wiley & Sons, Ltd.

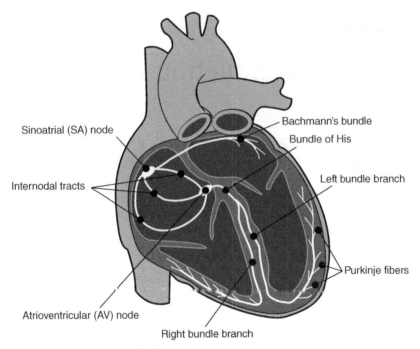

Figure 2.1 The conduction pathways in the healthy heart.

in turn, driven by electrolytes or positively and negatively charged ions (potassium, sodium, and calcium mainly), which are able to move in and out of the cardiac cells. A myocardial cell may be said to be polarized when in its resting state, that is, there is no electrical activity going on. In the resting state, the interior of the myocardial cell is somewhat more negatively charged that the outside. This state is called the resting state or sometimes phase 0 of the action potential.

An electrical stimulus changes the resting state abruptly. The electrical energy allows for the movement of ions to the point that the interior of the myocardial cell is now more positive than the outside. In other words, the charge reverses and the cell is said to be depolarized. When this happens, the cell contracts; when this happens to a large area of the myocardium, the heart muscle contracts. *Cardiac contraction occurs as a result of cellular depolarization.*

When the electrical stimulus moves past the myocardial cell, the ions move in reverse and the interior of the cell assumes its previous negative charge with respect to the outside. This process is called repolarization, and it brings the myocardial cell back to the resting state. When this happens, the cell relaxes. When a large area of the myocardium repolarizes, the heart resumes its previous shape (loses its contraction).

Intrinsic pacemakers

The healthy heart's *natural pacemaker* is the SA node, but the SA node is not the only area of the heart that can generate an electrical pulse. The SA node serves as the heart's pacemaker because it generates these pulses faster than other areas. In the healthy heart, the SA node can fire at around 60–100 times a minute, corresponding to a healthy heart rate. The AV junction can also fire, but it is much slower at around 40–60 times a minute. Even the Purkinje fibers (the ventricles) can act as a pacemaker, but they fire at only 20–40 times a minute. Thus, in a healthy individual, the SA node outpaces these other potential *pacemakers*. The AV junction and ventricles are sometimes called *backup pacemakers* because they take over the heart rate in the event that the SA node is not able to pace the heart. While these backup pacemakers may help keep the heart beating in the event of a dysfunctional SA node, they are slow and not as reliable as the SA node.

The healthy heart is able to pace itself because of a property called automaticity. Automaticity is an inherent property of individual cardiac conductive cells that allows them to depolarize spontaneously. In other words, some cells in the heart (such as the cells of the SA node) are able to generate an electrical stimulus on their own.

Refractoriness

Refractoriness refers to the temporary inability of a cardiac cell to respond to an electrical stimulus. Refractoriness can be the normal, appropriate, and expected behavior of cardiac cells. For example, immediately after electrical energy has passed through cardiac cells, they go through a phase where they are unresponsive to electrical energy, no matter how much voltage is delivered. This normal refractoriness is called the physiological refractory period, and it is very brief (it is measured in thousandths of a second). Of course, the exact duration of a refractory period is based in part on the heart rate; *the faster the heart rate, the shorter the refractory period and vice versa.*

Refractoriness may also occur when certain cells become dysfunctional, that is, cardiac cells may lose their ability to conduct properly. Furthermore, the heart's inherent pacemakers may change their rate; for instance, the AV junction may speed up and start to deliver impulses at 80 or 100 times a minute. When this happens—that is, when another pacemaker takes over the role of the SA node—that pacemaker is called a *usurping pacemaker* because it usurps the rightful role of the SA node. In the event that other pacemakers of the heart start to compete with the SA node, the fastest pacemaker always wins.

Conductivity

Conductivity is the cardiac cell's ability to transmit an electrical impulse to an adjacent cell. Typically, cardiac conduction is antegrade, that

is, it moves forward. Electrical impulses actually travel out in all different directions, but refractoriness prevents those cells that were just stimulated from depolarization. This keeps conduction moving in a single direction through the heart. Normal antegrade conduction in a healthy heart goes from SA node to atria to AV node over the bundle of His and down to the ventricles. Some individuals have the ability to conduct retrograde; retrograde conduction is abnormal but not uncommon.

Autonomic nervous system

The heart does not need direct stimulation from the nervous system to generate electricity and to beat, but that is not to say that the nervous system does not control the heart rate. The autonomic nervous system indirectly affects cardiac conduction by regulating how fast the heart will beat and how hard the heart muscle will squeeze (contractility). The autonomic nervous system communicates with the heart through a network of baroreceptors, which respond to chemical signals.

The autonomic nervous system of the body, like certain other physiological systems, exists as two systems in balance. The autonomic nervous system consists of a sympathetic system and a parasympathetic system. They both work together, and in a healthy individual, one may *overdrive* the other during specific times. The sympathetic nervous system is mainly associated with epinephrine (adrenaline), and it has the ability to speed the heart rate and increase cardiac contractility and can increase the speed by which electrical impulses can cross the AV node. The sympathetic nervous system takes over when we are stressed, frightened (*fight-or-flight* response), or exerting ourselves.

On the other hand, the autonomic nervous system also has a parasympathetic system that is associated with acetylcholine. This system can decrease the heart rate, decrease cardiac contractility, and cause impulses crossing the AV node to be slowed. The parasympathetic system might take over when we are sleeping or at rest.

The nuts and bolts of the cardiac conduction system

- The heart's natural pacemaker is the sinoatrial (SA) node, which generates an electrical impulse spontaneously about 60–100 times a minute in a healthy individual.
- The normal conduction path is from the SA node over the atria to the atrioventricular (AV) node and then via the bundle of His down the right and left bundle branches and into the Purkinje fibers.
- The AV node has the ability to slow down the electrical impulse. This serves two main purposes: it allows for atrial kick and it protects the ventricles from beating too rapidly.
- In the healthy heart, the right and left atria contract simultaneously, and then the right and left ventricles contract simultaneously.
- Depolarization and repolarization of myocardial cells are driven by positively and negatively charged ions, which cross the cell membrane. A resting cardiac cell is more negative on the inside than the surrounding media, but when it depolarizes, it becomes more positive on the inside relative to the surrounding media. Following depolarization, the ions move and the cell returns to being more negative on the inside than the outside in a process known as repolarization.
- Depolarization causes the cardiac cell to contract.
- The main ions involved in depolarization and repolarization are sodium, potassium, and calcium ions.
- Although the heart's natural pacemaker is the SA node, the AV junction and the Purkinje fibers (ventricles) can also assume (*usurp*) this role if the SA node cannot generate electricity properly. The AV junction and Purkinje fibers are not as reliable as a healthy AV node and typically generate electricity more slowly (the AV junction about 40–60 times a minute and the Purkinje fibers 20–40 times a minute).
- However, sometimes the AV junction or Purkinje fibers may generate electricity very quickly; this is abnormal. When they do, they may take over the heart. When pacemakers of the heart compete, the fastest one drives the heart.
- Automaticity is an inherent property of certain cardiac conductive cells to depolarize spontaneously. Not all cardiac conduction cells possess automaticity, but the SA node, AV junction, and Purkinje fibers possess automaticity.
- Refractoriness is the natural and expected behavior of cardiac conductive cells that makes them unresponsive to electrical impulses immediately after they have depolarized. The natural refractory period is very brief.
- The faster the heart rate, the shorter the refractory period; the slower the heart rate, the longer the refractory period.
- Refractoriness can also occur as a dysfunction.
- Conductivity is the cardiac cell's ability to transmit an electrical impulse to adjacent cells. Refractoriness means that cells that just depolarized will not depolarize again. This keeps conduction moving forward (antegrade conduction).
- Antegrade conduction is normal; retrograde conduction is abnormal but is not rare.
- The autonomic nervous system regulates the heart rate by controlling how fast the heart beats and how vigorously it contracts.
- The autonomic nervous system consists of a sympathetic and parasympathetic nervous system, which work together, but at certain times, one or the other is dominant. The sympathetic nervous system makes the heart beat faster and more vigorously; it takes over during times of stress, exertion, or *fight or flight*. The parasympathetic nervous system makes the heart beat slowly and less vigorously; it takes over during periods of rest.
- The neurotransmitters associated with these two systems are epinephrine or adrenaline (sympathetic nervous system) and acetylcholine (parasympathetic nervous system).

Test your knowledge

Please write in the landmarks of the cardiac conduction system. Select from the following (each is used only once).

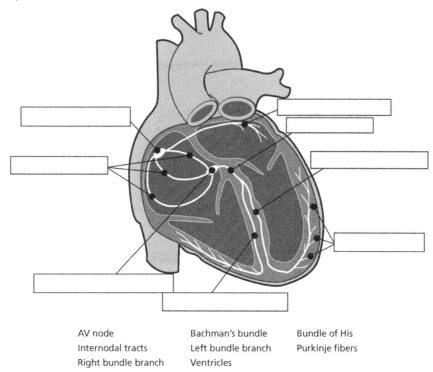

AV node   Bachman's bundle   Bundle of His
Internodal tracts Left bundle branch   Purkinje fibers
Right bundle branch Ventricles

1 Which of the following is not considered one of the heart's intrinsic pacemakers?
   A AV junction
   B SA node
   C Purkinje fibers
   D Aorta

2 Depolarization and repolarization involve the movement of charged ions across cardiac cell membranes. What types of ions are primarily involved?
   A Calcium, potassium, and sodium
   B Acetylcholine and epinephrine
   C Magnesium and folate
   D All of the above

3 Refractoriness refers to:
   A The ability of cardiac conduction cells to contract

   B The inability of cardiac conduction cells to respond to an electrical stimulus
   C The unique permeability of the cardiac cells
   D Abnormal cardiac conduction

4 When a cardiac cell depolarizes, the interior of the cell becomes what with respect to the surrounding media?
   A More positive
   B More negative
   C More acidic
   D Hotter

5 Fill in the blank. In the healthy heart, the faster the heart rate, the ___ the refractory period.
   A More vigorous
   B Less reliable
   C Longer
   D Shorter

6 Which specific part of the nervous system governs the *fight-or-flight* response and is associated with epinephrine (adrenaline)? (Pick the most exact answer.)

   A Autonomic nervous system

   B Parasympathetic nervous system

   C Sympathetic nervous system

   D Central nervous system

7 In normal antegrade conduction, the electrical impulse travels from the SA node, over the atria, to the AV node and to what structure before reaching the ventricles?

   A The intermodal tracts

   B The Purkinje fibers

   C The bundle of His

   D The ventricular apex

8 Which of the following is true about retrograde cardiac conduction?

   A Everyone has it.

   B It is perfectly normal and can be helpful in stressful situations.

   C It is abnormal but not uncommon.

   D It is impossible to diagnose definitively except in an autopsy.

9 What chemical is associated with the parasympathetic nervous system?

   A Acetylcholine

   B Potassium

   C Epinephrine

   D Dopamine

10 The stimulation of the myocardial cells of which of the following structures is most closely associated with ventricular depolarization?

   A SA node

   B AV junction

   C Bundle of His

   D Purkinje fibers

CHAPTER 3

The cardiac cycle and hemodynamics

Learning objectives

- Define basic terms in hemodynamics: stroke volume, cardiac output, systole, diastole, ejection fraction, preload, and afterload.
- Describe AV synchrony in simple terms and how it relates to hemodynamics.
- Calculate the cardiac output when the heart rate and stroke volume are known.
- Briefly explain how the autonomic nervous system affects the heart.

Introduction

The healthy heart beats about 70 times a minute or over 100 000 times a day. Each individual beat is a remarkable series of events known as the cardiac cycle. Each cardiac cycle involves atrial systole and ventricular diastole followed by atrial diastole and ventricular systole with the objective of having blood circulate efficiently through the body. Understanding terms like stroke volume and cardiac output helps us better measure the heart's pumping ability. Although the heart can act automatically, it is also greatly influenced by brain activity through the autonomic nervous system and neurochemicals. This chapter also reviews basic cardiovascular anatomy and the network of *pipes* that carry blood throughout the body.

Common terms related to hemodynamics

Hemodynamics describes the flow or movement of the blood and is an important component to understanding cardiac devices. Depolarization of the myocardial cells results in cardiac contraction, and repolarization results in their subsequent relaxation and return to the resting state. These two states relate to cardiac systole (contraction) and diastole (relaxing). During diastole, the heart's chambers fill with blood; during systole, the heart muscle contracts and pumps blood. The normal pattern of the cardiac cycle is atrial systole with ventricular diastole and atrial diastole with ventricular systole. A healthy heart has one atrial contraction for every single ventricular contraction, and atrial contractions do not occur at the same time as ventricular contractions. The pattern of one atrial contraction for each ventricular contraction is known as atrioventricular (AV) synchrony. AV synchrony is very important for health and well-being. When AV synchrony is disrupted, symptoms can occur and some of these patients may require pacing.

This pattern of atrial systole with ventricular diastole followed by ventricular systole with atrial diastole makes up the normal cardiac cycle. While we are tempted to think of the *heartbeat* as a single thing, the heart's pattern of beating is actually complex and encompasses both systole and diastole for the upper and lower chambers.

The Nuts and Bolts of Implantable Device Therapy Pacemakers, First Edition. Tom Kenny.
© 2015 John Wiley & Sons, Ltd. Published 2015 by John Wiley & Sons, Ltd.

In a healthy heart, the timing of systole and diastole is the same for the right side (right atrium, right ventricle) as the left side (left atrium, left ventricle).

The heart's job is to pump blood and an important measure of how well it is doing this job is the stroke volume, defined as the volume of blood pumped out of the heart during one cardiac cycle. For a healthy adult, this value usually falls between 70 and 100 milliliters (ml). This differs from another commonly used term in cardiology, cardiac output, which defines the volume of blood pumped by the ventricles in 1 min. Cardiac output values are much higher, normally around 4–8 l/min. Cardiac output is equal to the heart rate (beats per minute) times the stroke volume.

Stroke volume is only part of the picture. For a patient who weighs 95 pounds, a cardiac output of 6 l is different than the same cardiac output in a patient who weighs 495 pounds. The cardiac index is the cardiac output divided by the body surface area. Thus, cardiac index is probably the best value to measure the heart's actual pumping function. A healthy individual of normal weight has a cardiac index of around 2.4 l/m^2.

The ejection fraction compares how much blood is pumped out every time the left ventricle contracts compared to its total blood volume. For example, if the left ventricle contains 100 cc of blood and pumps out 65 cc of blood with one contraction, the ejection fraction would be stated as 65%. The ejection fraction is always measured from the left ventricle and is sometimes stated as the *left ventricular ejection fraction* or LVEF. No patient, no matter how perfect his cardiac health, has an LVEF of 100% because there is always some residual blood left in the ventricle. The LVEF and the cardiac output values are closely interrelated, that is, patients with a low cardiac output typically have a low LVEF. There remains some debate as to what constitutes a normal or healthy LVEF value, but most experts would agree that it falls in the range of 50–60%. An LVEF of 40% or lower is considered indicative of left ventricular dysfunction or systolic heart failure. The LVEF is good measure of the heart's pumping function. An LVEF value is typically obtained by an echocardiogram, which measures sound waves (echo) and assesses pumping ability.

The cardiac cycle

Stated simplistically, the cardiac cycle is a single *beat* of the heart (encompassing atrial systole/ventricular diastole plus atrial diastole/ventricular systole). For easy math, a person with a heart rate of 60 beats per minute (bpm) has a cardiac cycle length of 1 s (60 beats a minute = 1 beat per second). Clinicians typically use milliseconds (ms) to discuss cardiac cycle, so a person with a heart rate of 60 bpm has a cardiac cycle length of 1000 ms (=1 s). Diastole, when filling occurs, takes up about two-thirds of the total cardiac cycle, or in this case about 666 ms.

As the heart rate increases, the cardiac cycle length shortens. A heart rate of 100 bpm results in a cardiac cycle length of 600 ms. This, in turn, will reduce systole and diastole proportionally, but diastole still takes up about two-thirds of the total cardiac cycle duration. At a heart rate of 100 bpm and a cardiac cycle length of 600 ms, diastole will have a duration of about 400 ms.

In a healthy individual, the heart rate adjusts to activity levels, stress, and other factors (such as fever). Depending on age and fitness level, a healthy individual may have a resting heart rate of 60 bpm and rates during daily activities can run from 70 to 100 bpm. During exercise, heart rates may increase even more to 130 bpm. However, the heart requires a certain amount of time for diastole in order to fill adequately with blood. Just as there are heart rates too slow to support our body's function, heart rates can get too high for adequate cardiac filling, resulting in suboptimal cardiac output. The heart's maximum rate (above which it can no longer function efficiently) is determined by several factors, including age. The rule of thumb for determining the age-predicted maximum heart rate for a person is 220 minus the age in years (plus or minus about 11%). Eighty percent of the age-predicted maximum heart rate is the target heart rate zone for exercise (see **Figure 3.1**).

The heart rate also impacts cardiac output. For example, a patient with a resting heart rate of 70 bpm and stroke volume of 70 ml (converted to 0.07 l) has a cardiac output of 5 l/min ($70 \times 0.07 = 4.90$ l or ~5 l). However, if the heart rate increases to 195 bpm and the stroke volume increases to 0.113, these result in a cardiac output

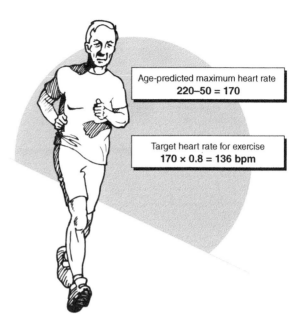

Age-predicted maximum heart rate
220−50 = 170

Target heart rate for exercise
170 × 0.8 = 136 bpm

Figure 3.1 Calculating target heart rate zones for exercise for a 50-year-old.

of 22 l/min ($195 \times 0.113 = 22.035$ l or roughly 22 l). That means that with a 2.5–3.5 increase in heart rate, the stroke volume increases 1.5 times, but the cardiac output increases 4- to 7-fold! From this simple equation, it is clear that heart rate has the more dramatic effect on cardiac output. To be sure, both stroke volume and heart rate influence cardiac output, but an increase in heart rate has the more pronounced effect. One of the reasons that heart rate has such a profound effect is that heart rate has a much wider range of variability, whereas stroke volume can only vary by small amounts.

Cardiac output

Cardiac output is influenced by stroke volume, which, in turn, is affected by three things: left ventricular end-diastolic pressure (LVEDP), systemic vascular resistance (SVR), and contractility.

LVEDP is the pressure in the left ventricle at the end of diastole or *preload*. Since volume creates pressure, it is clear that the LVEDP basically defines how much blood (volume) is in the left ventricle at the end of diastole, right before the ventricles contract. How much blood is pumped out is clearly related to how much blood is available within the left ventricle.

The SVR is also known as *afterload* and describes the resistance against which the left ventricle must pump, in other words, the pressure in the aorta that must be overcome by the left ventricle in order to pump blood out of the heart and into the body. One way to think of preload and afterload is to think of the aortic valve as a gate; preload is the pressure in front of the gate and afterload is the pressure on the other side of the gate.

Contractility is the ability of the muscle fibers in the myocardium to expand and contract, that is, how vigorously the muscle can squeeze to help pump out the blood. Contractility is governed by a principle known as Starling's Law. Contractility can be adversely affected by heart attack, cardiac ischemia, and cardiomyopathy, all of which may impair the heart muscle's ability to squeeze efficiently.

Systolic and diastolic pressures

Systole has to be vigorous and forceful because every systole must overcome the pressure on the other side of the cardiac valve. Left ventricular systole, in particular, must overcome the high pressures on the other side of the mitral and aortic valves. Pressure in the aorta is around 120 mmHg, so the left ventricle must overcome that pressure in order to force the aortic valve open and pump

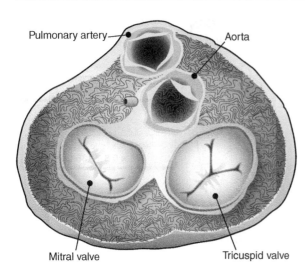

Pulmonary artery

Aorta

Mitral valve

Tricuspid valve

Figure 3.2 An overview of the heart showing the tricuspid (three-leaf) valve and the mitral valve (two cusps).

blood out into the aorta and into the rest of the body (see **Figure 3.2**).

Normal diastolic blood pressure is around 80 mmHg and is lower than systolic pressure. Blood pressure readings typically state the systolic and diastolic values, such as 120/80 mmHg. Hypertension refers to *high pressure* in the cardiovascular system and results in higher pressures in the aorta, which the left ventricle must overcome in order to force the aortic valve to open. For instance, if a hypertensive patient has 150/110 mmHg, it must work harder; at first, this extra work will make the heart larger and stronger, but eventually—like a rubber band stretched to the breaking point—the heart will be unable to keep up. A heart overworked over a long period of time will eventually fail. In other words, long-term high blood pressure is considered one of the causes of heart failure.

Systolic pressure is much lower in the right ventricle, around 12 mmHg (about one-tenth as great as the pressure in the aorta that the left ventricle must overcome). This pressure is measured in the pulmonary arteries and is stated as the pulmonary capillary wedge pressure (PCWP).

The nervous system and the heart

The heart's activities are regulated by the autonomic nervous system, specifically by way of the sympathetic and the parasympathetic nervous system. The brain regulates body activities through neurotransmissions that travel along certain predefined pathways. For example, there are pathways that help us feel heat or pain, and there are pathways that the brain uses so that we can control arm and leg muscles. Like these pathways, the brain has chemical pathways directly to the sinoatrial (SA) node and other areas of the heart. This is not to say that the SA node is incapable of firing independently; it has that property. However, in a healthy individual, the SA node is heavily influenced by the brain by way of these pathways in the sympathetic and parasympathetic nervous system.

The autonomic nervous system works via inputs from the sympathetic and parasympathetic nervous systems. Both systems are active and important and they control quite different things. The sympathetic nervous system is governed by the chemical adrenaline (also known as epinephrine, a potent catecholamine), and it becomes activated during periods of stress. The sympathetic nervous system is associated with our *fight-or-flight* response to perceived dangers. When the body is alerted, the sympathetic nervous system initiates a number of physical responses, including an elevated heart rate. It accomplishes this by speeding up cardiac conduction pathways, mostly at around the AV node. The sympathetic nervous system also increases cardiac contractility, allowing the heart to pump more vigorously. This increased contractility is the reason why we can sometimes feel our heart *pounding* during heavy exercise or when we are frightened.

In contrast, the parasympathetic nervous system runs on the brain chemical acetylcholine and it works to slow the heart rate, reduce conduction time through the AV node, and decrease cardiac contractility. Stimulating the vagus nerve (in the neck) has been shown to stimulate the body's parasympathetic nervous system. The parasympathetic nervous system is activated when we relax or rest.

In a healthy individual, the autonomic nervous system works by acting on messages from the dominant system, which changes over the course of the day, your activity, and your environment. You may feel very relaxed sitting in a recliner and watching TV (parasympathetic nervous system in control) but be suddenly frightened by a loud noise (sympathetic nervous system). The autonomic nervous system allows the body to respond seemingly instantly to the environment by shifting from parasympathetic to sympathetic inputs and vice versa. Thus, the autonomic nervous system constantly controls our heart rates and is the reason that our heart rate can increase when we are startled and decrease when we fall asleep.

The cardiovascular anatomy and hemodynamics

The nervous system not only affects the heart but influences the entire cardiovascular system (see **Figure 3.3**).

The heart rests in the body on a large muscle known as the diaphragm. When a pacing lead is placed in the apex of the right ventricle, it is actually quite close to the diaphragmatic muscle. The phrenic nerve is located in close proximity to the left atrium and left ventricle (see **Figure 3.4**). These anatomical considerations can be very important; during pacemaker implantation, the device should be tested to confirm that it does not stimulate the diaphragm. If a left ventricular lead is implanted, it is important to test to confirm that the lead does not stimulate the phrenic nerve.

The body's cardiovascular system consists of veins and arteries. These vessels range in size from very small to very large and all eventually flow back and forth from the heart (see **Figure 3.5**). During a pacemaker implant, the physician will

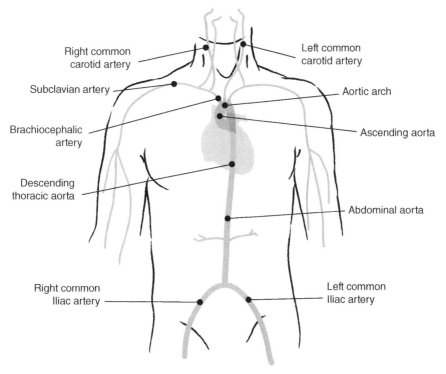

Figure 3.3 The cardiovascular system is centered around the heart; notice that the two primary destinations for blood from the left ventricle are upward to the head and brain and downward to the trunk and feet.

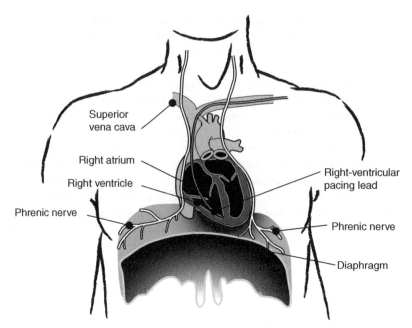

Figure 3.4 The heart rests on the diaphragm and a pacing lead placed in the apex of the right ventricle is anatomically close to the large diaphragm muscle.

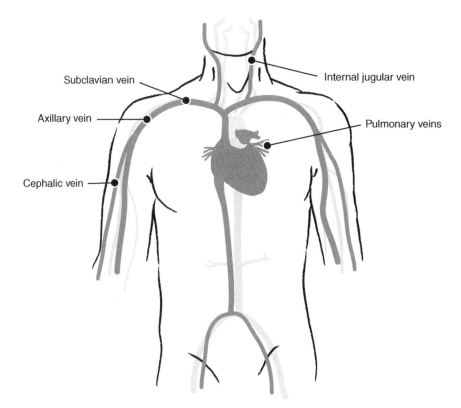

Figure 3.5 The cephalic vein flows into the axillary vein and then flows into the subclavian vein; the veins get progressively larger.

obtain venous access, that is, he or she will introduce a lead into a vein. Since the veins are an interconnected system, it is important to be able to visualize how they flow together and toward the heart.

Conclusion

Pacing specialists need to understand the flow of blood through the body and its relationship to the heart, because pacemakers regulate the heartbeat and thus, indirectly, control the body's hemodynamics.

The nuts and bolts of the cardiac cycle and hemodynamics

- Systole refers to the contraction of the heart muscle, while diastole refers to its relaxation. Blood pressure states systolic over diastolic pressure, such as 120/80 mmHg. The cardiac cycle consists of atrial systole/ventricular diastole followed by atrial diastole/ventricular systole.
- A healthy heart has one ventricular contraction for every atrial contraction. This is called AV synchrony and it allows for optimal blood flow through the body.
- The healthy heart pumps about 70–100 ml of blood in each heartbeat; this is the stroke volume.
- Cardiac output is the amount of blood pumped by the heart in 1 min and can be calculated as the stroke volume times the heart rate (beats per minute). Normal cardiac output is around 4–8 l/min.
- The cardiac index is the cardiac output divided by the body surface area.
- The ejection fraction is how much blood the left ventricle pumps out in a single contraction, stated as a percentage. A left ventricular ejection fraction (LVEF) of 50–60% is normal; nobody has an LVEF of 100%. An LVEF below 40% indicates left ventricular dysfunction.
- If a person has a heart rate of 60 beats per minute, his cardiac cycle length is 1 s or 1000 ms. Of this time, about two-thirds is diastole. As the heart rate increases, the cardiac cycle length shortens and the diastolic duration shortens as well.
- There is rate above which the heart can no longer beat efficiently, which relates to a person's age. The formula for calculating the age-predicted maximum heart rate is 220 minus the person's age in years, plus or minus about 11%.
- Cardiac output is influenced by heart rate and stroke volume, with heart rate far more influential.

- Cardiac output is also influenced by the left ventricular end-diastolic pressure (LVEDP), systemic vascular resistance (SVR), and contractility. Other terms for these are preload (LVEDP) and afterload (SVR). If you think of the aortic valve as a gate, preload is the pressure in front of the gate (trying to push it open), and afterload is the pressure behind the gate (trying to hold it shut).
- Contractility refers to the ability of the muscle fibers in the heart to contract and expand. Contractility determines how vigorously the heart can contract.
- Systolic pressure in the heart is about 12 mmHg in the right ventricle but 120 mmHg in the left ventricle, or 10 times as much on the left side.
- The autonomic nervous system influences the heart. The autonomic nervous system consists of the parasympathetic nervous system (regulated by acetylcholine and working by slowing the heart rate) and the sympathetic nervous system (which runs on adrenaline or epinephrine and speeds up the heart rate). This is why our heart rate goes up when we are startled or goes down when we are sleeping.
- The heart rests on the diaphragm, which anatomically is close to the right ventricular apex. When placing a pacemaker lead, testing should be done to assure it does not stimulate the diaphragm.
- The blood in the body flows through a network of veins and arteries; every vein (which carries blood toward the heart) has a corresponding artery (which carries blood away from the heart). Leaving the left ventricle, most blood takes one of two paths: toward the head or toward the feet. Note that veins and arteries are of varying sizes and run seamlessly into each other. For instance, the cephalic vein becomes the axillary vein and then becomes the subclavian vein.

Test your knowledge

1 If a person has a blood pressure reading of 150/90 mmHg, what does the 150 mean?
   A Beats per minute
   B Systolic pressure
   C Diastolic pressure
   D Cardiac output

2 What is AV synchrony?
   A The portion of the AV node that regulates conduction
   B The idea that the right and left sides of the heart beat at the same time
   C One atrial contraction for each and every ventricular contraction
   D A type of arrhythmia

3 What is a normal value for stroke volume for a healthy adult?
   A 100 ml
   B 50%
   C 2.4 l/m2
   D 81

4 Cardiac output is calculated as:
   A Heart rate times systolic blood pressure
   B 220 minus the person's age
   C Heart rate times stroke volume
   D The percentage of blood ejected from the left ventricle

5 Which of the following would be considered an impossible value for the left ventricular ejection fraction?
   A 8%
   B 40%
   C 60%
   D 100%

6 What is another name for the left ventricular end-diastolic pressure?
   A Preload
   B Afterload

   C Overload
   D Systemic vascular resistance

7 Pressure on the right ventricle is around 12 mmHg. What is the pressure in the aorta?
   A 1.2 mmHg
   B 12 mmHg
   C 120 mmHg
   D Heart rate times stroke volume

8 Which type of nervous system governs the body's *flight-or-fight* response and what is its primary neurochemical?
   A The parasympathetic nervous system and acetylcholine
   B The autonomic nervous system and dopamine
   C The sympathetic nervous system and epinephrine (adrenaline)
   D None of the above

9 A lead positioned in the right ventricular apex is anatomically in close proximity to what important structure that should not be stimulated?
   A The vagus nerve
   B The phrenic nerve
   C The myocardium
   D The diaphragm

10 What type of test is usually done to determine an LVEF?
   A Electrocardiogram
   B Stress test
   C Echocardiogram
   D Angiography

CHAPTER 4

Heart disease

Learning objectives

- Define and name differences between ischemic and nonischemic heart disease.
- State the incidence rates of coronary attacks.
- Explain why a myocardial infarction can be a risk factor for subsequent ventricular fibrillation.
- Name at least two disease processes that can result in arrhythmias.
- List four risk factors for coronary artery disease.
- Name at least two risk factors for nonischemic heart disease.
- Name the three main types of cardiomyopathy.

Introduction

Although a pacing clinicians needs to have a sound understanding of the healthy heart, he or she is not going to encounter too many healthy hearts in the clinic. Pacemaker clinicians deal regularly with patients with coronary artery disease (CAD) in reality, but as a matter of fact, device professionals do not ever treat CAD—instead, we treat the *consequences of CAD*, one of which is arrhythmia. This chapter offers a high-level overview of essential cardiac pathophysiology for device clinicians. Most cardiac rhythm disorders can be traced back to ischemic heart disease (CAD), nonischemic heart disease, and, in rarer instances, congenital abnormalities of the heart.

CAD

CAD is an ischemic heart disease. Ischemia refers to damage to the tissue caused by a lack of oxygen. In day-to-day clinical practice, the terms CAD and ischemic heart disease are virtually interchangeably. CAD is the main cause of arrhythmias that lead patients to get a pacemaker (or other implanted rhythm management device, such as a defibrillator); as a general rule of thumb, about 80% of device patients can be expected to have CAD. It is by far the most prevalent form of heart disease a device clinician will encounter in everyday practice.

CAD can be defined as the narrowing of the coronary arteries by atherosclerosis, a slow buildup of fatty deposits (called plaque) on the inside walls of the coronary arteries. Plaques are made up of cholesterol, fats, calcium, and other *cellular sludges* in the blood. Plaques are sticky, gooey substances that slowly start to adhere to the inner walls of the arteries, where they harden and progressively build up over time. When plaque forms in the coronary arteries, the heart is not able to get enough oxygen out of the blood; in other words, its demand for oxygen exceeds the available supply of oxygen (demand > supply). Over time, plaques calcify and become very stiff and rigid (see **Figure 4.1**).

A clinician examining a coronary artery cannot tell by the amount of plaques or the narrowing of the artery how long the patient has had CAD. However, CAD is a very slow disease, so a patient with any significant narrowing of the arteries has had CAD for some time, although the patient's exact history cannot be deduced from the degree of atherosclerosis (see **Figure 4.2**).

The Nuts and Bolts of Implantable Device Therapy Pacemakers, First Edition. Tom Kenny.
© 2015 John Wiley & Sons, Ltd. Published 2015 by John Wiley & Sons, Ltd.

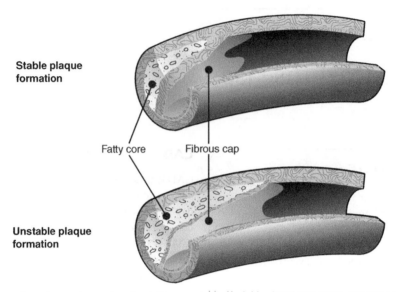

Figure 4.1 Plaque forms in an artery and can be stable or unstable. Unstable plaque formations are more prone to suddenly rupture and break off, posing the risk of a potentially life-threatening event.

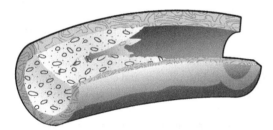

Figure 4.2 Blockage in a coronary artery that narrows the vessels and obstructs the flow of oxygen-rich blood.

Coronary heart disease is the most common type of heart disease in the United States. According to the Centers for Disease Control and Prevention in Atlanta, every year, about 715 000 Americans have a coronary attack (heart attack). For most of them (525 000), it will be a first heart attack, but 190 000 will experience a second or subsequent heart attack. About half of those who have a coronary attack (45%) will die from it.

Acute myocardial infarction (AMI) is generally considered to be a heart attack that occurred within the last three to seven days. After about a week, the myocardial infarction is considered old, but old is a relative term in that an *old* heart attack may have occurred last month or 2 years

ago. Patients who die of an AMI almost always die as a result of ventricular fibrillation (VF), a very dangerous rhythm disorder. Because AMI patients are vulnerable to VF, patients who have just had a heart attack should be treated in a coronary care unit (CCU) where they can be closely monitored and defibrillated if necessary. CCU patients are defibrillated promptly, ideally within about 30 s from onset of VF, to protect them from buildup of lactic acid in the blood, which causes the heart to become acidotic. The earlier a fibrillating patient can be rescued from fibrillation, the easier it is; as lactic acid builds up, it becomes increasingly more difficult to defibrillate them.

Patients who die of *old* myocardial infarction have two main modes of death: arrhythmic death or death from pump failure. The myocardial infarction leaves a scar or lesion of dead tissue in the heart; the size and location of this lesion depends on the location of the ischemia. This lesion is dead; it cannot contract or conduct. Myocardial infarction patients have electrical imbalance in their heart because they have areas of nonconducting, noncontracting tissue and areas immediately adjacent to those lesions that are electrically unstable. This sets the stage for sudden cardiac death, that is, an abrupt-onset VF. Such events can occur months or years after the myocardial infarction and trace back to the electrical instability around the scar(s) on the heart from the heart attack. Thus, heart attack survivors are at risk of VF even if they survive the heart attack and appear to otherwise be doing well.

Risk factors are characteristics or attributes that have been clinically proven to be associated with a disease or condition. Risk factors do not necessarily *cause* the problem but increase the statistical likelihood a person will have the problem. Risk factors are not always controllable. For example, men over the age of 45 are at increased risk for ischemic heart disease; for women, the risk starts at age 55 with a normal-onset menopause but at age 45 with early menopause. A family history of CAD or sudden cardiac disease puts a person at elevated risk for ischemic heart disease, particularly if CAD or sudden cardiac death occurred in a first-degree relative before he or she was age 55. Controllable risk factors include things like lack of exercise (sedentary lifestyle), obesity, and stress. Risk factors do not mean that a person will definitely get ischemic heart disease. In general, look at the combination of risk factors to help assess risk realistically.

Many women may underestimate their risk of ischemic heart disease, sudden cardiac death, and other heart diseases. Of the Americans who die every year of some form of cardiovascular disease, 53% are women. One in every three women will die of heart disease or stroke. More women die of heart disease than breast cancer and the other next six causes of death *combined*. All types of cancer combined kill 22% of American women, compared to 41% who succumb to forms of cardiovascular disease. Heart disease (not breast cancer) is the number one killer of American women, and it is only now starting to be recognized through campaigns like *Go Red!* by the American Heart Association. Despite these good efforts, more should be done to raise awareness in women about their risks of heart disease.

A very important and highly publicized risk factor for heart disease is hypercholesterolemia or high cholesterol. High cholesterol is generally defined by serum low-density lipoprotein (LDL) of <130 mg/dl and a high-density lipoprotein (HDL) level of <40 mg/dl for men or <50 mg/dl for women. While it is common to add these together to get a cholesterol number (such as 180 or 200), that total is less important than the ratio between LDL and HDL. LDL is *bad cholesterol*, while HDL is usually more stable and is considered *good cholesterol*. Patients with high cholesterol are first managed with lifestyle modifications, specifically diet and exercise. The next line of defense is statin therapy; statins are some of the most prescribed medications in America (see **Figure 4.3**).

Diabetes mellitus types I and II increase the risk of CAD by two- to eightfold. Diabetics have higher risk for kidney disease, eye problems, and pain in the lower legs. Diabetics are also at risk of developing peripheral neuropathy, a painful nerve disorder that often occurs in the hands and feet. Nerve damage in a long-term diabetic may make it hard for them to perceive pain in the chest that could indicate a heart attack. (When a heart attack occurs in a patient who does not have symptoms, it is sometimes called a *silent*

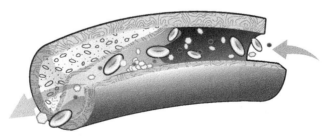

Figure 4.3 Cholesterol is a waxy fat in the blood made up of high-density lipoprotein (*good cholesterol*, shown here as the larger ovals) and low-density lipoprotein (*bad cholesterol*, shown here as the tinier *pellets*) that can build up inside the arteries.

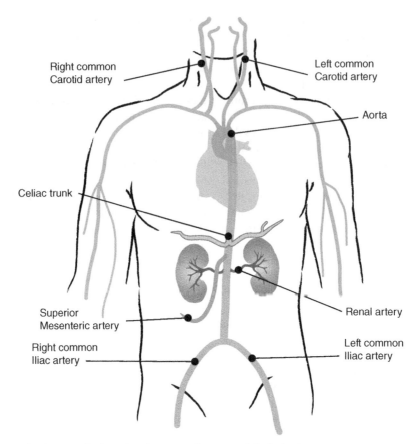

Figure 4.4 Vascular disease and atherosclerosis can occur in any vessels in the body.

heart attack.) Diabetics are at increased risk for infections and have high rates of amputations. Type II diabetes patients may be at particular risk for heart disease, because they often have two other risk factors for heart disease: obesity and a sedentary lifestyle. Today, we recognize that some people are *prediabetics*, that is, have insulin resistance and indications that full diabetes could develop. When such patients are aggressively treated with education and lifestyle modifications, it may be possible to delay or even prevent diabetes.

Hypertension or high blood pressure (defined as blood pressure reading > 140/90 mmHg) is a known risk factor for heart disease along with stroke and kidney disease. Hypertension has been called the *silent killer* because it is often asymptomatic. Regular blood pressure checks are important to determine

if this condition exists. Today, we recognize that some patients are at elevated risk for high blood pressure when they have blood pressure readings in the neighborhood of 120–139 mmHg systolic and 80–89 mmHg diastolic pressure. While technically not hypertension, this condition can be treated so that hypertension does not develop.

No discussion of risk factors is complete without mentioning smoking. Smoking is one of the leading causes of heart disease and stroke. Smoking is known to raise blood pressure and increase the risk of sudden cardiac death. Patients who smoke should be counseled that if they stop smoking, their risk of developing heart disease drops dramatically.

While we have focused our discussion on ischemic heart disease specifically in the coronary arteries, atherosclerosis can occur in any vessel, including the carotid artery, the aorta, the renal artery, and others. This disease can cause ischemia in other parts of the body, stroke, brain disease, pain, and dysfunction (see **Figure 4.4**). Atherosclerosis in the carotid may cause a stroke, for example. Ischemic disease is not unique to the coronary arteries and often builds up in multiple locations in a patient with atherosclerosis.

Nonischemic heart disease

Nonischemic heart diseases are far less common and may be defined as diseases of the heart muscle that are related to causes other than coronary disease. Nonischemic cardiac disease is often called cardiomyopathy, which simply means a disorder of the heart muscle. About 50 000 new cases of nonischemic heart disease are diagnosed every year in America. Risk factors for nonischemic heart disease include chronic or excessive alcohol intake (alcoholic cardiomyopathy) that can be reversed with abstinence. Toxins can damage the heart, for example, chemotherapeutic drugs can damage the heart. Other causes of nonischemic heart disease are valvular abnormalities; when the valves are misshapen or do not work properly, this can result in damage to the heart muscle. Hypertension is also a fairly common cause of cardiomyopathy. Although rare, viral infections can cause cardiomyopathy and have devastating effects on the heart muscle. In some cases, viral infections can be treated and may even resolve; in other cases, viral infections can be fatal. Lung diseases such as chronic obstructive pulmonary disease (COPD) can damage the heart muscle.

There are three main types of cardiomyopathy:
1 Dilated cardiomyopathy (congestive)
2 Hypertrophic cardiomyopathy
3 Restrictive cardiomyopathy
Dilated cardiomyopathy describes a heart that becomes enlarged, flabby, and floppy. A hypertrophic heart is more rigid and is sometimes called hypertrophic obstructive cardiomyopathy (HOCM) because most hypertrophic myopathy results in an obstruction, typically of the septum. Restrictive cardiomyopathy is very rare.

Patients with cardiomyopathy may develop arrhythmias as their hearts become increasingly less able to function optimally. Nonischemic heart disease can lead to left ventricular dysfunction, conduction abnormalities, and atrial as well as ventricular arrhythmias.

Congenital heart disease

Congenital heart disease refers a heart defect or malformation that is present at birth. About 40 000 babies are born every year with some kind of inborn cardiovascular defect. These defects vary greatly in severity, and there are at least 35 distinct defects recognized by cardiologists. Some of the more common congenital heart conditions include ventricular septal defect (VSD), valvular abnormalities, and abnormal connections between the heart and vessels. While some congenital heart disease patients will require cardiac pacing, this population of pacemaker patients is actually relatively small compared to patients with ischemic and even nonischemic heart disease (see **Figure 4.5**).

Actually, about 25% of American adults actually have a form of septal defect (although this might not necessarily be termed a true form of congenital heart disease). As a baby develops in the womb, there is a hole between the right and left atrium called the foramen ovale so that blood can flow directly between these two upper chambers. The foramen ovale helps circulate the blood, but this hole is supposed to close up when the baby is born. In about a quarter of people, the hole never closes and is described as a patent foramen ovale (PFO). Most people with PFO have no symptoms and may never know they have a septal defect. However, PFO puts an individual at elevated risk for stroke. Some patients opt to have a surgical procedure to close the PFO.

The term heart *murmur* can be very confusing because it is widely used and means different things. A murmur is a sign of turbulent blood flow through the heart. Broadly speaking, there are innocent and pathological murmurs. Most children have innocent murmurs that resolve as they grow. Persistent murmurs can be pathological and indicate the presence of a more severe congenital abnormality.

Risk factors for congenital abnormalities include maternal alcohol or drug abuse, genetic defects, or congenital abnormality, and some people with congenital abnormalities never know they have them, either because they have no symptoms or they are never properly diagnosed. Arrhythmias may develop in such patients; this can happen in the immediate postoperative period or it may occur years later, when scar tissue from the surgery results in conduction disorders and electrical instability. Moreover, sometimes congenital abnormalities of the heart are surgically corrected in a way that damages or removes the SA node or otherwise impairs the heart's ability to conduct normally. Such patients often are implanted with a pacemaker during or right after surgery.

Conclusion

Device patients have some form of heart disease, most frequently ischemic cardiac disease (CAD) but sometimes cardiomyopathy (nonischemic heart disease) or, even less frequently, a congenital cardiac abnormality. Understanding these disease processes and their risk factors are important for device clinicians in treating the whole patient and in identifying the types of cardiology patients who may benefit from an implanted pacemaker. Risk factors for heart disease are important for treating patients but not all risk factors can be controlled (age, genetics, gender). When considering risk, it is important to keep the big picture in mind: patients at highest risk are those with the most numerous and most severe risk factors.

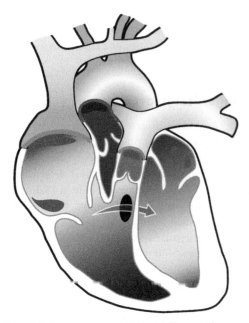

Figure 4.5 A common congenital heart disease is the ventricular septal defect or VSD, which is an abnormal hole connecting the right and left ventricle. Like many other congenital heart abnormalities, VSD can be surgically repaired in many patients.

a viral infection transmitted to a child in the womb. However, in most cases, congenital abnormalities of the heart occur in children with no known risk factors (idiopathic etiology).

Congenital abnormalities cannot be treated with drugs or devices, but in many instances, they are amenable to surgical repair. Some patients opt to live with a known but mild

The nuts and bolts of heart disease

- Coronary artery disease (CAD) is a form of ischemic heart disease; in fact, the terms are often used interchangeably in the clinic. Ischemic heart disease refers to damage to the heart muscle caused by deprivation of oxygen.
- Most pacemaker patients have CAD.
- Other types of heart disease that can cause a patient to need a pacemaker are nonischemic heart disease and congenital heart abnormalities (structural heart disease).

- Nonischemic heart disease is often called cardiomyopathy. There are three types of cardiomyopathy: dilated cardiomyopathy, hypertrophic cardiomyopathy, and restrictive cardiomyopathy.
- Hypertrophic cardiomyopathy is often called hypertrophic obstructive cardiomyopathy (HOCM) because typically the septum becomes thickened and stiffened and creates an obstruction of the outflow tracts.

- CAD is caused by a buildup of *sludge* in the blood that sticks to the inside walls of the vessels, creating plaque buildup and atherosclerosis. People with CAD often have atherosclerotic buildup in other vessels in the body, too.
- CAD is associated with heart attack or myocardial infarction (MI). The first few days after an MI is the acute phase; acute MI (AMI) patients are at very high risk for potentially fatal ventricular fibrillation. That's why most AMI patients are treated in a coronary care unit where they can be closely monitored for ventricular fibrillation and quickly defibrillated, if necessary. Ideally, such patients should be defibrillated within 30 s of onset of ventricular fibrillation, when it is easiest to rescue them from this arrhythmia.
- After a few days, the MI is considered *old*. Patients who have survived an MI are at risk for arrhythmias because the MI has left lesions (scars) on their heart. The lesion neither contracts nor conducts electricity, and the area around the scar is electrically unstable.
- There are known risk factors for ischemic heart disease including noncontrollable factors (men over 45, women over 55 or over 45 with early-onset menopause) and genetic factors as well as controllable factors, such as obesity, sedentary lifestyle, smoking, hypertension, high cholesterol, and diabetes.
- Women and even clinicians probably underestimate a woman's chances of getting heart disease. Heart disease is the number one killer of women, and women with heart disease often have poorer outcomes than men. This is likely due to the fact that heart disease in women is underdiagnosed and therefore goes untreated.
- High cholesterol is a known risk factor for heart disease. Cholesterol should be <130 mg/dl of low-density lipoproteins (LDL or bad cholesterol) and <40 (men) or <50 mg/dl of high-density lipoproteins (HDL or good cholesterol). Rather than the overall number, it is the ratio between these numbers that is important. High cholesterol is treated first with lifestyle modifications (diet and exercise) and then with statin therapy.
- Diabetes (both type I and type II) increases risk of CAD by two- to eight fold and also increases the risk of stroke, infection, and peripheral neuropathy.
- Hypertension (>140/90 mmHg) is a risk factor for CAD as well as for stroke and kidney disease.
- Nonischemic heart disease is not as commonly seen in device clinics as ischemic heart disease.
- Risk factors for nonischemic heart disease include excessive drug or alcohol use, toxins (such as chemotherapy drugs), viruses, and valvular abnormalities.
- Congenital heart defect is a structural abnormality of the heart that is present at birth. About 40 000 babies a year are born with a congenital heart defect. There are many different types of congenital heart defects, and some more severe than others. These conditions cannot be treated with lifestyle modifications or drug therapy, but many are amenable to surgical repair.
- Patients with congenital heart defects may have rhythm disorders, or they may require surgery that results in arrhythmias and thus require pacing.
- Risk factors for congenital heart defects include maternal drug and alcohol abuse, genetic defects, or a viral infection passed to the baby in the womb. Most congenital heart defects are of unknown origin (idiopathic).

Test your knowledge

1 Why would an acute myocardial infarction patient be treated in the coronary care unit?
  A To prevent a congenital defect
  B To monitor the patient and defibrillate him if necessary
  C To provide intravenous statin therapy
  D To prevent ischemic heart disease

2 What is the number one killer of women in America?
  A Breast cancer
  B Lung cancer
  C Ovarian cancer
  D Heart disease

3 The most common type of heart disease found in pacemaker patients is:
  A Coronary artery disease
  B Hypertrophic cardiomyopathy
  C Diabetes
  D Valvular disorders

4 Which of the following is *not* a risk factor for coronary artery disease?
  A High cholesterol
  B Stress
  C Viral infection
  D Hypertension

5 Alcohol abuse is considered a risk factor for which type of heart disease?
  A Cardiomyopathy
  B Defect of the mitral valve
  C Ventricular septal defect
  D Coronary artery disease

6 Patients who survived a heart attack for a year or more have two primary modes of death. One of these is arrhythmic death. What is the other?
  A Stroke
  B Kidney failure
  C Pump failure
  D Peripheral neuropathy

7 What increases a person's risk of CAD by two- to eightfold?
  A Mild hypertension
  B Male gender
  C Ventricular septal defect
  D Diabetes

8 Which disease is sometimes called the *silent killer* because it is often asymptomatic?
  A Hypertension
  B Hypercholesterolemia
  C Patent foramen ovale
  D Myocardial infarction

9 If a patient had a severe congenital heart defect, how would it most likely be treated?
  A Lifestyle modification (diet and exercise)
  B Drug therapy
  C Surgery
  D Pacemaker therapy

10 According to the Centers for Disease Control and Prevention, how many Americans who suffer a heart attack will die from it?
  A 10%
  B 45%
  C 80%
  D All of them

CHAPTER 5

Cardiac medications related to cardiac rhythm management devices

Learning objectives

- Name five of six common categories of heart medication, their effects on the heart, and the potential complications associated with their use.
- Name two or three types of drugs most frequently used by cardiac rhythm management device patients.
- Briefly list heart drugs commonly used in emergencies.
- Define the terms inotropic, chronotropic, and dromotropic.

Introduction

Patients who come to a device clinic frequently take multiple medications; in fact, it is rare to see a pacemaker patient who is not on a drug regimen. Although device clinicians may want to perceive themselves as *device experts*, pacemaker patients are ultimately patients. The pacemaker clinic does not manage pacemakers; it manages patients who happen to have pacemakers. Thus, our clinical concerns always have to be centered on the patient, that is, based on optimal management of the whole person. This typically involves both drug and device therapy.

Cardiac drugs and certain other types of drugs can affect the heart rate and rhythm. Understanding these effects is important for device therapy. In some cases, the drugs a patient takes may require certain modifications to the pacemaker's programmable settings. There are even cases where a necessary drug therapy results in an iatrogenic (*physician-induced*) bradycardia that requires pacing. Thus, device clinicians need to have a good basic knowledge of pharmacology and the heart.

Drug actions and interactions

Cardiac drugs exert three main types of action on the heart:
- *Inotropic drugs* increase or decrease the force of cardiac contractility.
- *Chronotropic drugs* increase or decrease the rate of contraction.
- *Dromotropic drugs* increase or decrease the rate of cardiac conduction.

Many cardiac drugs are complex in that they exert more than one type of action on the heart. Their effects can be mild to severe.

Drug–drug interactions occur when two drugs exert an influence on each other apart from the intended effect. Drug–drug interactions are not at all uncommon and may be mild to severe, even life threatening. Any time a patient takes more than one drug, the clinicians should be sure that these drugs do not interact with each other. Drug–drug interactions can result in one or both of the drugs being stronger (potentiation) or weaker than it

The Nuts and Bolts of Implantable Device Therapy Pacemakers, First Edition. Tom Kenny.
© 2015 John Wiley & Sons, Ltd. Published 2015 by John Wiley & Sons, Ltd.

would be if taken alone. It is beyond the scope of this section to discuss drug–drug interactions in detail, but clinicians can use information in the drug's package insert or from reputable online sources to determine if two drugs have the potential to interact.

Drug–device interactions can occur as well. In such cases, it is more common for the physician to alter the drug therapy (such as reducing the dose or changing the medication) than to alter the device, but there are times when pharmacological therapy may necessitate alterations to a pacemaker's programmed settings.

Ten of the most frequently encountered cardiac drugs for pacemaker patients

Pacemaker patients and candidates for pacing therapy often take cardiac medications. In fact, it is unusual to encounter pacemaker patients who do not take some form of cardiac drug. Ten of the most commonly encountered drugs for pacemaker patient will be presented here. Bear in mind that this list is not exhaustive.

Cardiac glycosides

Cardiac glycosides are drugs that increase the efficiency of the heart by making the cardiac contraction of the heart muscle more vigorous, thus exerting an inotropic effect on the heart. The best-known of these agents is digitalis or digoxin (marketed as Lanoxin); dobutamine is an intravenous (IV) cardiac glycoside. Cardiac glycosides slow cardiac conduction through the SA and AV nodes (producing what is known as a *negative dromotropic effect*) but also increase the forcefulness of the cardiac contraction (resulting in a *positive inotropic effect*). One effect of these agents is that they slow the heart rate. Cardiac glycosides are typically prescribed to treat heart failure because of their effect on cardiac contraction; cardiac glycosides are also prescribed to treat atrial fibrillation, atrial flutter, and paroxysmal atrial tachycardia, but in these cases, they are prescribed to slow cardiac conduction.

When digoxin is prescribed to treat an arrhythmia, it is generally used to slow conduction.

A potential side effect of digoxin is digitalis toxicity, which may cause weakness, dizziness, nausea,

and even arrhythmias. When digitalis toxicity is suspected, a serum blood test must be performed to assess blood levels of the drug (>2 is digoxin toxic). In such cases, a drug known as Digibind may be used to help bind the digitalis and lower serum levels to nontoxic levels.

Cardiac glycosides such as digoxin lower the heart rate to the point that patients should be instructed to take their pulse prior to taking their dose. In some cases, the patient may be told that if his or her pulse rate is below a certain number (such as 50 bpm), the patient should refrain from taking the drug and instead contact the clinic for further advice.

Clinicians should monitor the potassium levels of their patients taking cardiac glycosides.

Antianginal drugs

As the name implies, antianginal drugs are given to patients who have angina, that is, patients with symptomatic forms of coronary artery disease (CAD). There are three main categories of antianginal drugs, that is, drugs used to fight angina:

- Calcium-channel blockers
- Vasodilators
- Beta-adrenergic blockers (also called beta-blockers)

Calcium-channel blockers work on the smooth cardiac and vascular muscles. These muscles rely on the flow of extracellular calcium in and out of the cell to contract. These extracellular calcium ions travel through permeable smooth muscle cells via *calcium channels*. As the name implies, a calcium-channel blocker inhibits the ability of calcium ions to move through these calcium channels, which, in turn, inhibits contractions of the cardiac and vascular muscles. The net effect of a calcium-channel blocker is inotropic, in that it decreases contractility and inhibits vascular contractions, resulting in dilation of coronary and peripheral arteries.

Like any drug, calcium-channel blockers confer on patients both risks and benefits. The most common side effect associated with calcium-channel blockers is a swelling of the ankles or feet, which may be at least partially relieved by elevating the feet. Less common side effects include difficulty breathing, dizziness, erratic heartbeat, dyspnea, and a tightness in the chest.

Vasodilators may also be prescribed to treat angina; these drugs relax the smooth muscle layer of blood vessels, allowing for dilation of those vessels, which, in turn, improves blood flow through the vessels. Vasodilators decrease preload, afterload, and myocardial oxygen consumption.

Side effects associated with vasodilators are uncommon, but the following is a partial list of side effects that have been reported: abnormal heart sounds, body aches, blood in the urine or pain while urinating, chest tightness or discomfort, confusion, headache, itchiness, light-headedness, and loss of appetite.

Beta-adrenergic blockers or beta-blockers are another type of antianginal drug that work by decreasing the activity in certain tissue of the sympathetic nervous system. Beta-blockers slow conduction (dromotropic effect), lower the heart rate (chronotropic effect), decrease contractility (inotropic effect), and thus decrease the workload on the heart. Beta-blockers may be prescribed for any number of conditions, and they are frequently prescribed to treat hypertension. Beta-blockers may also be prescribed to treat angina or for certain types of cardiac arrhythmias.

Beta-blockers may produce side effects, the most commonly reported of which include blurred vision; chest pain or discomfort; confusion; diarrhea; dizziness; erratic heart rate; light-headedness; nausea and vomiting; dyspnea; sweating; swelling of face, hands, and lower legs; fatigue; and wheezing. Although side effects are not necessarily rare with beta-blockers, many are mild and will resolve without medical attention over time. For that reason, beta-blockers are usually started at a low dose and progressively increased as the patient tolerates them. However, moderate to severe side effects should be clinically treated. It is possible to overdose on beta-blockers; signs of beta-blockade toxicity include anxiety, cold sweats, coma, cool and pale skin, nightmares, no heart rate, seizures, shakiness, and slurred speech.

Names of some of the most commonly prescribed and frequently encountered antianginal agents appear in **Table 5.1**, but this table is by no means exhaustive. Note that some of these drugs may be available in sublingual formulations, IV formulations, transdermal patches, and so on.

Table 5.1 Antianginal drugs by group with a few of the most commonly used generic and brand names

Group	Main actions	Generic name	Brand name
Calcium-channel blockers	Inhibit movement of calcium ions and thus decrease contractility, lower heart rate, and dilate coronary and peripheral arteries	Amlodipine Diltiazem Nifedipine Verapamil	Norvasc® Cardizem® Procardia®, Adalat® Calan®
Vasodilators	By relaxing smooth muscle layer of blood vessels, they dilate vessels and improve blood flow	Nitroglycerin	Nitro-Bid®, Nitro-Dur®, Nitrol, Nitrolingual® Pump Spray, and others
		Isosorbide dinitrate (sometimes called just *nitrates*)	Isordil®
		Isosorbide mononitrate (also a *nitrate*)	Imdur®
Beta-blockers	Decrease activity of the sympathetic nervous system, lower heart rate, and decrease contractility	Atenolol Sotalol Esmolol Nadolol Metoprolol	Tenormin® Betapace® Brevibloc® Corgard® Lopressor® Toprol® and Toprol-XL®
		Propranolol	Inderal®

Brand names are trademarks or registered trademarks of their owners.
Note that this table is not intended to be exhaustive.

Antiarrhythmics

Antiarrhythmic agents (sometimes called *antidysrhythmics* or abbreviated AAAs) are drugs intended to prevent and/or treat cardiac arrhythmias. Antiarrhythmic drugs work by altering the action potential of the heart. The action potential (phase 0 through 5) is a graphic depiction of the electrical activity of the myocardial cells. Most antiarrhythmic drugs work in the *plateau* region of the action potential but actually may work at any point in changing the action potential. AAAs work by slowing conduction through the cardiac cells, depressing automaticity (the heart's ability to generate electrical impulses spontaneously), and increasing resistance to premature stimulation of cardiac cells.

Like any powerful drugs, AAAs have risks as well as benefits. The main risk associated with AAAs seems paradoxical: they are proarrhythmic, that is, they can induce arrhythmias. AAAs affect the cardiac action potential, as we will see in the next sections, and altering the action potential can both inhibit or provoke arrhythmic events. Virtually all of the AAAs available can be proarrhythmic, although some may be more proarrhythmic than others. For this reason, care should be taken when prescribing these agents; they require careful dosing and consistent monitoring. Of particular concern is the patient with a benign arrhythmia who is given some of these drugs and winds up with a potentially dangerous rhythm disorder! While these drugs have a rightful place in the care of patients with arrhythmias, it cannot be stressed enough that these drugs have proarrhythmic effects and must be prescribed prudently by experienced clinicians and monitored closely. This monitoring may include lab testing, measuring of QT intervals and other ECG parameters, and evaluating the patient for side effects.

AAAs can be grouped by classes and even subclasses, which helps to better characterize their effects. Class I AAAs block the fast sodium channels of the myocardial cells that results in a slightly delayed depolarization, which, in turn, slows the heart rate. Class I AAAs are further subdivided into classes IA , IB, and IC, which have different effects on the action potential (see **Figure 5.1**).

An antiarrhythmic class IA drug causes a modest depression of phase 0 of the action potential and, in that way, prolongs both depolarization and repolarization. This prolongs the patient's native QT interval, which should be clinically monitored as it may put the patient at risk for potential ventricular rhythm disorders. Although not used frequently today, quinidine is an example of an antiarrhythmic class IA agent. Quinidine can prolong the QT interval in patients, and many years ago, this effect was called *quinidine syncope* rather than prolonged QT interval, resulting in ventricular tachyarrhythmia. Patients on quinidine with *quinidine syncope* frequently got dizzy and light-headed or even passed out. Because of these proarrhythmic effects, quinidine is not used often today, and when used, it must be carefully monitored. Other class IA

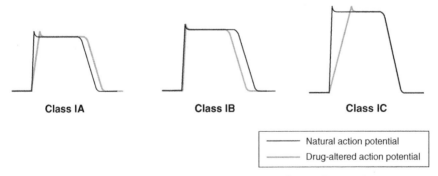

Class IA   Class IB   Class IC

———— Natural action potential
———— Drug-altered action potential

Figure 5.1 The different subclasses of class I antiarrhythmic agents have different effects on the action potential. Class IA agents delay the onset of depolarization slightly and prolong the duration of depolarization, while class IB agents shorten the duration of depolarization. Class IC antiarrhythmics markedly affect phase 0 of the action potential but have no effect on depolarization. Note that these agents may have proarrhythmic effects; for example, class IA agents prolong the patient's QT interval, which can set the stage for possible ventricular arrhythmic events.

antiarrhythmics are procainamide and disopyramide, both of which may also prolong the QT interval.

An antiarrhythmic class IB agent causes a modest depression of phase 0, shortens depolarization, and decreases the duration of the action potential. Lidocaine is a class IB antiarrhythmic, which also is sometimes used as a local anesthetic. Administered intravenously, lidocaine can suppress ventricular ectopic activity. Its mechanism of action involves sodium-channel blockade, mostly in ventricular cells. Thus, lidocaine may be considered a good treatment specifically for ventricular (not atrial) arrhythmias. An oral formulation of lidocaine used to treat arrhythmias is marketed as mexiletine.

A class IC AAA provokes a strong depression of phase 0 but has no effect on depolarization. A good example of a class IC antiarrhythmic is flecainide, which was originally developed as a local anesthetic. Flecainide slows conduction in all areas of the heart and inhibits abnormal automaticity. Flecainide can be an effective treatment for atrial arrhythmias, such as atrial flutter and atrial fibrillation, but it is not used by some physicians owing to some negative scrutiny on the drug as a result of the clinical CAST. Another class IC AAA is propafenone, which likewise slows conduction in all parts of the heart, offers a weak beta-blockade, and blocks some calcium-channel activity.

The class II antiarrhythmics can be generally described as the beta-blockers. There are two types of beta-adrenergic effects, with beta-1 involving more cardiac activities and beta-2 more pulmonary activities. Beta-blockers have two main mechanisms of action that can be simply described as blocking the myocardial beta-adrenergic receptors and stabilizing the membrane effect of sodium channel blockade. Beta-blockers for cardiac arrhythmias should selectively work on the beta-1 system. Beta-blocker generic names end in *olol*, and drugs in this class include propranolol, metoprolol, atenolol, and carvedilol, among many others. Beta-blockers slow the SA node and can block arrhythmias, particularly arrhythmias brought on by exertion. In fact, beta-blockers are often prescribed for patients with exercise-induced arrhythmias. (Patients with exercise-induced arrhythmias experience a blast of adrenaline during exertion that brings on the arrhythmia; the beta-blocker is able to blunt the force of that adrenaline and keep it from affecting the heart rate.)

Class III AAAs are potassium-channel blockers that were originally developed because some patients did not tolerate sodium-channel blockers. A class III agent delays repolarization (see **Figure 5.2**), which results in a prolonged refractory period. These agents are not used a great deal with the exception of amiodarone, a drug that prolongs the action potential by delaying the outflow of potassium ions from myocardial cells. Other class III agents include ibutilide, bretylium, and dofetilide. Amiodarone is often used to treat atrial tachyarrhythmias and can be effective in the treatment of certain ventricular arrhythmias as well. Interestingly, amiodarone's effect on atrial tachyarrhythmias is that it can convert the rhythm back to normal sinus rhythm, that is, it is a *rhythm* rather than *rate* control drug for atrial tachycardia. However, amiodarone has been associated with a number of dose-related side effects and other adverse events. It has a long half-life and can build up in the body over time, so amiodarone should be carefully dosed and monitored.

Class IV AAAs are calcium-channel blockers and work by slowing the rate of AV conduction, particularly in the setting of atrial fibrillation. Calcium-channel blockers can be used to treat angina but are effective as AAAs as well. Examples of calcium-channel blockers that treat arrhythmias are verapamil and diltiazem.

A summary of the AAAs appears in **Table 5.2**.

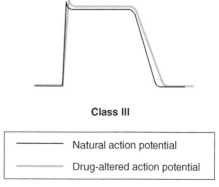

Class III

————	Natural action potential
-----------	Drug-altered action potential

Figure 5.2 Class III antiarrhythmic agents, such as amiodarone, prolong the refractory period.

Table 5.2 Antiarrhythmic agents by class and subclass with a few of the most commonly used generic and brand names

Class/subclass	Main actions	Generic name	Brand name
Class IA	Slightly depresses phase 0 of the action potential and prolongs depolarization and repolarization and thus the QT interval. All class I agents inhibit the sodium channel	Quinidine Procainamide	Generic only Procan® Procanbid® Pronestyl®
		Disopyramide	Norpace®
Class IB	Causes a modest depression of phase 0, shortens depolarization, and decreases the duration of the action potential	Lidocaine Phenytoin	Xylocaine® Dilantin® Phenytek®
		Mexiletine	Mexitil®
Class IC	Provokes a strong depression of phase 0 but has no effect on depolarization, slows conduction in all areas of the heart and inhibits abnormal automaticity	Flecainide Propafenone Moricizine	Tambocor® Rythmol® Ethmozine®
Class II	Beta-blockers that suppress the sympathetic nervous system, can be particularly useful in treating exercise-induced arrhythmias	Atenolol Sotalol Esmolol Nadolol Metoprolol	Tenormin® Betapace® Brevibloc® Corgard® Lopressor® Toprol® Toprol-XL®
		Propranolol	Inderal®
Class III	Potassium-channel blockers that delay repolarization and thus prolong the refractory period	Amiodarone Ibutilide Dofetilide Dronedarone	Cordarone® Corvert® Tikosyn® Multaq®
Class IV	Calcium-channel blockers that slow the rate of AV conduction, particularly in atrial fibrillation	Verapamil	Calan® Covera-HS® Isoptin® Verelan®
		Diltiazem	Cardizem® Cartia® Dilacor® Dilt® Diltia®

Brand names are trademarks or registered trademarks of their owners.
Note that this table is not intended to be exhaustive.

Angiotensin-converting enzyme inhibitors

Angiotensin I is converted in the body by way of an enzyme to angiotensin II and, in so doing, causes strong vasoconstriction. An angiotensin-converting enzyme (ACE) inhibitor prevents angiotensin I from converting into angiotensin II and, in so doing, promotes vasodilation.

ACE inhibitors are often prescribed to treat hypertension but are also appropriate for virtually all heart failure patients. ACE inhibitors block aldosterone, which prevents sodium and water retention; in this way, ACE inhibitors increase blood flow to the kidneys, lower blood pressure, and reduce both preload and afterload. ACE inhibitors are frequently prescribed to patients, and clinicians in device clinics will encounter them; ACE inhibitor names usually end in *il* and include captopril, monopril, prinivil, and accupril, among many others.

Like any other powerful drugs, ACE inhibitors are associated with certain adverse events, including angina, tachycardia, hypotension, rash, gastric ulcers, liver toxicity, renal insufficiency, urinary frequency, neutropenia, and hemolytic anemias.

Clinicians in device clinics should expect to encounter patients taking ACE inhibitors in practice. When appropriately prescribed, dosed, and monitored, ACE inhibitors are a safe and effective agent for patients with left ventricular dysfunction.

Analgesics

Analgesics are pain relievers, and for arrhythmia patients, these drugs are mainly prescribed to treat chest pain. The typical dosing regimen of an analgesic agent is to start low and titrate upward slowly to the point that the patient's pain is relieved. In this connection, it should be noted that complete pain relief may not be possible for every patient, so in some cases, analgesics help to control but do not entirely eliminate pain. Typical analgesics for ischemic heart disease patients include nitroglycerin (a powerful vasodilator) or morphine.

Morphine is an interesting drug for myocardial infarction patient. Known best as a narcotic pain reliever, morphine vasodilates and thus decreases workload of the heart, in addition to relieving both pain and anxiety in the patient. For these reasons, IV morphine is often administered to in-hospital myocardial infarction patients. Morphine is associated with numerous side effects, including dizziness, nausea, vomiting, constipation, and itchiness, which may be mild to intolerable. In some cases, side effects of morphine can be managed, such as giving the patient antiemetic drugs to control nausea and vomiting. Morphine in this setting would be used only in-hospital to manage acute pain.

Diuretics

Diuretics work in the tubules of the kidney cells (nephrons) to increase the secretion of water and electrolytes from the body. Diuretics are widely prescribed and can be effective in treating heart failure, fluid overload, certain endocrine disorders, kidney dysfunction, and liver disease. There are several different types of diuretics including loop diuretics (Lasix[1], Bumex, Edecrin, Demadex), osmotic diuretics (mannitol), potassium-sparing diuretics (Aldactone, Dyrenium), thiazides (Diuril, Lozol), and carbonic anhydrase

inhibitors, which are not used for cardiac conditions but rather to treat glaucoma or ocular edema in patients with heart failure.

Patients with heart failure should be treated with diuretics, and these drugs are widely prescribed among arrhythmia patients. A potential problem with long-term diuretic use is that patients excrete electrolytes, in particular potassium. Low serum potassium levels are known as hypokalemia, which can lead to arrhythmias. For that reason, potassium-sparing diuretics were created, which allow for diuretic action without the loss of large amounts of potassium. Heart failure patients taking loop diuretics may be prescribed a potassium supplement to help compensate for the loss of potassium and prevent hypokalemia.

Although diuretics are widely prescribed, clinicians should be aware that these familiar drugs are associated with side effects and should be monitored. Diuretics can lead to hypotension, electrolyte imbalances (typically hypokalemia, but hyperkalemia may occur in patients treated with potassium-sparing diuretics), and nausea and vomiting. Elderly patients, diabetics, and those with renal dysfunction may be particularly vulnerable to these effects. Since electrolyte imbalances are associated with arrhythmias, patients on diuretics should be carefully monitored.

Anticoagulants

Anticoagulants are prescribed to prevent the formation and spread of thrombi. A thrombus or blood clot can form anywhere in the body; if a thrombus dislodges, it becomes an embolus; the embolus is carried along in the circulation and may clog a vessel. Depending on where the clog occurs, this event can precipitate a stroke, a heart attack, or a pulmonary embolism. Thrombi may develop anywhere; of particular concern are the so-called deep vein thrombi, which occur deep within the circulatory system. Heart attack survivors are particularly vulnerable to thrombi and are routinely treated with anticoagulants. Patients with atrial fibrillation are also prone to develop thrombi because a relatively large amount of the blood in their heart remains stagnant and may clot. Thus, anticoagulants are prescribed chronically to atrial fibrillation patients and are routinely administered in the hospital setting for acute myocardial infarction and other conditions.

---

[1] Product names, company names, and proprietary feature names are trademarks or registered trademarks of their owners.

Coumadin, sometimes known as warfarin, and a newer agent known by the trade name Pradaxa® are oral anticoagulants intended for long-term use in patients who have or are at risk for deep vein thrombus, patients with atrial fibrillation, heart attack survivors, and those who have had valve replacement surgery. Coumadin is a very useful drug but may interact with other agents, including nonsteroidal anti-inflammatory drugs (NSAIDs) and beta-blockers.

Heparin is an anticoagulant intended for acute use, typically in the hospital setting. Heparin may be administered subcutaneously or intravenously.

Thrombolytics

A thrombolytic agent dissolves a thrombus (blood clot) and can help to reopen blood vessels. These drugs are sometimes nicknamed *clot busters*. Thrombolytics are administered in the hospital for acute use, and patients must be closely observed for signs of potentially dangerous bleeding. Thrombolytics can be highly effective when administered in the first six hours following myocardial infarction. Thrombolytics are typically administered intravenously, and they work by inhibiting fibrin, a fibrous substance in the body used to form clots. Some common names of thrombolytics are Activase, Retavase, and streptokinase.

Another type of thrombolytic drug is ReoPro, which acts on the platelets in order to prevent clots from forming. ReoPro is given intravenously during certain cardiac procedures and may be used with heparin and aspirin in patients with unstable angina or acute myocardial infarction.

Antiplatelet agents

Antiplatelet agents, including aspirin and brand names such as Plavix®, Persantine®, Ticlid®, and ReoPro®, are commonly prescribed to patients immediately following stroke or myocardial infarction. They prevent platelet formation, which can form plaque and contribute to thrombi. Antiplatelet agents are typically used because of their effect in the arterial circulatory system, where anticoagulants are less effective. Antiplatelet agents can be prescribed long term for patients at high risk for stroke or cardiovascular events associated with thrombi.

Antihyperlipidemics

Cholesterol is a waxy substance in the circulatory system that is composed of high-density lipoproteins (HDL), low-density lipoproteins (LDL), and triglycerides. The human body produces these naturally, but a high-fat diet, sedentary lifestyle, and genetic predisposition can cause some people to have unusually high serum lipid levels. This condition, known as hyperlipidemia, is widespread and is thought to contribute to heart attack and other cardiovascular events. Lipid-lowering drugs are called antihyperlipidemics or statins. The goals of statin drugs are to lower serum cholesterol levels overall and to bring about a more optimal ratio of HDL to LDL. The best-known brand of statin drug is Lipitor®, but other statin drugs include Zocor®, Lescol®, Lopid®, Crestor®, and many others.

Emergency drugs

There are a number of drugs that are routinely administered for cardiovascular emergencies.

Atropine increases the heart rate and increases conduction across the AV node. It is administered for patients in asystole or with profound bradycardia.

Dopamine is a vasopressor agent, meaning that it increases the blood pressure and cardiac output. A surgeon may order a dopamine drip if the patient's blood pressure drops during a procedure.

Isuprel increases both contractility and heart rate, and it is used in emergency situations to stimulate the heart rate.

Nipride or sodium nitroprusside is a very powerful vasodilator and would be administered to help lower hypertension in an emergency situation.

Sodium bicarbonate is administered intravenously to treat an acidotic heart. Cardiac acidosis occurs when there are not enough sodium or bicarbonate ions in the blood.

Calcium chloride is not a first-line drug for cardiac care, even in emergencies, but in case of a cardiac arrest when nothing else has worked, calcium chloride may be used to stimulate muscle contractions. Calcium chloride may protect the heart muscle from high levels of sodium and can also be used to treat calcium-channel blocker toxicity.

Dobutamine is an inotropic medication used for heart failure, and following cardiac surgery, it increases cardiac contractility.

Catecholamines include epinephrine and would be administered for cardiac arrest or asystole.

Levophed is a potent vasoconstrictor, stimulates muscles, and increases flow to the coronary artery. This would be given to surgical patients with precipitous drops in blood pressure.

Conclusion

Drugs play an important role in the care of most modern cardiac patients and pacemaker patients are no exception. Even when a clinician concentrates on device therapy, it is important to recognize the main types of cardiac agents and how they can potentially influence device therapy. AAAs work by altering the action potential at the myocardial cellular level, and while they can have antiarrhythmic effects, their work in changing the action potential can sometimes lead to proarrhythmic effects as well. For that reason, antiarrhythmic drugs should be used with caution and carefully dosed and monitored. Beta-blockers are used for many indications, including heart failure and hypertension, and they slow the heart. Sometimes, patients taking beta-blockers for a noncardiac indication (such as hypertension) may develop a beta-blocker-induced bradycardia necessitating pacemakers. Beta-blockers are very common drugs in the pacing clinic, and most heart failure patients take them along with an ACE inhibitor. Amiodarone, a class III AAA, can inhibit ambient tachyarrhythmias but is associated with toxicity and has a very long half-life (measured in months!). Device clinicians should have a working knowledge of the main types of drugs cardiac patients may take for two main reasons. First, knowing the type of drugs the patient takes can shed light on the patient's cardiac condition. Second, understanding the effects of these drugs can allow for better device programming.

The nuts and bolts of medications related to cardiac rhythm management devices

- Most device patients take one or more medications, including cardiac drugs. Cardiac drugs are powerful agents that affect the heart and may possibly influence device programming selections.
- Cardiac drugs may have inotropic effects (increase/decrease vigorousness of cardiac contractility), chronotropic effects (increase/decrease rate of contraction), or dromotropic effects (increase/decrease rate of cardiac conduction). Some drugs, such as beta-blockers, have more than one type of effect.
- Digoxin or digitalis is a cardiac glycoside that makes the contraction of the heart more vigorous (positive inotropic effect) and slows conduction (negative dromotropic effect). Patients who take digoxin often have a slowed heart rate.
- Antianginal drugs are agents that help patients manage angina or chest pain as a result of coronary artery disease (CAD). There are three main types of drugs that treat angina: calcium-channel blockers, vasodilators, and beta-blockers.
- Calcium-channel blockers inhibit the flow of calcium ions through the cardiac cell, decreasing contractility (negative inotropic effect) and resulting in dilation of coronary and peripheral arteries.
- Vasodilators, as the name suggest, dilate the coronary and peripheral vessels and improve blood flow through the vessels, decreasing preload, afterload, and myocardial oxygen consumption.
- Beta-blockers inhibit the sympathetic nervous system and have multiple effects: they slow conduction (negative dromotropic effect), reduce the heart rate (negative chronotropic effect), decrease contractility (negative inotropic effect) and, in that way, reduce the heart's workload. Beta-blockers are prescribed for heart failure but may also be indicated to treat hypertension and other conditions.
- Antiarrhythmic agents are grouped into four classes and there are three subclasses (A, B, and C) of class I. These are complex agents that alter the action potential at the myocardial cellular level, and while they can prevent or inhibit arrhythmias, they may sometimes have proarrhythmic effects. For this reason, they should be prescribed prudently and monitored closely.

Continued

Continued

- Class I antiarrhythmics are sodium-channel blockers that slow the heart rate.
- Examples of subclass of class I are as follows: class IA, quinidine; class IB, lidocaine; and class IC, flecainide.
- Drugs have various routes of administration; some are administered orally, some are administered subcutaneously or intravenously, and there are even transdermal patches or nasal spray formulations (of nitroglycerin).
- Many drugs are used in multiple settings. For example, lidocaine is a local anesthetic but can be administered intravenously to fight ventricular ectopic activity. It is considered a class IB agent.
- Beta-blockers suppress activity of the sympathetic nervous system and are routinely administered to heart failure patients. They also can be prescribed to inhibit exercise-induced arrhythmias in that they blunt the force of adrenaline. Beta-blockers also are antihypertensives.
- Patients who take beta-blockers may have a slowed heart rate; in some cases, this may be beneficial. However, patients who take beta-blockers for noncardiac reasons (such as high blood pressure) and deal with a slowed heart rate as a side effect of the drug may need a pacemaker.
- Beta-blockers are class II drugs.
- Calcium-channel blockers are class III drugs (as well as class IA drugs when taken to manage angina). Calcium-channel blockers delay repolarization and prolong the refractory period. They are less commonly prescribed than class II agents. The best-known class III drug is amiodarone, which can inhibit or reduce both atrial and ventricular tachyarrhythmias.
- Amiodarone is associated with toxicity and has a long half-life, meaning that the drug levels can accumulate and build up in the body over time.
- Angiotensin I is converted in the body via an enzyme into angiotensin II, and in this transformation, a strong vasoconstrictive force occurs. Angiotensin-converting enzyme (ACE) inhibitors prevent this transformation and promote vasodilation. ACE inhibitors are prescribed for high blood pressure and are routinely administered to heart failure patients.
- There are two main analgesic (pain-relieving) agents for chest pain. Nitroglycerin is given to help manage ischemic chest pain. In-hospital patients with chest pain or recovering from myocardial infarction may be given intravenous morphine, which not only relieves pain and anxiety but also has a vasodilative effect.
- Diuretic agents are given to reduce fluid retention in the body and may be loop diuretics (such as Lasix) or potassium-sparing diuretics. Since diuretics promote water excretion from the body, they result in electrolyte depletion. Patients taking loop diuretics should be monitored so that they do not become hypokalemic. Potassium-sparing diuretics (e.g., Aldactone) allow a diuretic effect without depleting the body of potassium. It is important not to supplement potassium in a patient taking a potassium-sparing diuretic, in that they may become hyperkalemic.
- Anticoagulants help prevent emboli or blood clots. An embolus is a blood clot lodged in position; when it dislodges and can potentially clog a vessel, it is called a thrombus and may be treated by a thrombolytic (or *clot-busting*) drug.
- Coumadin (warfarin) is a common anticoagulant, which is nicknamed a *blood thinner*. Patients taking these drugs can bleed copiously from even small cuts. Coumadin has multiple drug interactions and should not be taken by patients who are also taking beta-blockers or nonsteroidal anti-inflammatory drugs (NSAIDs).
- Thrombolytics can be very effective when administered within the first six hours after a myocardial infarction.
- Antiplatelet agents (such as Plavix) prevent platelet formation that can contribute to plaque and thrombi. They are often prescribed to patients after heart attack or stroke.
- Patients with high cholesterol are often prescribed antihyperlipidemics or statin drugs if diet and exercise cannot control their serum cholesterol levels.
- In an emergency, there are many powerful drugs that may be administered to increase the heart rate (atropine, Isuprel), increase blood pressure (dopamine, Levophed), decrease blood pressure

(Nipride), stimulate cardiac contractions (calcium chloride), increase contractility (dobutamine), and treat cardiac acidosis (sodium bicarbonate) or cardiac arrest (catecholamines).

• Pacemaker specialists treat patients not pacemakers, so it is important for device experts to understand cardiac drugs and how they may affect the patient's condition and possibly interact with the pacemaker. Most drug–device interactions are handled by changing the drug dose or type of drug, but sometimes, the pacemaker's programmed settings can be adjusted to accommodate drug therapy. Most device patients are also drug patients, and clinicians need to be mindful of both types of therapies.

Test your knowledge

1 Beta-blockers are often prescribed to patients:
   A Who have just had a stroke
   B Who have heart failure
   C Who have dangerously low blood pressure
   D All of the above

2 What is a potentially dangerous side effect of most antiarrhythmic agents?
   A They can be proarrhythmic.
   B They are potentially addictive.
   C They may cause blindness.
   D They cause hypertension.

3 Amiodarone is a:
   A Class IA antiarrhythmic drug
   B Class II antiarrhythmic drug
   C Class III antiarrhythmic drug
   D Class IV antiarrhythmic drug

4 Intravenous morphine may be given to an in-hospital acute myocardial infarction patient for what reason?
   A To manage pain
   B To help reduce anxiety
   C To help dilate vessels
   D All of the above

5 Drugs that increase or decrease cardiac contractility have what kind of effect?
   A Inotropic
   B Chronotropic
   C Dromotropic
   D None of the above

6 Which of the following is an example of a thrombolytic agent?
   A Plavix®
   B Coumadin
   C Activase®
   D Lipitor®

7 Why would a patient be prescribed an antihyperlipidemic drug?
   A To lower hypertension
   B To control pain
   C To reduce serum cholesterol
   D To prevent thrombosis

8 Which of the following is a loop diuretic agent?
   A Lasix®
   B Aldactone
   C Carvedilol
   D Brevibloc®

9 ACE inhibitors such as captopril are often and appropriately prescribed to patients with:
   A Diabetes
   B Tachycardia
   C Bradycardia
   D Heart failure

10 Which of the following drugs is a class IV antiarrhythmic agent that blocks calcium channels, slows AV conduction, and is often prescribed to patients with atrial fibrillation?
   A Atenolol
   B Verapamil
   C Lidocaine
   D Propafenone

6 CHAPTER 6

The basics of ECG and rhythm interpretation

Learning objectives

- Explain how cardiac activity is *translated* into waveforms on an ECG.
- Describe Einthoven's triangle and how it relates to the placement of limb leads I, II, and III.
- Outline a systematic approach for analyzing an ECG tracing and name the main types of waveforms.
- Using standard ruled ECG paper, determine the rate and waveform amplitude of an ECG.
- Name three methods for determining the heart rate on an ECG.
- Identify and be able to measure key ECG landmarks such as the PR interval and the QRS width.

Introduction

The electrocardiogram (abbreviated both ECG and EKG) is a graphic depiction of the electrical activity of the heart. As the heart muscle cells depolarize (leading to contraction) and then repolarize (leading to relaxation), they produce electrical signals. The size and strength of these electrical signals can be picked up using electrodes on the skin, allowing a tracing or waveform to be created. The ECG quickly became an important tool in medicine, particularly cardiology, because they are quick, easy, and painless to produce and they reveal a wealth of information about the patient's heart rate and rhythm. While most clinicians need to have a basic understanding of the ECG, pacing specialists will find that the ECG is essential to effective practice. In this chapter, we'll learn about the ECG of a patient without a pacemaker or other cardiac rhythm management device. Later on, we'll learn how to interpret paced ECGs.

When dealing with ECGs, it may be helpful to remember that we are measuring electrical activity, which reflects depolarization and repolarization. In other words, we are not measuring the cardiac contraction; we are assessing the electrical changes that lead to the cardiac contractions. When there is no electrical activity, there is just a flat line known as the isoelectric line. Electrical energy will show up as deflections from that isoelectric line or baseline.

Einthoven's triangle

Willem Einthoven, a Dutch physician born in what today is Indonesia, invented what we today know as the ECG in 1903; he won the Nobel Prize in medicine in 1924 for this crucial discovery. Around 1900, it was known that the heart produced electrical signals as it beat, but there was no way to record these signals except by attaching electrodes directly to the heart. The electrical activity from the heart actually traveled to the skin, but these tiny signals were too small to be detected until Einthoven invented something known as a string galvanometer (a wire and electromagnets), which later evolved into an ECG that could amplify these

The Nuts and Bolts of Implantable Device Therapy Pacemakers, First Edition. Tom Kenny.
© 2015 John Wiley & Sons, Ltd. Published 2015 by John Wiley & Sons, Ltd.

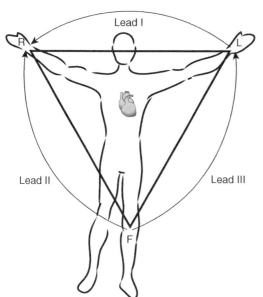

Figure 6.1 Einthoven's triangle required placement of electrodes on the limbs. This concept is still crucial to understanding the ECG today. These limb leads allow for the depiction of the vector or travel of the electrical activity through the heart.

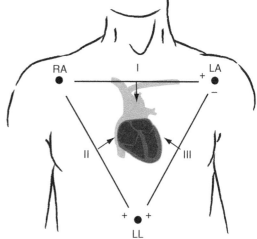

Figure 6.2 In an ECG, a lead is an electrical circuit with a positive and a negative pole. Leads I, II, and III are standard configurations for an ECG. As electrical energy from the heart moves toward the positive pole, it results in a positive waveform; as it moves away from the positive pole, it results in a negative waveform.

tiny signals and render them graphically. To make an ECG work, Einthoven placed electrodes at three points on the body, which form an inverted triangle. Einthoven's triangle, as it came to be known, found the ECG worked best with electrodes placed on the limbs, that is, the right and left hands and left knee. **Figure 6.1** shows how Einthoven's triangle *surrounds* the heart.

Today, an ECG still uses Einthoven's triangle but uses shoulders and solar plexus regions rather than wrists and knees. The ECG is an electrical device and, as such, relies on an electrical circuit with a positive and a negative pole. A good way to think of how the ECG is created is to think of the positive pole as a camera, and when electrical energy from the heart travels toward the camera, it results in a positive graphic depiction; as the electrical energy travels away from the positive pole, it results in a negative waveform. (In this case, positive means the waveforms deflect upward from the baseline; negative deflect downward.) Thus, a three-lead ECG has three cameras in position to help the ECG to draw the tracing. Moving the electrodes changes the camera position. When clinicians talk about

Lead I, Lead II, or Lead III on an ECG, they are talking about standard positions for these *cameras*. Leads could be placed at any number of locations, but Leads I, II, and III are familiar and standard positions (see **Figure 6.2**).

Lead configurations: leads I, II, and III

In a pacing clinic, it is most typical to use three to five electrodes for the surface ECG, which can be depicted using a pacemaker programmer or an ECG monitor. In reality, the ECG is being created from only two electrodes at any one time. Leads I, II, and III are probably the most important lead configurations for an ECG (see **Figure 6.3**).

Lead II is probably the most common electrode configuration as an ECG, and again, it results in primarily a positive ECG (see **Figure 6.4**). In fact, Lead II ECGs are so common clinicians ought to assume that a rhythm strip is from a Lead II configuration unless otherwise stated. Although it is described as using the right shoulder and the left leg, the left-sided electrode may not literally be placed on the leg. Instead, it may be placed on the left side of the abdomen or the left side; it may also be placed on the left thigh or lower leg.

The Lead III configuration involves moving both electrodes to the left side of the body, one on

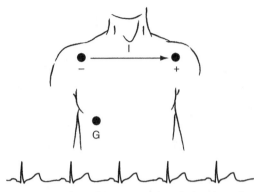

Figure 6.3 Lead I configuration involves placing electrodes on the right and left shoulders with the left shoulder serving as the positive pole. Note that the resulting ECG will be mostly positive as the electrical activity is moving toward the positive pole (think of it as a *camera*).

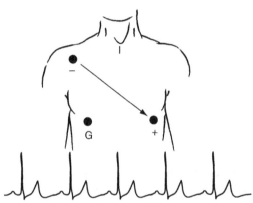

Figure 6.4 Lead II configuration, the most commonly used, results in a strongly positive tracing.

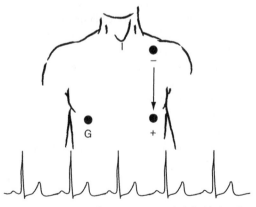

Figure 6.5 Lead III configuration is entirely left sided and also results in a positive tracing.

top (the shoulder area) and the other on what is called the left leg but which may be anywhere from the left abdomen to the left lower leg (see **Figure 6.5**).

Waveform landmarks

Willem Einthoven not only invented the ECG, but he also invented some of the terminology we still use today. The individual portions of the ECG are identified by the letters P, Q, R, S, and T. Cardiologists are also interested in certain intervals, such as the QRS complex, the PR interval, and the QT interval (see **Figure 6.6**). By the way, these letters have no particular medical meaning; it appears that Einthoven simply selected some letters from the middle of the alphabet.

The P-wave is created by the atrial depolarization. Typically, the right and left atria depolarize simultaneously, creating a rounded P-wave. Atrial dyssynchrony may result in a bit of a bump in the P-wave. Because the atria are much smaller chambers than the ventricles, the P-wave is relatively small compared to the other waveforms. Once the atria depolarize, there is a short pause in the ECG evidenced by the isoelectric line. This shows that for a short moment, there is no movement of electrical potential; it corresponds to the heart's being at rest.

The Q-, R-, and S-waves represent the electrical activity of the ventricles and are usually described as one unit, the QRS complex. The QRS presents a graphic depiction of electrical energy through the AV node, the bundle of His, and the bundle branches and then down the ventricles in the Purkinje fibers. The ventricles are much larger chambers than the atria and create larger waveforms. In a healthy heart, the left ventricle actually contracts faster than the right ventricle by a matter of a few milliseconds. This means that the electrical waveform actually proceeds from left to right and then from right to left. When ventricular depolarization is complete, the isoelectric line reappears, demonstrating that there is a brief pause in electrical activity.

Before the heart can depolarize again, it must now repolarize. Ventricular repolarization is depicted in the ECG in the T-wave. The atria must also repolarize, but this occurs during ventricular depolarization and the much larger amount of

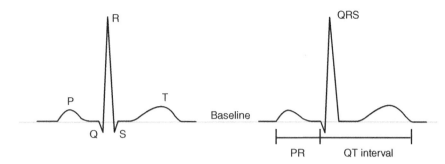

Figure 6.6 The landmarks on an ECG tracing.

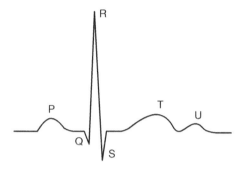

Figure 6.7 Although not commonly seen on the ECG, the U-wave can be a small waveform following the T-wave that may relate to the repolarization of the papillary muscles or Purkinje fibers.

ventricular depolarization energy overwhelms the atrial repolarization to the point that it does not show up on an ECG. It does happen—it just is too small to compete with simultaneous ventricular depolarization. At the end of the T-wave, the isoelectric line emerges, showing a cessation of movement of electrical potential.

On some but not all ECGs, you may find a small wave that appears after the T-wave but before the next P-wave. Designated the U-wave, it is actually not entirely clear what this waveform depicts. It has been theorized this may be the repolarization of the Purkinje fibers of the ventricle or perhaps the repolarization of the papillary muscles. While these are certainly reasonable theories, the question must be asked as to why the U-wave does not routinely appear on most ECGs. It is much more common to see a U-wave in the ECG of patients with electrolyte imbalances, such as hypokalemia (low serum potassium) (see **Figure 6.7**).

The QRS complex depicts ventricular depolarization, and although it is talked about as one

thing, it is typically composed of three distinct waveforms. When it appears, the Q-wave is always a negative waveform that precedes the larger R-wave. However, in clinical practice, it is not unusual to see variations in the QRS complex such that there is no distinct Q-wave or S-wave (see **Figure 6.8**). Regardless of the actual waveforms present, this section of the ECG is called the QRS complex and it depicts ventricular depolarization.

Systematic rhythm strip analysis

The rhythm strip is an ECG used specifically to analyze the heart's rhythm and rate. Rate is the speed at which the heart beats, while rhythm might best be described as the pattern in which it beats. There is probably no greater *secret* to rhythm strip analysis than the fact that clinicians must develop a systematic or step-by-step approach. It is less important what system a clinician uses than the fact that he or she regularly and consistently uses a valid system. Think of this system as your checklist. This checklist system does two important things: it assures that nothing is ever overlooked, and it keeps us as clinicians from *eyeballing* a rhythm strip and jumping to conclusions. Following is my system for rhythm strip analysis.

Calculate rate

There are actually several ways to measure rate on a rhythm strip. When a rhythm strip is printed out on standard ECG paper at the standard speed (25 mm/s), you can use the large and small boxes on the paper to assess the rate. Every small box on the ECG is equivalent to 40 ms. The small boxes

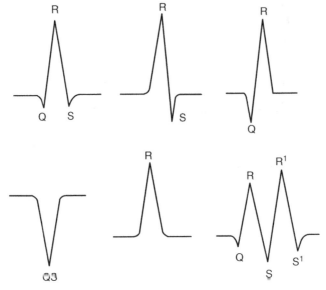

Figure 6.8 The QRS complex may or may not be depicted with clearly discernible Q-, R-, and S-waves; many variations are possible. In a textbook-perfect ECG, the Q- and S-waves are smaller negative waveforms that surround a larger positive R-wave. In clinical practice, the QRS complex may take a variety of appearances. In some cases, R- or S-wave may have two *points* and be designated as R and R1 or S and S1.

are grouped on the paper into larger boxes (5 × 5 small boxes make a big box). The larger box is equivalent to 200 ms. While using ECG paper to calculate rate is not the most accurate method, it is fast and easy and gives reliable approximations (see **Figure 6.9**). While cardiologists often talk in beats per minute (bpm), pacemakers report rates and intervals in milliseconds. The formula to convert them is simple:

$$\text{Interval (ms)} = \frac{60\ 000}{\text{Rate (bpm)}}$$

$$\text{Rate (bpm)} = \frac{60\ 000}{\text{interval (ms)}}$$

Another way to determine rates and intervals is to use a special tool called a *rate ruler* that maps out the various values so you can look up one value to find the other. Pacemaker manufacturers often make rate rulers available to pacing clinicians. While rate rulers are very practical and extremely common in clinical practice, they are often forbidden in pacing exams, so pacing clinicians should be familiar with all rate calculation methods!

Using the grid paper, the easiest way to calculate rate is to find an R-wave (or other landmark) that starts on a bold line. If you have such a landmark, this becomes your reference. Then count the boxes. The first box is 40 ms or a rate of 300 bpm. The second box is 80 ms or 150 bpm. The third box is 120 ms or 100 bpm. The fourth box is 160 ms or 75 bpm. The fifth box is 200 ms or 60 bpm. The sixth box is 240 ms or 50 bpm (see **Table 6.1**). This method is both more time-consuming and more accurate, and it requires some memorization—but it is a good way to get reasonably accurate results from a rhythm strip (see **Figure 6.10**).

Sometimes, the top of the ECG paper will also have small markers that indicate intervals of 3 s, which can also be used in rate calculations. Simply take 6 s worth of the rhythm strip (two 3-s intervals) and then calculate the rate by multiplying by 10; for example, if there are five R-waves in the 6 s, the patient's heart rate is 50 bpm (5 × 10). Using this method, all of your results will be multiples of 10 (50, 60, 70 bpm), so it should be considered an approximation. While this method is not the most exact, it is the method to use when the patient has an irregular rhythm.

The best tool for measuring rate is a pair of calipers; simply place one pin on the calipers on one

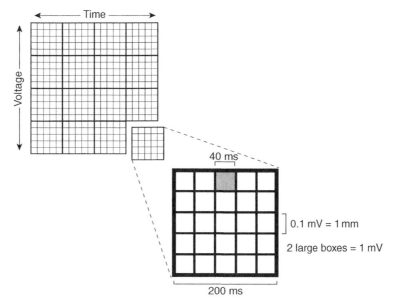

Figure 6.9 Standard ECG paper is divided into large (200 ms) and small boxes (40 ms) to facilitate calculation of rate. You can also measure the waveform amplitude in mV on ECG paper; one small box equals 0.1 mV and 2 large boxes equals 1 mV.

Table 6.1 Using the ECG grid to calculate rate from a reference point

Small box	Duration (ms)	Rate (bpm)
1	40	300
2	80	150
3	120	100
4	160	75
5	200	60
6	240	50

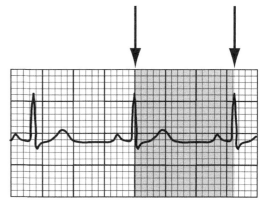

Figure 6.10 Using the ECG grid paper to calculate rate. Start with an R-wave that falls on the line (shown here by the arrow). Then calculate the small boxes using Table 6.1. In this case, the next R-wave occurs after the third and before the fourth box for a rate between 100 and 75 bpm.

of the landmarks, expand the calipers as necessary, and place the other pin on the other landmark. Then remove the calipers and place them on a clean section of ECG paper, starting at the beginning of a large box. Calipers are easy to use and provide a reasonably accurate way to measure rates.

Rate can be assessed by measuring the RR interval, that is, the time period from one R-wave to the next R-wave. This will determine the patient's ventricular rate. It is also possible to measure the PP interval to calculate the patient's atrial rate. Knowing that a normal heart rate ranges from about 60 to 100 bpm, this must be calculated into intervals or milliseconds. A patient with a heart rate of 60 bpm has a heart that beats once per second or once every 1000 ms. To keep the math easy, 1000 ms equals a heart rate of 60 bpm.

When measuring the R-wave, consistently use the same area of the R-wave, whether it's the onset of the R-wave, the peak, or the end. I recommend measuring from the top of the R-waves simply because these are easier landmarks to see. Whichever area you use, be consistent.

In actual practice, sometimes clinicians will encounter very rapid or very slow rates. In such cases, it is more important to treat the patient than to fuss over whether the heart rate is 280 or 290 bpm. It is also possible to encounter abnormal rates that the patient tolerates relatively well, such as a patient who gets around even though his heart is only beating 40 bpm. Rate can be a particularly important analysis and very extreme results should result in immediate medical attention rather than further ECG analysis.

Determine regularity

Rate can be measured by a single complex, but regularity requires measurement of rate over several complexes to determine if the rate is consistent or variable. If you are using calipers, you can *walk* the calipers to see if the distance between landmarks remains consistent in interval after interval. You can also measure multiple intervals and compare the results.

Regularity is a relative concept; even healthy patients will not have a perfectly regular heart rhythm. As a rule of thumb, a heart rhythm is considered to be regular if it does not vary by more than 600 ms (three small boxes) from the shortest to the longest intervals. Regular rhythms are typically sinus-driven rhythms. If the patient has an atrial arrhythmia, such as atrial fibrillation, the rhythm is considered *regularly irregular*, meaning it is irregular but in a consistent pattern. Some rhythms are considered *irregularly irregular*, which might be described as chaotic or without a discernible pattern.

Assess the P-waves

It is not always easy in real-life clinical practice to identify the P-wave on a rhythm strip. These are small waves that precede the QRS complex. The P-waves should be present and positive (positive P-waves indicate normal sinus rhythm). Patients with so-called silent atria or atrial disorders may not have P-waves on the rhythm strip or P-waves may be irregular and intermittent.

Next, the clinician should evaluate whether the P-waves all look the same. An occasional or single unusual-looking P-wave may represent differences in electrical activity that should be noted.

In the healthy heart, there is one P-wave for each and every QRS complex. One-to-one AV synchrony describes a healthy heart rhythm in which there is one P-wave for each QRS complex. Many rhythm disorders will result in rhythm strips without a P-wave for each QRS complex.

Determine the PR interval

The PR interval can be calculated in the same manner as the rate, using ECG paper or calipers. A normal PR interval ranges from about 120 to 200 ms (three to five small boxes).

The PR interval depicts the time it takes for the atria to depolarize and for the electrical impulse to reach and then cross the AV node. Measure the PR interval by starting at the onset of the P-wave and going to the onset of the QRS complex. Although the PR interval is named for the P-wave and R-wave, in reality, its duration is from the beginning of the P-wave to whatever wave initiates the QRS complex—often the Q-wave. Do not be fooled by the fact that it is not called the PQ interval!

Determine the QRS duration

Using the same calculation methods, the QRS duration can be calculated using the boxes on the ECG paper or calipers. The QRS interval is measured from its onset (typically but not always the Q-wave) to the end of the complex (typically but not always the S-wave). A normal QRS interval is less than 120 ms, usually in the range of 40–120 ms (one to three boxes).

Although clinicians rarely measure P-wave and T-wave duration, the typical values would be 60–110 ms and 160 ms, respectively. A measurement that may be relevant for some patients is the QT interval, measured from the onset of the QRS complex until the completion of the T-wave. In a healthy heart, the QT interval should be under 400 ms; it is considered abnormally long when it exceeds 450 ms (males) or 470 ms (females).

Putting it all together

Using this system, a clinician can take a rhythm strip and state:
- Rate
- Regularity
- P-waves and AV synchrony
- PR interval
- QRS duration

When all of these things fall in the normal range, the patient has a normal sinus rhythm. When abnormal results occur, these can be reported and diagnosed further. Abnormal results might include very high or very low rates, irregular rhythms, lack of P-waves, too many P-waves, or loss of 1:1 AV synchrony, too-long or too-short PR and QRS intervals (indicating conduction problems).

Refractory periods

The refractory period is a cardiac interval during which time the heart cannot depolarize, regardless of the level of stimulation it receives. The refractory period prevents the heart from depolarizing too soon after the prior depolarization and contraction. Refractory periods can be further subdivided into the absolute refractory period (during which time no depolarization can occur at all) and the relative refractory period (during which time the heart resists depolarization but might be depolarized in the presence of sufficient energy) (see **Figure 6.11**).

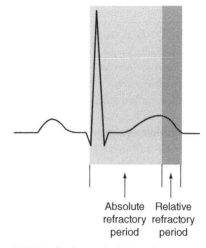

Absolute refractory period   Relative refractory period

Figure 6.11 The absolute and relative refractory periods map onto the QRS complex and the T-wave, depicting ventricular depolarization and repolarization. The absolute refractory period, which starts during the QRS complex and extends into the first portion of the T-wave, precedes the relative refractory period, which occurs during the latter portion of the T-wave.

Conclusion

The rhythm strip reveals a great deal to the systematic clinician about the patient's rhythm (but virtually nothing about other disease states, such as ischemia or infarction). It is important to approach every rhythm strip systematically and go through a sequence of steps rather than glance at it to notice a prominent feature (and possibly overlook other important elements). Clinicians must calculate rate, determine if the rhythm is regular, assess the P-waves, calculate the PR interval, and calculate the QRS duration. There are many ways to calculate the rate, including using standard ECG grid paper (one small box equals 200 ms, one large box equals 1000 ms). Rate and interval are two ways of stating the

same thing and can be *translated* one from another using a rate ruler or a math formula. Clinicians should learn to calculate rate by ECG grid paper, using calipers, and using three-second markers on ECG paper. Rhythms should also be assessed for whether or not they are regular, for example, how much variation in rate occurs over the strip. Some degree of irregularity is normal; the difference between the longest and shortest intervals should not exceed 600 ms. The clinician should also identify P-waves; positive or upward-deflecting P-waves indicate sinus rhythm. There should be one P-wave for each and every QRS complex. The PR interval and the QRS duration should be in normal range; abnormal values suggest conduction problems.

The nuts and bolts of basic ECG and rhythm interpretation

- The rhythm strip from an ECG is a simple but powerful tool that can provide a wealth of information to the pacing clinician.
- The ECG measures electrical activity from the heart on the skin's surface using an electrical circuit (positive pole and negative pole). These circuits are called leads. An ECG should be assumed to be Lead II (from the right shoulder to the left leg or lower abdomen) unless otherwise noted.
- The positive pole can be thought of as a camera that measures the electrical energy coming toward it in a positive way (upward deflection from baseline).

Continued

Continued

- On an ECG, the P-waves indicate atrial depolarization. You can measure the atrial rate by measuring the interval between one P-wave and the next P-wave.
- The QRS complex consists of three waves (Q, R, and S), which may or may not be individually discernible on the rhythm strip. Taken as a unit, the QRS complex represents the ventricular depolarization.
- The isoelectric line or baseline (flat line) is the section of the rhythm strip where no electrical activity is recorded. On a normal rhythm strip, expect to see an isoelectric line after the P-wave and before the QRS complex as well as after the T-wave.
- Sometimes, particularly in patients with electrolyte imbalances, a small U-wave occurs after the T-wave. It is important not to confuse U-waves with P-waves.
- The T-wave represents ventricular repolarization.
- Despite its name, the PR interval is measured from the onset of the P-wave to the beginning of the QRS complex. It is normally from 120 to 200 ms long.
- When measuring the ventricular rate, measure from one R-wave to the next (peak-to-peak is a good way). When measuring the atrial rate, measure from one P-wave to the next.
- There are several ways to measure rate. Using ECG grid paper, one small box equals 200 ms and one large box equals 1000 ms (or 1 s). Some ECG has three-second markers at the top; you can measure the number of R-waves in 6 s and multiply by 10 for an approximate beats-per-minute (bpm) rate. You may also use calipers and grid paper to calculate rate.
- Intervals (ms) and rates (bpm) are simply two different ways to say the same thing. Most pacemakers rely on intervals. You can calculate intervals and rates using a formula or you can use a rate ruler (chart).
- When evaluating an ECG, it is crucial to approach it systematically rather than eyeballing it. You should calculate rate, determine regularity, assess the P-waves, and then measure PR and QRS intervals.
- Regularity is a relative term; nobody has a perfectly regular heart rate like a metronome. As a rule of thumb, the variation between the shortest and longest intervals in rate should not exceed 600 ms (three small boxes).
- Heart rhythms can be described as regular (this is the best), regularly irregular (such as occurs with atrial fibrillation), and irregularly irregular (chaotic).
- A textbook-perfect rhythm strip will have one P-wave for each and every QRS complex. This is 1:1 AV synchrony. In clinical practice, not all patients will exhibit regular P-waves and some may not have P-waves at all (silent atria), while others may have too many P-waves (atrial arrhythmias). Many rhythm disorders will result in abnormal AV synchrony.
- The QRS duration describes how long it takes for the ventricles to depolarize. It is normally from 40 to 120 ms long and should not be longer than 120 ms.
- The refractory period defines the time during which the heart will not depolarize. There is an absolute refractory period (which occurs during the QRS complex and to the beginning of the T-wave) when the heart will not depolarize at all, regardless of how much energy it receives. There is also a relative refractory period (second half of the T-wave) during which the heart resists depolarization but may depolarize in the presence of sufficient energy.
- If you know the patient's interval and want to figure out the rate, divide 60 000 by the interval. For example, if the patient's ventricular interval is 1 000 ms, then his rate is 60 bpm (60 000 divided by 1 000 = 600). On the other hand, if you know the rate and want to calculate the interval, then divide 60 000 by the rate. For example, if the patient's heart rate is 120 bpm, the interval is 500 ms (60 000 divided by 120 is 500).

Test your knowledge

1 The patient's ventricular rate is 55 bpm. What interval does that correspond to?
   A 1091 ms
   B 550 ms
   C 400 V
   D None of the above

2 From what landmarks do you measure the PR interval?
   A From the start of the P-wave to the start of the R-wave
   B From the end of the P-wave to the end of the R-wave
   C From the peak of the P-wave to the peak of the R-wave
   D From the start of the P-wave to the onset of the QRS complex

3 The QRS complex corresponds to what electrical phenomenon?
   A The repolarization of the ventricles
   B The depolarization of the ventricles
   C The passage of electrical energy through the AV node
   D Atrial depolarization

4 On standard ECG paper at the regular speed of 25 mm/s, one small box on the grid equals:
   A 100 ms
   B 200 ms
   C 500 ms
   D 1000 ms

5 Using 3-s markers on ECG paper, if you find that six R-waves occur in 6 s, approximately what rate is the patient's heart beating?
   A 60 bpm
   B 150 bpm

   C 65 bpm
   D 90 bpm

6 What is the best way to measure the patient's ventricular rate?
   A From R-wave to R-wave
   B From P-wave to P-wave
   C From R-wave to T-wave
   D From R-wave to P-wave

7 Looking at an ECG, where would does the absolute refractory period fall?
   A On the P-wave
   B From the end of the P-wave to the end of the T-wave
   C From the onset of the QRS complex to the beginning of the T-wave
   D Immediately after the T-wave

8 A clinician should assume what lead configuration for an ECG if none is stated?
   A Lead I
   B Lead II
   C Lead III
   D Lead IV

9 What is a normal QRS duration?
   A About 10 ms
   B Less than 50 ms
   C More than 800 ms
   D Less than 120 ms

10 What would be an example of a *regularly irregular* rhythm?
   A Bradycardia
   B Atrial fibrillation
   C Brady–tachy syndrome
   D Ventricular fibrillation

CHAPTER 7

Arrhythmia analysis

Learning objectives

- Define normal sinus rhythm and name two types of sinus-related arrhythmias.
- Explain how to differentiate between a sinus pause and sinus exit block on an ECG in terms of both cause and appearance.
- Describe the three types of premature beats and how to differentiate them on an ECG.
- State the key ECG landmark for differentiation among the four main types of AV block.
- Describe AV conduction in the four main types of AV block.
- Define premature atrial contraction (PAC) and explain how it differs from normal sinus rhythm.

Introduction

The term arrhythmia can be defined as a collective term to describe any type of cardiac rhythm that is different from normal sinus rhythm (NSR). Arrhythmias are described by where they originate; atrial arrhythmias are arrhythmias originating in or near the atria and may affect both the atria and ventricles. Supraventricular arrhythmias originate at some point *above* (supra) the ventricles and thus include atrial arrhythmias but also others. Ventricular arrhythmias originate in or around the ventricles. Many arrhythmias occur because of conduction disorders resulting from poor or no conduction over the AV node. One of the biggest mistakes clinicians make in dealing with these types of arrhythmias is to evaluate the ECG too quickly. The ECG must be approached systematically for the specific clues needed to pinpoint the type of rhythm disorder. Clinicians who just glance at an ECG or eyeball a rhythm strip without measuring intervals can miss important evidence that can identify arrhythmias definitively.

In this section, we are going to evaluate the main types of arrhythmias that occur in pacemaker patients: sinus arrhythmias and AV block. While it is not out of the question for one patient to have both types of rhythm disorders, most pacemaker patients will have at least one of them. Pacemaker consultants must have expertise in identifying and differentiating these main arrhythmias.

Interpretative challenges

Textbook ECGs are always *perfect*, but they are rarely what real-life clinicians see in the field. Patients who move around or fidget during an ECG may create a rhythm strip with a wandering baseline. As long as the clinician can identify the key waves and landmarks (P-waves, PR interval, QRS complex, T-wave), this twisting or irregular baseline should not be a cause for much concern. Sometimes, artifacts or noise can show up on the ECG, which can lead to misinterpretation. For example, a patient with muscle tremors may have an ECG with bumps all along the baseline, tempting the clinician to see atrial activity that is not really there. Irregular ECGs can also occur when electrodes are not properly affixed. Depending on the configuration, waveforms may be disproportionately large or small, such as a rhythm strip with a T-wave that is larger than the QRS complex. As long as we can recognize the various

The Nuts and Bolts of Implantable Device Therapy Pacemakers, First Edition. Tom Kenny.
© 2015 John Wiley & Sons, Ltd. Published 2015 by John Wiley & Sons, Ltd.

landmarks, the rhythm strip can still be ana-lyzed, and the relative sizes of the various wave-forms do not matter and should not influence our interpretation.

Arrhythmias that originate in the sinus node

An abnormal sinoatrial (SA) node or abnormal SA node activity can result in a sinus arrhythmia, which may manifest as a too-slow rate (sinus bradycardia, typically <60 beats per minute (bpm)) or a too-fast rate (sinus tachycardia, typi-cally over 100 bpm). NSR, that is, a normal heart rhythm driven by the SA node, falls in the rate range of 60–100 bpm. While the SA node is the heart's natural pacemaker, it, in turn, is influ-enced by the autonomic nervous system. In a healthy individual, the autonomic nervous system regulates the heart rate in such a way that it can optimally meet that individual's metabolic demands. This accounts for the heart's ability to speed up or slow down as the body exercises or rests, for instance. When the sympathetic ner-vous system is stimulated, the heart rate increases (chronotropic response), the AV conduction rate increases (dromotropic response), and contrac-tility increases (inotropic response). By the same token, when the parasympathetic nervous system is stimulated, rate (chronotropic), conduction (dromotropic), and contractility (inotropic) decrease.

In the healthy heart, the SA node generates a regular electrical impulse that drives the heart rate. NSR can be described as having a regular rhythm, a rate of around 60–100 bpm, normal P-waves (all the same morphology or shape) with one P-wave preceding each QRS complex, a PR interval of about 120–200 ms, and a QRS duration less than 120 ms. When interpreting ECGs, the key is to determine how the presenting rhythm differs from NSR; in other words, how does this rhythm deviate from normal? (see **Figure 7.1**)

Sinus tachycardia
Arrhythmias originating from the sinus node can be too fast (tachycardia) or too slow (bradycardia). A sinus tachycardia is actually a sinus rhythm with one simple exception: it's too fast. Sinus tachycardia originates in the SA node, produces normal-looking positive P-waves, and maintains 1 : 1 AV synchrony (one P-wave for each and every QRS complex), but it is faster than normally, typically falling in the range of 100–150 bpm. The causes of sinus tachycardia can be a normal response to workload, for example, your heart may enter sinus tachycardia when you jog. That added workload may be physiologic (exercise) or it may be pathological, that is, a result of heart failure or other strains on the heart that cause it to work harder. In general, sinus tachycardia tends to start and stop gradually, that is, there are a *warm-up* period as the rate increases and a *cooldown* period as the rate returns to normal. Sinus tachycardia

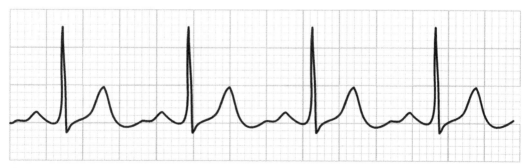

Figure 7.1 A good example of NSR with P-waves appearing before each QRS complex and every beat (P-waves and QRS complexes) having a similar size and shape (morphology). The positive (or upward-deflecting) P-waves indicate sinus rhythm. The similar morphologies indicate that each electrical impulse driving the heart starts in the same place and conducts across the atria, through the AV node, and into the ventricles at the same speed and following the same electrical pathways.

occurs when the sympathetic nervous system is stimulated and/or the parasympathetic nervous system is depressed. Examples of such situations include exercise or exertion, fever, pain, anxiety, and myocardial infarction. Sinus tachycardia can be very dangerous, even life threatening, in acute myocardial infarction patients because the coronary arteries are already blocked, which can lead to an imbalance between coronary oxygen supply and demand.

Sinus tachycardia is defined as a sinus rhythm that is normal in all respects except for rate—it's too fast. However, as sinus tachycardia increases in rate, abnormalities in the P-waves will start to show up. Typically, as sinus tachycardia accelerates, P-waves may be more difficult to discern on the ECG.

Sinus bradycardia

Sinus bradycardia, on the other hand, is a sinus rhythm that is normal in all respects except for its rate—it's too slow. By standard definition, sinus bradycardia ranges from 40 to 60 bpm, although clinicians may see it at even lower rates than that. When we rest, relax, or sleep, the healthy heart slows down. To some extent, sinus bradycardia is normal; for instance, it may be perfectly normal for a healthy individual to have a heart rate of 55 bpm while sleeping. Highly trained athletes often have sinus bradycardia in that their resting heart rates may be 50 bpm. For that reason, it may be useful to consider what is called *relative bradycardia* rather than textbook definitions. For example, a marathon runner can have a resting heart rate of 40 bpm and not have an arrhythmia. A pediatric patient, whose heart rate should normally be around 90–100 bpm, may have sinus bradycardia at 70 bpm. Thus, when evaluating sinus bradycardia as an arrhythmia, consider the patient and the context. When treating patients with sinus bradycardia, symptoms must be considered—asymptomatic sinus bradycardia patients do not require treatment. Symptomatic sinus bradycardia (leading to symptoms such as dizziness, light-headedness, fatigue, presyncope, and syncope) is typically treated pharmacologically with atropine, which accelerates heart rate and increases conduction speed across the AV node.

Sinus bradycardia is driven by stimulation of the parasympathetic nervous system and/or depression of the sympathetic nervous system. Vasovagal reactions (neurocardiogenic syncope), acute inferior wall myocardial infarction, and so-called sick sinus syndrome (abnormal SA node) can all cause sinus bradycardia.

Sinus arrhythmia

Technically, a sinus arrhythmia is a sinus rhythm with some degree of irregularity, and as such, it is actually quite normal. Irregularities of sinus rhythm often occur simply with respiration, with heart rate increasing in many individuals with inhalation. This is more common in children than adults but occurs in a large number of individuals, most of whom never know they have this arrhythmia.

An irregular rhythm is defined as one with a variation of more than 120 ms (three small boxes) between the longest and the shortest RR intervals. Note that this regularity is measured between longest and shortest intervals, not one RR interval to the next. When encountering such a sinus arrhythmia, it is a good idea to approximate rate by using the six-second method (counting the number of R-wave peaks in six seconds and multiplying by 10). Such sinus arrhythmias are often cyclical in nature because they are related to changes in intra-thoracic pressure associated with the patient's respiratory cycles (inspiration, expiration) (see **Figure 7.2**). When calculating the rate, it's best to count the number of R-waves in six seconds and multiply by 10. Sinus arrhythmia at a normal rate looks very much like a *normal* rhythm (see **Figure 7.3**). In some cases, sinus arrhythmia may result in apparent *pauses* on the ECG. If you can view both patient and monitor at the same time, pauses may correlate with exhalations.

Sinus arrest and SA exit block

Sinus arrest and SA exit block look alike but are actually different phenomena. Sinus arrest occurs when the SA node does not fire consistently, that is, there is a problem with impulse formation. Sinus exit block occurs when the SA node fires consistently but some of the impulses do not conduct properly. Both sinus arrest and sinus exit block can be collectively called *sinus pauses*.

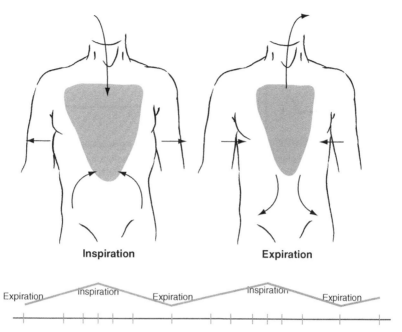

Inspiration   **Expiration**

Figure 7.2 Sinus arrhythmia is quite common and is often associated with the patient's respiratory patterns.

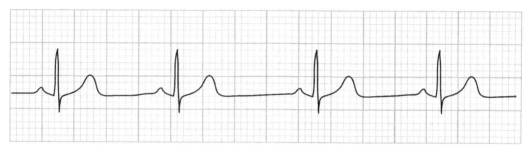

Figure 7.3 An example of sinus arrhythmia, an irregular rhythm driven by the SA node. Note that the heart rate is normal, around 60 bpm, and the PR interval is 120–140 ms and the QRS duration ranges from 60 to 80 ms. Sinus arrhythmia usually coordinates with the respiratory cycle.

Sinus pauses should be evaluated just like any other pause—the clinician needs to study the rhythm strip to see what is missing. In some cases, it will be just the P-wave; in other cases, it will be the P-wave plus the QRS complex and T-wave. In sinus arrest, the P-wave and the following QRS complex and T-wave will be absent.

In sinus arrest (problem with impulse formation), the rhythm strip will look normal except for the pause. That is, the clinician will see an underlying rhythm that is mostly regular, an underlying rate that is either normal or slow, and normal positive P-waves and 1 : 1 AV synchrony, except for the

pause. The *missing parts* of the ECG are the P-wave and QRS–T complex. Sinus arrest happens when the SA node fails to fire. The next time the SA node delivers an impulse, it resets its timing so it does not result in a properly timed beat. On the rhythm strip, this shows up as a gap or pause (see **Figure 7.4**).

Sinus exit block (also called SA block) has a similar appearance but is the result of improper conduction. In sinus exit block, the sinus node is not reset, so it means that although a pause occurs, the R-waves will be timed to each other. Taking calipers, the R-waves should be associated in sinus

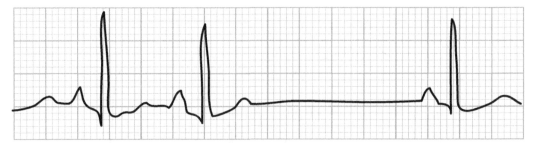

Figure 7.4 Sinus arrest is caused by a failure of the SA node to deliver an electrical output; this resets the SA node and when it fires again, it resets its own timing, resulting in a pause on the ECG. Sinus exit block has a similar appearance but the R-waves will come back on cycle, despite the pause.

exit block; that is, despite the pause, the R-wave will come in the proper time. In sinus arrest, there is no such relationship as the sinus node resets its timing cycle. To help remember this, think that you can *walk* (your calipers) around the block!

It is important to remember that sinus arrest is a problem of *impulse formation*, while sinus exit block is a problem of *impulse conduction*. When the rhythm comes back, sinus arrest is reset and will not be timed to the preceding events. Sinus exit block, on the other hand, does not reset timing and the next R-wave will come in at the appropriate interval. That's because with sinus exit block, the impulses were always forming but they just did not always conduct properly. Either of these conditions may be caused by increased vagal tone, acute inferior wall myocardial infarction, sick sinus syndrome, or metabolic disorders. In cases where it is impossible to differentiate sinus arrest from sinus exit block (for instance, when the next event after the pause is not a sinus beat but premature ventricular contraction (PVC)), it is appropriate and accurate to call the arrhythmia a *sinus pause*. Sinus pause includes both sinus arrest and sinus exit block.

Arrhythmias that originate in the atria

Atrial tachyarrhythmias
In NSR, the SA node fires and the wave of depolarization it generates spread out through the atria, over the AV node, to the bundle of His, and to the bundle branches so that the ventricles depolarize. On an ECG, NSR appears with P-waves, QRS complexes, and T-waves. A healthy NSR is regular, that is, the intervals between P-waves are regular

and, likewise, the intervals between R-waves are regular. One reason the SA node acts as the body's natural pacemaker in healthy individuals is that it is the fastest impulse-generating source and its speed does not allow other areas of the heart to *take over* and control the heart. However, when an ectopic area of the heart does take over and fires too early, the wave of depolarization that results will cause the tissue to contract early. If that ectopic area is within the atrial region, the resulting premature contraction is called a premature atrial contraction (PAC) or an atrial premature beat (ABP). A PAC generally has a different morphology than a normal P-wave on the ECG because the contraction resulted from a different area of the heart. This may appear wider or look distorted compared to the other P-waves. If the ectopic focus is particularly low, the P-wave may be biphasic, that is, partly positive and partly negative; in fact, it is possible that some PACs appear on the ECG to be partially or fully inverted (see **Figure 7.5**).

PACs may occur in patterns, such as every other beat (bigeminal PACs), or in some other sequences. Such rhythms are sometimes described as *occasionally irregular*, meaning that they are predominantly regular but have short periods of irregular activity. The degree of irregularity can be an important point when discussing atrial arrhythmias as we will learn shortly.

PACs occur because an ectopic focus, which in this case is nothing more than a small area of atrial cells, is able to form an impulse that is then conducted normally through the AV node and down into the ventricles. Atrial irritability—which occurs at the cellular level—is the condition that makes the heart susceptible to PACs and other types of

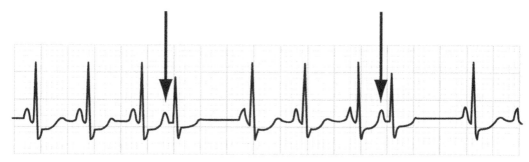

Figure 7.5 The two atrial events highlighted have occurred too early or prematurely in the rhythm. Their P-wave morphology differs slightly but noticeably from that of the other properly timed atrial contractions. These are premature atrial contractions (PACs). QRS morphology is typically not affected by PACs. The PR interval after a PAC is at least as long as the normal PR interval and may be somewhat prolonged.

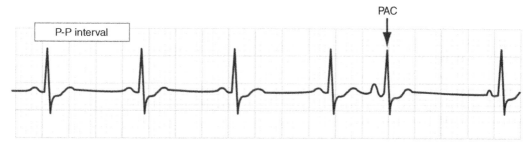

Figure 7.6 Note the PAC interrupts a run of NSR activity. One might expect the next normal P-wave to occur timed to the preceding normal P-wave (not the PAC). Instead, in some patients, the next normal P-wave after a PAC occurs after a pause.

atrial arrhythmias. Pulmonary disorders, including chronic obstructive pulmonary disease (COPD), as well as heart failure are associated with atrial irritability and thus set the stage for potential atrial arrhythmic activity. In fact, the sudden development of PACs in a patient who did not have them previously should at least suggest to the clinician the possibility that the patient may be developing heart failure or a pulmonary disorder.

In patients with frequent PACs, clinicians may often observe in their rhythm a noncompensatory pause, also called a *less-than-compensatory* pause (see **Figure 7.6**). When a PAC occurs to *interrupt* normal NSR activity, the next NSR P-wave is not timed to the preceding normal P-wave but occurs after a pause.

The heart has a physiologic refractory period during which time it does not respond normally to depolarization.

In this context, it is important to be aware of something called a nonconducted PAC. A nonconducted PAC is usually evident on a rhythm strip

by a pause. Whenever a clinician is trying to determine the causes of pauses, he or she needs to study the ECG to determine what is missing. If a PAC occurs followed by a pause and then a normal P-wave, the missing element to the strip is the QRS complex. This event occurs when a PAC occurs but fails to conduct properly over the AV node and into the ventricles. This results in an absence of ventricular depolarization, which is evident on the ECG as a missing QRS complex. Nonconducted PACs leave pauses on the ECG that can be easily mistaken for heart block, but there is a fast way to differentiate it: the clinician should determine if the P-wave preceding the pause is properly timed to the preceding P-waves (then it's heart block) or if that P-wave came in too early with respect to preceding P-waves (then it's a nonconducted PAC).

PACs can be benign and asymptomatic in patients, but they are important for clinicians to note because PACs can often originate other atrial or supraventricular arrhythmias. (A supraventricular arrhythmia is any arrhythmia that originates above the ventricles and would include atrial tachycardia (AT) as well as sinus tachycardia.) AT are usually paroxysmal, that is, they are characterized by a sudden or abrupt onset. Sinus tachycardia is a too-fast heart rhythm driven by the SA node, which usually ramps rate up gradually; a good example of a sinus-driven fast rate is an exercise-related rate where the heart *warms up* by raising the rate from 60 to 70, 80, 90 bpm, and so on. In contrast, some supraventricular arrhythmias literally transition from 60 to 100 bpm in a couple of beats or in a matter of seconds. Such paroxysmal high-rate activity would be called AT or an atrial tachyarrhythmia. A good way to distinguish AT from sinus tachycardia or other types of arrhythmias is to look on the ECG to determine if the beat that originated it can be identified. If the ECG looks relatively normal and regular at the outset and then a PAC occurs followed immediately by a run of high-rate activity, that is AT.

Sudden-onset rapid rates may be called paroxysmal supraventricular tachycardia (PSVT) or paroxysmal AT (PAT). Such rhythms are often caused by atrial irritability and are characterized by good conduction. On an ECG, this will result in a normal-looking QRS morphology. A PSVT or PAT can also be caused by abnormal conduction in the AV node in the form of *reentry*, resulting in what is called reentrant AV nodal tachycardia. On a rhythm strip, P-waves can sometimes be obscured in fast supraventricular tachycardias (SVTs). On a rhythm strip, look for QRS morphology as a clue: normal QRS morphology suggests that the rhythm is an SVT. Moreover, if the rhythm strip confirms abrupt onset, it is a PSVT.

A special form of AT is known as atrial flutter, characterized by a *sawtooth* pattern on the ECG. These triangular-shaped waves are also sometimes called F-waves. Atrial flutter is a type of reentrant tachycardia in the right atrium that commonly occurs at 300 bpm. Atrial flutter is often easy to identify on an ECG because of the P-wave morphology. Sometimes, the strip consists of all F-waves, but it is not unusual to see certain P-waves conducting to the ventricle in a regular pattern (see **Figure 7.7**). However, it is possible to have atrial flutter with a varying ventricular response. In atrial flutter, the atrial rate (P-wave rate) will always exceed the ventricular rate (R-wave rate), and the QRS morphology will look normal. In atrial flutter, there are no PP intervals

Atrial flutter is associated with right atrial reentrant activity and is more common in patients with heart failure or pulmonary disease.

Atrial fibrillation (AF) is characterized by an *irregularly irregular* ventricular rate. In fact, in AF, the ventricular rate is always irregular and can sometimes even be described as *chaotic*. AF occurs when multiple supraventricular focal points start firing and literally bombard the AV node with rapid-fire impulses. These multiple sites may be in the atrium, but recent research suggests they can also be found in or around the pulmonary veins, which are over by the left atrium. Since multiple sites of origin are involved, the rhythm is fast but completely uncoordinated. With all of those impulses

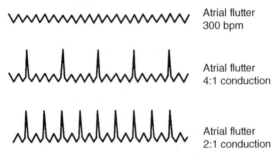

Atrial flutter
300 bpm

Atrial flutter
4:1 conduction

Atrial flutter
2:1 conduction

Figure 7.7 Atrial flutter with AV nodal conduction and the characteristic *sawtooth* appearance. P-waves in atrial flutter are sometimes called F-waves. In 4:1 atrial flutter with an atrial rate of 300 bpm, the ventricular rate can be calculated to be 75 bpm. The bottom rhythm (2:1 conduction) is one that is easy to misinterpret because the second flutter wave is buried in the QRS complex. Clinicians should be suspicious of atrial tachycardias that occur at exactly or very close to 150 bpm—they may really be 2:1 atrial flutter with an obscured flutter wave.

hitting the AV node, the AV node conducts an impulse, has a refractory period, and keeps getting hit by electrical impulses. Thus, the AV node responds as best as it can, allowing some but not all of those impulses that occur outside the refractory period to cross the node and depolarize the ventricles. The AV node actually works as a protection mechanism during AF by not allowing the very high atrial rate to commandeer the ventricular rate entirely. However, AF can involve a rapid ventricular response (RVR), and it is the RVR that is responsible for most of the symptoms typical of AF (dizziness, light-headedness, fainting or nearly fainting, and so on). RVR is typically defined as a ventricular rate greater than 100 bpm, while lower ventricular rates, for example, 60–99 bpm, are called AF with *controlled ventricular response*. Drug therapy for AF often aims at controlling the ventricular response. In some patients, you may see AF with a slow ventricular response, defined as a ventricular rate under 60 bpm. (If that patient is symptomatic, AF with slow ventricular response can be an indication for a pacemaker.)

One challenge in identifying AF on rhythm strips is that it has many different types of appearances. The commonality in AF is that all of these rhythms are *irregularly irregular*. There is never a discernible regular pattern in AF! Some clinicians look for a lot of bumps in the baseline to indicate erratic high-rate atrial activity; this is sometimes called a *wandering baseline*. While it is true, a wandering baseline will show up in some AF rhythm strips but it is not always present. The key criterion for identifying AF is an *irregularly irregular* ventricular rate (and QRS complexes tend to look normal or near normal and are of normal duration). The atrial rate in AF can be 350 bpm or even higher and is sometimes impossible to determine specifically (see **Figure 7.8**).

One of the risk factors for AF is unavoidable: advancing age. AF is relatively uncommon in people under age 60, but by age 80, it may affect as much as 10% of the population. Among seniors hospitalized for a rhythm disorder, the number one arrhythmia involved is AF. AF can be caused by enlargement of the atrium, particularly the left atrium, and multiple reentrant circuits. AF may be caused by ischemia or atrial irritability and can be triggered by PACs; AF is characterized by multiple focal points and multiple micro reentry *wavelets*.

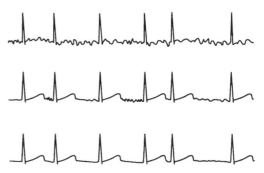

Figure 7.8 AF is characterized first and foremost by an irregularly irregular ventricular rate. A bumpy or *wandering* baseline sometimes appears, but this can be deceiving because it is not always discernible on an ECG. AF strips with a bumpy baseline may be described as *coarse* AF (see top strip) compared to the *fine* AF at the bottom. Note that AF has a distinct appearance that differs from atrial flutter.

Arrhythmias that originate in the AV junction

Junctional rhythms

The AV junction is the area of tissue that surrounds the AV node. In the event that the heart's SA node becomes depressed or dysfunctional, the AV junction can act as the heart's pacemaker by generating an electrical output pulse. In an otherwise healthy heart, the junctional beat represents the heart's *backup system* to fire and keep the heart going even when the SA node is out of commission. However, in abnormal situations, the AV junction can attempt to compete with and usurp the role of the SA node and take over control of the heart rhythm.

A junctional rhythm is one that originates in the AV junction, that is, in the proximity of the AV node. On the ECG, this will make the PR interval very short or even nonexistent. If you do see a P-wave before a junctional beat, it is going to be inverted (going downward from the baseline) on Lead II (see **Figure 7.9**).

Premature beats on an ECG are complexes that show up *too soon* in a rhythm strip. For instance, on a strip with several normal-looking beats at an appropriate rate, any beat that occurs too soon and out of sync with the rest of the strip would be considered a premature beat. There are three main types of premature beats: PACs, PVCs, and premature junctional contractions (PJCs). They are named based on the place in the heart that fired to

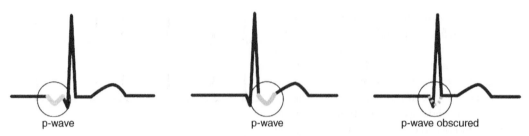

p-wave   p-wave   p-wave obscured

Figure 7.9 Identifying junctional beats using P-waves involves locating the P-wave and then determining if it is inverted. The P-wave may appear before the QRS but with an abbreviated PR interval, or it may appear slightly after the QRS (these can be harder to locate). In some cases, the P-wave will occur simultaneously with the QRS interval and not be evident on the ECG complex.

Premature junctional contraction

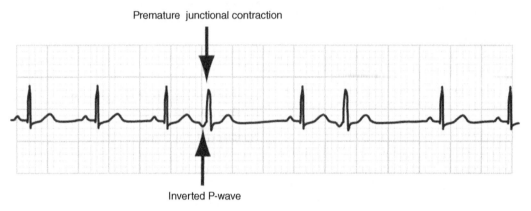

Inverted P-wave

Figure 7.10 Premature junctional contraction (PJC) is a premature beat fired from the AV junction. On the ECG, it will show up *too soon* on an otherwise normal strip, have a morphology similar to other QRS complexes, and be preceded by an inverted P-wave on Lead II. Note that in some cases, the inverted P-wave may immediately follow the QRS complex.

generate the premature activity. As a general rule of thumb, a PVC has wide and bizarre-looking QRS complexes. If you have a tracing with multiple complexes, the PVC will stand out because the QRS has a clearly aberrant look. If you can rule out a PVC, the premature beat will either be a PAC or a PVC. A PAC is a premature beat that is preceded by a positive or biphasic P-wave on Lead II. If the premature beat has the same morphology as the other QRS complexes and there is an inverted P-wave on Lead II (provided, of course, that the P-wave is visible at all), it is a PJC (see **Figure 7.10**).

Sometimes, a beat originating from the AV junction will show up late in the cycle, that is, instead of being *too* early, they occur *too late* and after a pause. This kind of junctional beat is called an *escape beat*, although it is a PJC in all other respects. There are two main types of escape beats: junctional escape beats and ventricular escape beats. A junctional escape beat may be preceded or immediately followed by an inverted P-wave on Lead II, and the QRS morphology will be similar to the normal QRS complexes on the strip.

Sometimes, more than an isolated PJC occurs and the patient's rhythm reverts to a junctional rhythm, sometimes called a junctional escape rhythm. Junctional rhythms are typically in the range 40–60 bpm, have regular PP and RR intervals, and show a normal QRS duration. But like with an isolated PJC complex, the P-wave is going to occur right before or right after or be buried within the QRS complex and be inverted on Lead II (see **Figure 7.11**). A junctional rhythm is a backup rhythm and occurs in patients with sinus

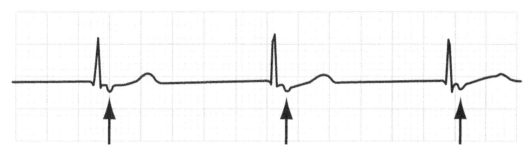

Figure 7.11 An example of junctional rhythm, a sequence of AV junctional beats. Note that the rhythm is slow (while junctional rhythms are typically in the range of 40–60 ppm, this one is even slower at 33 bpm) but regular with consistent PP and RR intervals. QRS duration is in the normal range. The P-wave, if it is visible at all, will appear right before or right after the QRS complex and be inverted on Lead II.

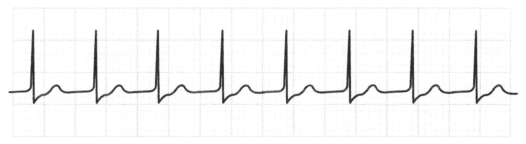

Figure 7.12 An accelerated junctional rhythm may look—at first glance—very much like a normal rhythm strip. In this strip, the rate is 65 beats per minute and the PR interval is around 80–100 ms. The PP and RR intervals are regular, the PR interval is short, and the P-waves are inverted. The regularity and inverted P-waves are the clues that this is actually a junctional rhythm and that the AV junction is usurping the role of the SA node.

node dysfunction, hypoxia, increased parasympathetic or vagal tone, or third-degree AV block or as a side effect of certain cardiac drugs, such as beta-blockers.

An accelerated junctional rhythm occurs when what is otherwise a typical junctional rhythm occurs at a rate in the range of 60–100 bpm. It can be identified in that it has all of the classic characteristics of a junctional rhythm (regularity and inverted P-waves on Lead II) but at a more rapid rate (see **Figure 7.12**). An accelerated junctional rhythm occurs in those situations where the AV junction has taken over and usurped the role of the SA node. This might be caused by ischemia of the AV junction, hypoxia, digitalis poisoning, inferior wall myocardial infarction, or rheumatic fever.

A rapid accelerated junctional rhythm may be as fast as 90 or even 100 bpm or more. Sometimes,

clinicians confuse accelerated junctional rhythms with AF, but there is an easy way to distinguish them. Accelerated junctional rhythms are regular in terms of RR intervals, while AF is irregular. When a junctional rhythm breaks the speed limit and exceeds 100 bpm, it is called junctional tachycardia (and it would be a type of SVT). A junctional tachycardia is the same thing as an accelerated junctional rhythm except at a faster rate. One of the most common types of SVT is a rhythm disturbance called AV nodal reentry tachycardia (AVNRT).

Most PJCs are benign. When they occur frequently—which is more than 10 per minute—they can lead to the formation of arrhythmias. Frequent PJCs might be a sign of underlying organic heart disease or some other problem. Patients with frequent PJCs should be closely observed for potential heart disease and arrhythmias.

Patients who experience junctional rhythms have a slower-than-normal heart rate that can reduce cardiac output, may lead to angina, and result in syncope, hypotension, or altered mental states. Patients in these too-slow junctional rhythms may be treated pharmacologically with atropine or with oxygen. Many patients with junctional rhythms are asymptomatic.

Accelerated junctional rhythms may be more apparent to the patient but are usually well tolerated. Since ischemia is a potential cause, patients should be closely observed for the possible cause of the accelerated junctional rhythm. If the patient is taking digitalis, digitalis toxicity should be considered as a possible cause of the arrhythmia.

Junctional tachycardia may be well tolerated in younger, strong, healthy patients without underlying disease, although they may be aware of its symptoms. For older patients, the frail, and those with underlying heart disease, junctional tachycardias may result in more symptoms and be more dangerous. For individuals with ischemic heart disease, junctional tachycardia may cause palpitations, a sense of a pounding or racing heart, reduced cardiac output, angina, heart failure, hypoxia, and hypotension. Junctional tachycardia can be treated with drug therapy, chemical or electrical cardioversion (to convert the rhythm back to normal), or vagal maneuvers, a physical technique to slow the heart. A patient with AVNRT who becomes symptomatic may require radio-frequency ablation.

Arrhythmias that originate in the ventricles

Ectopic ventricular rhythms

Ventricular contractions that occur in isolation are one of the more common types of ectopic rhythms (the other are atrial contractions). When a ventricular ectopic beat occurs *too soon* in the timing of the rhythm strip, it is called a PVC. Occasional PVCs are common and often benign. On a surface ECG, a PVC will exhibit a very wide QRS complex (>120 ms) that looks bizarre in comparison with the morphology of the other QRS complexes. This bizarre appearance owes to the fact that a PVC originates in the ventricular region and conducts in an entirely different way than a ventricular contraction that occurs as a result of an impulse fired by the SA node and conducted via the AV node into the ventricles. A P-wave may not appear before the PVC (see **Figure 7.13**).

PVCs may be unifocal (having one focus point) or multifocal (with more than one focus point). A unifocal PVC has one ectopic focus and will look the same in the same lead on the ECG because the focus depolarizes the ventricles consistently in the same way. A multifocal PVC (sometimes called multiform PVC) may look different because each of the different focus points depolarizes the ventricles in different ways. Generally speaking, multifocal PVCs may be more dangerous for the patient as they indicate that there are multiple sites of irritability within the ventricles.

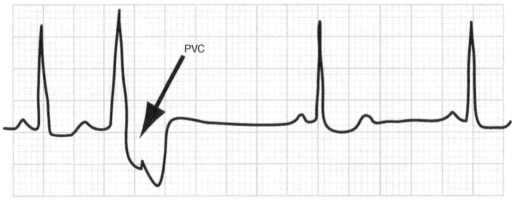

Figure 7.13 A premature ventricular contraction (PVC) is an ectopic beat that appears *too soon* on the ECG. Characteristics of a PVC are long QRS duration (>120 ms), a bizarre-looking morphology compared to the other QRS complexes, and a T-wave that is opposite of the other T-waves, that is, if most T-waves are positive, the PVC will likely have a negative T-wave and vice versa.

Interpolated
PVC

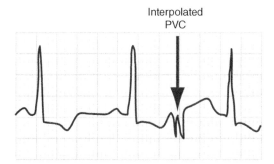

Figure 7.14 An interpolated PVC that occurs between two normal sinus beats in such a way that the rhythm is not interrupted.

R-on-T PVC

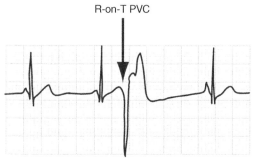

Figure 7.15 The most dangerous form of PVC is the R-on-T PVC, which can cause a ventricular tachyarrhythmia. An R-on-T PVC is a PVC that occurs at the same time as the T-wave or repolarization.

PVCs may occur in isolation (this is actually not unusual), but some patients will exhibit distinct patterns of PVC activity. When two PVCs occur in a row, this is called a couplet. When every other beat is a PVC, for example, the rhythm is described as ventricular bigeminy. Ventricular trigeminy is a rhythm where there are two sinus beats and then one PVC in a consistent pattern. Likewise, ventricular quadrigeminy describes a rhythm where every fourth beat is a PVC. Fortunately, the terminology ends there although you may in practice see patients where every fifth or sixth beat is consistently a PVC.

Sometimes, a PVC will occur between two normal sinus beats in such a way that the PVC does not interrupt or reset timing of the sinus rhythm. This is relatively rare and is known as an interpolated PVC (see **Figure 7.14**).

The rule of thumb is that more than 10 PVCs a minute constitute *frequent PVCs*. Frequent PVCs may cause symptoms, be distressing to patients, and be indicative of future arrhythmic problems. By far, the most dangerous type of PVC is the PVC that occurs at the same time as the T-wave, sometimes called R-on-T. During the cardiac repolarization (represented on the ECG by the T-wave), there is an absolute refractory period followed by a relative refractory period or the vulnerable period. A PVC that occurs during the absolute refractory period will not depolarize the heart, but if the PVC occurs during the relative refractory period, it can depolarize the heart too soon, which, in some cases, can trigger a potentially dangerous ventricular tachyarrhythmia (VT) (see **Figure 7.15**).

PVCs occur because one or more ventricular cells are depolarizing too early and that depolarization

is conducting through the ventricles. Stimulants, ischemia, hypoxia, electrolyte imbalances, and myocardial infarction are all associated with PVCs.

VT

A run of three or more PVCs in a row constitutes ventricular tachycardia (VT, sometimes called V-tach), which has a ventricular rate of over 100 bpm. VT originates in the ventricles and has a characteristic look: the complexes look like PVCs, but they make up the rhythm rather than interrupt it, the T-wave polarity is opposite that of the QRS complex, the QRS complex is wide (>120 ms) and can be described as *bizarre*, and the P-waves disappear from the rhythm strip (so it is impossible to measure PR intervals). As a general rule, VT tends to be regular. The clinical implications of VT can be severe: the patient has lost 1 : 1 AV synchrony and the benefits of *atrial kick*, which, in turn, means a loss of cardiac output. The faster the VT, the more likely it is that the patient will suffer hemodynamic decompensation. Like many other tachyarrhythmias, the most common cause of VT is a reentry pathway in the heart, that is, cardiac conduction gets stuck on an *endless loop*.

A more dangerous form of VT is described as polymorphic, which means that the VT is originating from more than one site (*poly*) in the ventricles, which means the QRS complexes will have different shapes (*morph*). A well-known form of polymorphic VT is called *torsades de pointes* (French for *twisting of the points*) because the tracing takes on the twisted appearance of a helix.

Although rare, sometimes, polymorphic VT is called ventricular flutter. In polymorphic VT, there are multiple different QRS morphologies, all of which are wide and bizarre; the rate is very fast (>250 bpm), and the tracing takes on a sawtooth appearance because it is no longer possibly to distinguish the QRS complex from the T-wave. Polymorphic VT is a serious and potentially life-threatening arrhythmia.

While VT can be a dangerous rhythm in and of itself, one of the greatest dangers facing patients with VT is that such rhythms can often deteriorate into ventricular fibrillation (VF). VF is characterized by a chaotic rhythm strip at a rate that can be almost unmeasurable (>300 bpm). There are no discernible P-waves, QRS complexes, or T-waves on the strip; instead, the tracing shows a chaotic series of wide, rapid, extremely irregular events. When the ventricles try to beat at very high rates, they can no longer effectively contract and relax; instead, they just quiver. The result is that the blood is not pumped through the heart and cardiac output drops quickly. VF tracings are sometimes called *coarse* (low-amplitude waveforms) that usually precede *fine* VF (very low-amplitude waveforms that can look like a flat line).

Idioventricular rhythm

Some rhythms that originate in the ventricles are escape rhythms and do not have high rates. Known as idioventricular rhythms, these arrhythmias have a low ventricular rate (20–40 bpm); a wide, bizarre QRS complex (>120 ms); and no discernible P-waves. The difference between monomorphic VT and idioventricular escape rhythms is rate: monomorphic VT is fast, idioventricular rhythms are slow.

A particularly interesting arrhythmia is the accelerated idioventricular rhythm. It is an escape rhythm originating from the ventricles, but it may occur in the normal rate range of, say, 60–80 bpm. Thus, when assessing rhythms originating from the ventricles:

• If they are slow (20–40 bpm), they are idioventricular or escape rhythms.
• If they are fast (>100 bpm), they are VT.
• If they are in between, they are accelerated idioventricular rhythms.

It is important to be able to clinically distinguish an accelerated idioventricular rhythm (which is an arrhythmia and of concern) from NSR. To make this distinction, it is important to observe QRS morphology (wide, bizarre) since rate is not helpful here.

Ventricular standstill

Ventricular standstill occurs when there is no ventricular activity; on the rhythm strip, the clinician may still see P-waves, but there will be no ventricular activity in response (ventricular asystole). When no atrial or ventricular activity occurs at all, this is cardiac standstill or asystole. Both of these conditions can be fatal in a matter of minutes.

AV block

The sinus arrhythmias described earlier all involve intact conduction from the atria to the ventricles, resulting in 1:1 or nearly 1:1 AV synchrony. By contrast, AV block (sometimes called heart block) is a broad term for several different types of arrhythmia in which the relationship of the atria to the ventricles is disordered. AV block involves a delay or interruption of electrical conduction from the atria to the ventricles, so that the key to understanding AV block resides in the PR interval. AV block is divided into three main types, defined as degrees or grades. First- and second-degree AV block may be considered partial or incomplete heart block; conduction from the upper chambers to the lower chambers is delayed but not entirely blocked. Third-degree AV block is the most severe form of AV block and involves total or complete block. Third-degree AV block is sometimes called complete heart block. In a patient with third-degree AV block, impulses from the atria do not conduct to the ventricles at all so that there is complete dissociation of the upper and lower chambers.

First-degree AV block

In first-degree AV block, the PR interval is longer than 200 ms; by contrast, in a normal heart rhythm, the PR interval will be less than 200 ms. First-degree AV block is otherwise a regular rhythm with a P-wave occurring before each and every QRS complex (1:1 AV synchrony). In first-degree AV block, the PR interval is prolonged (>200 ms) but is

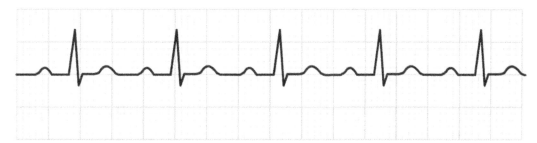

Figure 7.16 First-degree AV block is a regular rhythm with a P-wave appearing before each QRS complex but with a prolonged but regular PR interval of 200 ms or more. Note in this strip that the PR intervals are consistent at 260 ms.

consistent (see **Figure 7.16**). First-degree AV block may also occur in patients with concomitant sinus bradycardia.

In many ways, a rhythm strip from a patient with first-degree AV block will appear at first glance to be like NSR, which is why rhythm strips should be systematically approached rather than glanced at!

First-degree AV block occurs when the AV node—which normally slows conduction from the atria to the ventricles—is slowing conduction down too much. This excessive slowing over the AV node may be related to an electrolyte imbalance, drugs (such as beta-blockers), myocardial ischemia, and inferior wall myocardial infarction and increased vagal tone.

Second-degree AV block

In second-degree AV block, the PR interval and the relationship of atrial to ventricular activity begins to change. There are two types of second-degree AV block: Mobitz type I (sometimes called Mobitz type I, Type I, or Wenckebach) and Mobitz type II (sometimes called type II).

Mobitz type I or Wenckebach

Second-degree heart block type I or Mobitz I is characterized by a PR interval that gets progressively longer until eventually a QRS complex is dropped. At this point, 1:1 AV synchrony is lost. However, in patients with Mobitz I, another P-wave will occur followed by a short PR interval and a QRS complex. The cycle starts again with a gradual lengthening of the PR interval until, finally, a P-wave appears without a QRS wave. An important characteristic of Mobitz I is that after the pause, the first PR interval is shorter—perhaps not short

enough to be considered normal (<200 ms) but markedly shorter than the preceding few PR intervals. When describing Mobitz I, it is typical to refer to the pattern of P-waves to R-waves or a P–R ratio, such as 3:2 or 4:3. This pattern often repeats itself consistently in the arrhythmia, but some patients exhibit variable conduction with Mobitz I. Following the pause in the rhythm, the next PR interval will be markedly shorter than its predecessor. The lengthening of the PR interval in Wenckebach arrhythmias is not always prolonged by regular increments, that is, the PR intervals may vary somewhat. The key in identifying Mobitz I is to look at the PR interval after the pause and assess whether it is shorter than the preceding PR interval. Because of the pauses, Wenckebach arrhythmias may be described as irregular (see **Figure 7.17**).

From a clinical standpoint, it is important to think of what Mobitz I does to cardiac output and for that, the P–R ratio is required. For example, a patient with an atrial rate of around 90 bpm and 3:2 Wenckebach will have a ventricular rate of around 60 bpm. However, if that same patient had an atrial rate of 60 bpm and 3:2 Wenckebach, the ventricular rate is going to be much slower at around 40 bpm. Thus, the same arrhythmia may provoke different symptoms depending on the P-to-R relationship and the patient's underlying atrial rate. Thus, when caring for a patient with Wenckebach arrhythmias, determine what the ventricular rate is when those Wenckebach pauses occur.

Mobitz I typically is caused by disease or ischemia at or around the AV node. Anything that slows conduction over the AV node, such as drug therapy, ischemia, or infarction, may potentially result in Mobitz I arrhythmias.

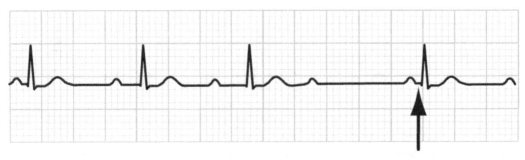

Figure 7.17 Second-degree heart block type I (also known as Mobitz I or Wenckebach) is an irregular rhythm with a prolonged PR interval and eventual dropout of the QRS complex. Note that the first PR interval after the pause (shown by arrow) is shorter than the previous PR interval.

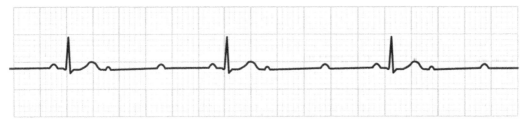

Figure 7.18 Mobitz II is a sinus rhythm characterized by regular PR intervals and then a sudden dropout of the QRS complex, resulting in a pause in the strip. The next PR interval after the pause will be shorter than the previous PR interval, although it may still be longer than normal (>200 ms).

Mobitz II

Second-degree heart block type II or Mobitz II exhibits a sudden dropout of the QRS complex but without the progressive lengthening of the PR interval. Like Mobitz I, Mobitz II can also be described with a P–R ratio, such as Mobitz II with a ratio of 2 : 1 (two P-waves for each QRS complex). When observing a Mobitz II strip, PR intervals— when they appear—will be consistent. In other words, when there is atrial conduction to the ventricle, it is stable.

In the clinic, sometimes, Mobitz II with a 3:2 ratio is confused with Mobitz I. Without a systematic approach to ECG analysis, it is easy to look at the dropped QRS and pronounce it Mobitz I, but the key is to examine the PR interval. In Mobitz I, the PR interval lengthens progressively until the QRS drops out, but in Mobitz II, the PR interval is stable and then suddenly—almost unexpectedly—the QRS drops out. Check the PR interval before determining if an arrhythmia is Mobitz I or II! While Mobitz II may be described as a regular rhythm (it looks regular and PP intervals will be regular), the RR intervals will be irregular (see **Figure 7.18**).

Mobitz II may be associated with moderate to severe symptoms. To understand this, look at the PR interval and determine the patient's ventricular rate. For example, in a patient with an atrial rate of around 80 bpm and 2:1 Mobitz II, the ventricular rate drops to 40 bpm.

Unlike Mobitz I, which is associated with inferior wall myocardial infarction, Mobitz II is more likely to be the result of anterior wall myocardial infarction. With Mobitz II, the patient will alternately exhibit intact normal conduction and then no conduction. This may owe to damage or dysfunction in the AV node or, more usually, the bundle of His (slightly below the AV node). Mobitz II may be caused by drug therapy, ischemia, or anterior wall myocardial infarction.

Third-degree AV block

Third-degree or complete heart block may be described as the complete dissociation of the atria from the ventricles. The atrial rate is regular

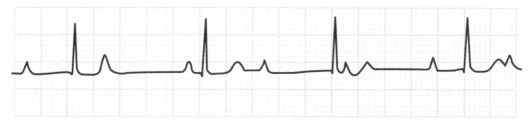

Figure 7.19 Third-degree or complete AV block exhibits dissociated atrial and ventricular rates. In this particular example, the PP interval is regular and appears normal, the RR interval is regular, and the QRS complexes are narrow and look normal—but the atrial rate is faster than the ventricular rate and is not synched to it. Since atrial and ventricular rates are independent of each other, the PR intervals are always different; in fact, one could even argue there is no *PR interval* in the usual sense.

Table 7.1 A summary of key characteristics of different types of AV block

Name	PP interval	RR interval	PR interval	Conduction
1st degree	Regular	Usually regular	>200 ms, consistent	1:1 P–R
2nd degree Mobitz I or Wenckebach	Regular	Irregular	Progressive lengthening of PR interval until 1 P-wave is blocked and QRS drops out	Some P-waves conduct
2nd degree Mobitz II	Regular	Usually regularly irregular	Constant on conducted beats	
3rd degree	Regular	Regular	Not constant; P-waves are independent of QRS complexes	P-waves do not conduct at all

although it can fast, slow, or normal— but the atrial rate and the ventricular rate have no relationship to each other. Sometimes, this type of arrhythmia is described as AV dissociation.

Since none of the atrial beats conduct over the AV node to stimulate the ventricle, some other area of the heart (a so-called backup pacemaker) must be causing the ventricles to depolarize. This may be the AV junction or the ventricles themselves, and the resulting rate is often slow. If the QRS complexes on the ECG look normal, the escape rhythm is likely a junctional escape rhythm. If the QRS complexes look wide or bizarre, it is likely a ventricular escape rhythm (see **Figure 7.19**).

The main characteristic of complete AV block is that no atrial beats conduct to the ventricle, resulting in an atrial rate that is independent of the ventricular rate. This type of arrhythmia usually originates at the AV junction or bundle of His and may be associated with myocardial infarction or other conditions that disturb AV conduction.

Summary of AV block

The key to understanding AV block is to assess the PR interval to determine the relationship of the atrial rate to the ventricular rate. **Table 7.1** provides a short summary of key landmarks to evaluate on the surface ECG to differentiate the types of AV block.

Conclusion

There are few subjects more important to pacemaker clinicians than being able to readily and confidently evaluate rhythm disturbances. Sinus arrhythmias include sinus bradycardia and sinus tachycardia, both of which maintain 1:1 AV synchrony. Typically, sinus bradycardia looks like what would otherwise be an *NSR* except the rate is too slow—around 40–60 bpm. Sinus arrhythmia occurs when there is some irregularity in the sinus rhythm with 1:1 AV synchrony, a subtle and surprisingly common type of arrhythmia that is often asymptomatic, and requires no treatment. Sinus arrest occurs when the SA node fails to fire and there is a *missing beat* on the ECG, that is, a P-wave and related QRS complex do not occur. When sinus arrest occurs, the next beat will reset the timing so that the next beat is not timed to preceding PP or RR intervals. This differs from sinus exit block, which also results in a *missing beat*, but this beat is missing because the atrial beat occurs but fails to conduct. With sinus exit block, a P-wave appears without the resulting QRS and the RR intervals will be regular. One way to think of distinguishing these is *you can walk around the block* (walk the calipers RR through sinus exit block) but *you can't get arrested* (you can't walk calipers RR through sinus arrest).

AV block involves conduction delays or blocks between the atria and ventricles. AV block is described by degrees and can be distinguished on the surface ECG by evaluating the PR interval. First-degree AV block involves a longer-than-normal PR interval (>200 ms) but otherwise is a regular *normal-looking* sinus rhythm. In second-degree AV block, dropouts occur. In second-degree AV block type I (also called Mobitz I or Wenckebach), the PR interval progressively lengthens until one QRS complex drops out, and then the rhythm is

restored and the pattern repeated. The key to identifying Mobitz I (and Mobitz II, below) is to evaluate the PR interval of the first beat after the pause—it should be markedly shorter than the last PR interval. Second-degree AV block type II (also called Mobitz II) exhibits a sudden dropout of the QRS but without progressive lengthening of the PR interval. In 2:1 Mobitz II, for example, every other P-wave will exhibit a dropped QRS complex, resulting in potentially dangerous rates such as an atrial rate of 60 bpm with a corresponding ventricular rate of 30 bpm. Third-degree AV block (also called complete heart block) involves no conduction at all between the atria and ventricles, such that the atrial and ventricular rates (which may be regular, that is, regular PP and regular RR) are dissociated. In such cases, the SA node drives the atrial rate, but either the AV junction or the ventricles drive the ventricular rate (this is an *escape rhythm* and is characteristically slow).

The nuts and bolts of arrhythmia analysis

- Arrhythmias are named from the areas where or near where they originate. An atrial arrhythmia originates in or near the atria but may also affect the ventricles. In fact, some atrial arrhythmias produce symptoms not because of their effects on the atria but because they affect the ventricles.
- Sinus tachycardia is a rapid heart rhythm that originates in the SA node and occurs because the SA node fires too quickly; AV conduction is normal and there is 1:1 AV synchrony. Sinus tachycardia tends to start and stop gradually. The typical rate range for sinus tachycardia is 100–150 bpm, but this range may vary depending on the patient's age, health, and fitness level.
- Sinus bradycardia is a too-slow heart rhythm that exhibits normal AV conduction and 1:1 AV synchrony. Sinus bradycardia is usually described as falling between 40 and 60 bpm, but this rate is relative since it depends on the patient's age, health, and fitness level. Sinus bradycardia occurs when the SA node fires too slowly but cardiac conduction is normal. Sinus bradycardia can be an indication for a pacemaker.
- Sinus arrhythmia describes an irregular rhythm that originates in the sinus node and involves

normal 1:1 AV conduction. An irregular rhythm is defined as one with a variation of >600 ms between the longest and shortest RR intervals. Sinus arrhythmias are surprisingly common and may be asymptomatic. They often vary with the patient's respiratory rhythms.
- Sinus arrest and sinus exit block look deceptively similar on an ECG, but they are caused by two different things. Sinus arrest occurs when the SA node does not fire; sinus exit block occurs when the SA node does fire but does not conduct. Both will exhibit long pauses on the surface ECG. The way to tell them apart is that sinus arrest *resets* the timing cycles so the first beat after the pause will not be timed out to the preceding beat. Sinus exit block will exhibit regular timing so you can *walk* calipers through the RR or PP intervals and get consistent timing.
- A premature ventricular contraction (PVC) typically has a wider-than-normal QRS complex (>120 ms) and a bizarre morphology compared to the other normally conducted ventricular beats. PVCs are common—everybody has them occasionally—but may be dangerous when they

occur too frequently (>10 per minute) or when they fall on the T-wave. This is called an R-on-T PVC and may trigger a potentially dangerous ventricular tachycardia.

- Junctional rhythms are those that originate in the AV junction, the tissue surrounding the AV node. Junctional rhythms will exhibit a P-wave that appears very close to the QRS complex—either right before or immediately following it. In some cases, the P-wave will not be evident on the surface ECG because it is *buried* within the QRS. When a P-wave is evident on a Lead II surface ECG of a junctional rhythm, it will be inverted.

- An occasional junctional beat may occur in an otherwise normal rhythm. If it occurs too soon with respect to the other beats, it is called a *premature beat*. If it occurs too late, it is called an *escape beat*.

- If a patient has occasional premature junctional contractions (PJCs), the condition may be benign, produce no or very mild symptoms, and require no particular treatment. In fact, occasional PJCs are not that uncommon.

- Junctional rhythms occur when the patient has mainly or only junctional beats. A junctional rhythm is a backup rhythm based on the firing of the AV junction rather than the SA node. As such, junctional rhythms are typically slower, often in the range of 40–60 bpm. Junctional rhythms exhibit the same P-wave morphology as junctional beats.

- Sometimes, a junctional rhythm can occur at rates of 60–100 bpm; this is known as an accelerated junctional rhythm and is attributed to an AV junction that is trying to take over and usurp the role of the SA node.

- Do not confuse an accelerated junctional rhythm with atrial fibrillation (AF). Accelerated junctional rhythms will display regular RR intervals, but AF will not.

- AV block is always a form of conduction disorder between the atria and ventricles. The key to assessing the different types or degrees of AV block is to evaluate the PR interval.

- There are three degrees of AV block: 1st-degree (in which AV conduction is delayed), 2nd-degree (in which AV conduction is alternately delayed and blocked), and 3rd-degree or complete AV block (in which there is no AV conduction at all). Second-degree AV block is further subdivided into Mobitz I (or Wenckebach) and Mobitz II.

- In 1st-degree AV block, the PR interval is abnormally long (>200 ms) but is consistent and the rhythm is otherwise regular.

- In 2nd-degree AV block type I or Mobitz I, the PR interval lengthens progressively from one complex to the next until one QRS complex drops out. Then the rhythm is restored. The key to identifying Mobitz I on an ECG is to look at the PR interval of the first beat after the pause; it should be clearly shorter than the previous PR interval.

- In 2nd-degree AV block type II or Mobitz II, the PR interval is abnormally long but does not lengthen—but sudden pauses occur in the ECG where a QRS complex drops out. Again, the PR interval after the pause should be noticeably shorter than the previous PR interval.

- In both Mobitz I and II, it is typical to describe it using the ratio of P-waves to R-waves, such as 3:2 or 2:1. This ratio can help the clinician identify the atrial and ventricular rates, for instance, a patient with an atrial rate of 100 bpm and 2:1 Mobitz II will have a ventricular rate of 50 bpm.

- The most severe form of AV block is 3rd-degree or complete AV block in which the atrial rate and the ventricular rate are completely independent of each other. In 3rd-degree AV block, there are no consistent PR intervals; in fact, a true PR interval does not occur because no atrial events are conducted to the ventricle!

- Atrial tachycardia is a collective term for too-fast arrhythmias that originate in the atria specifically; an even broader term is supraventricular tachycardia, which is any tachycardia that originates *above* (supra) the ventricles. Atrial flutter and AF are two commonly occurring types of atrial tachycardia.

- Atrial flutter is characterized by a sawtooth pattern of the atrial waves, while the main criterion for identifying AF on a rhythm strip is an *irregularly irregular* ventricular rate.

- A premature atrial contraction (PAC) is a type of ectopic beat that, like the PVC, appears too early on the rhythm strip and suggests cardiac irritability.

Test your knowledge

Quiz 1

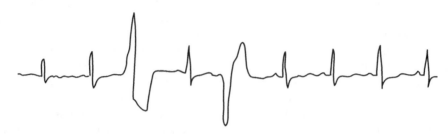

1 Looking at the rhythm strip above, how would you describe this rhythm?
  A Sinus tachycardia
  B Multiform PVCs in normal sinus rhythm
  C Mobitz I
  D Complete heart block

2 Which of the following statements is most true for sinus arrhythmias?
  A They occur mainly in geriatric patients.
  B They are exceedingly rare.
  C They often coordinate to the respiratory rate.
  D They can trigger potentially dangerous ventricular tachycardias.

3 Sinus tachycardia can be physiologic or pathologic. What is a good example of a physiologic sinus tachycardia?
  A A high-rate sinus rhythm that occurs during sleep.
  B A high-rate sinus rhythm that occurs during fever.
  C A high-rate sinus rhythm that occurs during exercise.
  D There is no such thing as a physiologic sinus tachycardia.

Quiz 2 (Relates to Question 4)

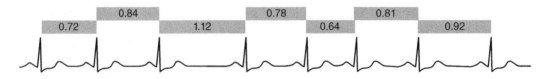

4 Note the RR intervals in the above strip. How would you best describe this rhythm?
  A Sinus arrhythmia
  B Sinus bradycardia
  C Sinus tachycardia
  D Atrial fibrillation

5 What is the difference between sinus arrest and sinus exit block?
  A Nothing, they are the same thing.
  B Sinus arrest is a problem with impulse formation and sinus exit block is a problem with impulse conduction.
  C Sinus arrest is the more severe form of sinus exit block.
  D Sinus arrest means the atria do not beat at all; sinus exit block means the ventricles do not beat at all.

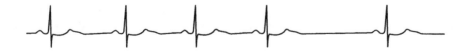

6 Is the above ECG an example of sinus arrest or sinus exit block and why?

   A It's sinus arrest because the pause is more than 200 ms.

   B These cannot be differentiated from a rhythm strip.

   C It's sinus exit block because the QRS comes in on the same timing cycle.

   D Sinus arrest and sinus exit block are the same thing.

7 For AF, what is the rate range for describing *rapid ventricular response*?

   A > 60 bpm

   B 60–100 bpm

   C >100 bpm

   D >300 bpm

8 Which of the following occurs in Mobitz I?

   A Progressive lengthening of the PR intervals until a QRS is dropped

   B Progressive shortening of the PR intervals

   C Complete dissociation of atrial and ventricular activity

   D Abnormally short PR intervals followed by a dropped QRS complex

9 What is the single most crucial *clue* to identifying a rhythm strip as atrial fibrillation?

   A A bumpy or wandering baseline

   B A very fast atrial rate

   C Irregularly irregular ventricular activity

   D Very fast ventricular activity

10 Which best describes ventricular trigeminy?

   A Two sinus beats and then one PVC.

   B An extended pause following every third beat.

   C An inverted P-wave on every third beat.

   D It is any type of accelerated junctional rhythm.

CHAPTER 8

Electricity 101

Learning objectives

- Understand and be able to correctly use electrical terminology common in pacing, such as conductor, anode, cathode, current, and resistance.
- Be able to state the advantages and disadvantages of unipolar and bipolar systems.
- State Ohm's law and explain why it is important in terms of lead impedance values.
- Describe how lead impedance values might be affected in the event of a lead fracture as well as an insulation breach.
- Define basic electrical terms used in pacing: pulse amplitude, pulse duration, and interference.

Introduction

Electric management of cardiac rhythm disorders is nothing new. In 1786, Luigi Galvani observed that dissected frog muscles could be made to twitch by application of electrical energy. The *first defibrillator* was arguably invented in 1788 by Charles Kite who found that electrical energy could resuscitate a drowned person. The first patented *artificial cardiac pacemaker* dates back to 1931, and it is not a device any of us today would recognize as a pacemaker. (It was not implantable—you had to crank it to generate electricity!) Today, we understand more than ever about electrical energy, and this knowledge is vital to understanding cardiac pacing. This chapter will present key electrical concepts and their specific application to cardiac pacing; the goal is to give practical knowledge relevant to cardiac rhythm management.

Electricity basics

For device clinicians, electricity is best defined as the energy that is made available when an electric charge flows through a conductor. Conductors are often wires (found in pacing leads), but they can be anything that readily conducts electricity. To be a little more scientific, electricity is a physical phenomenon associated with stationary or moving electrons and protons. To go back to your chemistry class, electrons are tiny particles that carry a negative charge, while protons carry a positive charge. The proton is situated in the nucleus of the atom, is very stable, and possesses a positive charge equal to the negative charge of the less stable electron that orbits around the nucleus. (The nucleus also contains neutrons that are neutral, i.e., have no charge.)

It is the electricity in the heart that causes the myocardial cells to depolarize. Depolarization refers to a change in polarity (negative to positive or vice versa). When myocardial cells depolarize, the cells contract, and this, in turn, leads to a cardiac contraction. Thus, the purpose of delivering electrical energy through the pacing lead (conductor) and into the heart is to make the heart muscle depolarize and, in that way, to cause the heart to beat.

Electricity is delivered to the myocardial cells by a pacemaker using leads. A lead is an insulated wire with one or more electrodes at the end. When talking about pacing leads, it is important

The Nuts and Bolts of Implantable Device Therapy Pacemakers, First Edition. Tom Kenny.
© 2015 John Wiley & Sons, Ltd. Published 2015 by John Wiley & Sons, Ltd.

to differentiate the anode (positive electrode) from the cathode (negative electrode). For example, on a typical ventricular pacing lead with a tip electrode and a ring electrode, the tip electrode is the cathode (negative) and the ring electrode is the anode (positive). Electricity always travels in a circuit

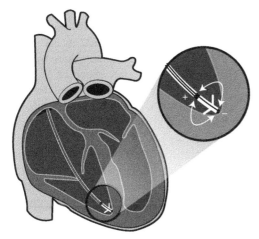

Figure 8.1 Electrical energy in this bipolar lead travels from the tip to ring electrode (cathode to anode) to form an electrical circuit. The tip electrode is the cathode and the ring electrode is the anode.

(circle). The pacing lead in the heart sends energy out, but that electrical energy must have a return path to the lead in order to form its circuit. Using the same example, the tip electrode (cathode, negative pole) sends out electrical energy that travels through the cardiac tissue and closes its circuit by returning to the ring electrode (anode, positive pole) (see **Figure 8.1**). In any pacing system (or, as a matter of fact, in any electrical system), there has to be a positive and negative pole; without them, the electricity cannot form a circuit.

Unipolar and bipolar systems

Pacing systems are often described as unipolar or bipolar systems, but there are important distinctions. While both unipolar and bipolar leads use a tip electrode as the cathode (negative pole), what distinguishes them is the anode (positive pole). In a unipolar system, the pacemaker can itself serve as the anode. In a bipolar system, the ring electrode on the lead is the anode. Both of these systems work well, but the *antenna* or area that the electricity has to travel in order to form its circuit is much larger in the unipolar system than the bipolar system (see **Figure 8.2**). While unipolar and bipolar

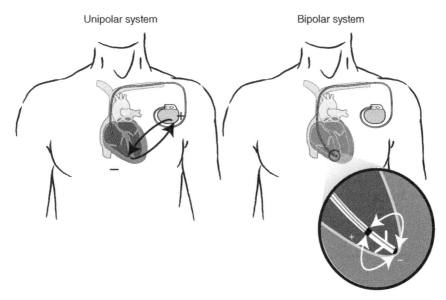

Figure 8.2 The unipolar pacing system uses the tip electrode on the lead as the cathode and the pacemaker itself as the anode; this creates a large body area described as the *antenna*. On the other hand, a bipolar pacing system uses the tip electrode as the cathode and a ring electrode on the lead as the anode, creating a much smaller antenna.

Table 8.1 A fast comparison of unipolar (single conductor) and bipolar (two conductors) leads

	Thickness of lead	Robust design	Redundancy	Familiar
Unipolar	Thinnest	Simpler design	No	Becoming rare
Bipolar	Today may be nearly or as thin as a unipolar lead	More complex design (two coils)	Yes, can be programmed to unipolar in the event of coil fracture	By far the more common lead in clinical practice today

systems will both be seen in clinical practice, bipolar systems are much more common.

The term unipolar pacing system is a bit misleading because it suggests there is only one pole. Electricity will not conduct unless there are two poles—a positive and a negative. The name *unipolar* derives from the fact that there is only one pole *on the pacing lead*. A bipolar system has *both poles on the pacing lead*. But both unipolar and bipolar systems require a positive and negative pole!

A bipolar lead is designed with two conductor coils, one coil going to the tip electrode and the other going to the ring electrode. (A unipolar lead only needs one coil.) Unipolar leads are therefore thinner and less mechanically complicated. Thin leads pass more easily through veins and are less likely to obstruct blood flow. Historically, physicians preferred the unipolar design because it offered them a substantially thinner lead. Technological advances have made today's bipolar leads just as thin or nearly as thin as unipolar leads. With these design advancements, the bipolar leads have rapidly gained popularity. Bipolar leads offer a redundancy advantage as well, in that if the outer conductor should fracture, the lead can still be used by programming the system to unipolar. Obviously, if a unipolar lead suffers conductor fracture, it cannot be reprogrammed to bipolar! If a unipolar lead loses its one conductor, it can no longer function (see **Table 8.1**).

Pacemaker battery

Pacemakers contain a battery within the case and they use that battery to produce electricity. The battery is able to do that because it contains several primary or secondary cells arranged in parallel or in series. Implantable devices also contain capacitors. Capacitors are specialized components that store electrical energy. A good analogy for a capacitor is a bucket; think of electricity as a flow of water pouring into a large bucket. When the bucket is full, it can be tipped over and all of its stored-up contents are dumped out at once. Capacitors are necessary in pacemakers because most pacemaker batteries are about 2.8 V. For a pacemaker to pace at 5 V, it needs to store up electrical energy to be able to deliver 5 V—that is the role of the capacitor. Capacitors allow pacemakers to use very small batteries and still work effectively, contributing to the small size of most devices today. Capacitors are also used in implantable cardioverter–defibrillators (ICDs), but they have a somewhat different design.

Ohm's law

Pacemakers rely on Ohm's law in terms of how they manage their energy, and device clinicians should have a good grasp of Ohm's law to understand device function. In a nutshell, Ohm's law states that the electrical current in any system is directly proportional to voltage and inversely proportional to resistance. There are a few ways to write out the formula for Ohm's law, but it is clearest for device clinicians to state that voltage = current times resistance or $V = IR$ (in this case, I stands for *current*).

Voltage is scientifically defined as the difference in electrical potential between two points, but for device clinicians, we can think of voltage as the *push* or force that causes electrons to move through a circuit. In cardiac pacing, voltage can be programmed and is often referred to as *amplitude* because it helps define the size of the pulse amplitude on the ECG or intracardiac electrogram. Volt is abbreviated V, but when talking about pacing voltage, it is typically written as $\bar{V}$. This symbol means that voltage is constant. In pacemakers (unlike certain other systems), voltage (the *push*) is constant.

Current is the flow of the electrical charge and is typically measured in milliamperes or mA. Milliamperes is a unit of measure whereby

1 ampere (A) equals 1000 mA. Because pacing deals with very low values in this area, devices typically report electrical parameters in milli-amps or mA. In the equation for Ohm's law, current is represented by the letter I; do not let that confuse you. *The letter I stands for current!*

Resistance is the opposition to the current flow. Think of voltage pushing current along a conductor; resistance is the force that current has to overcome to flow. Resistance is measured in units called ohms, which are sometimes written with the symbol Ω, which is the Greek letter omega. To an electrical engineer, there is a difference between *resistance* and *impedance*, but in cardiac pacing, these two terms can be used interchangeably. This creates a problem for Ohm's law because we, device clinicians, naturally want to make the I in the equation stand for impedance when it actually stands for current. The formula for Ohm's law is *voltage equals current times resistance*. If the letters $V = IR$ trip you up, then remember the formula as words. You can also think of it even more simply: *push equals flow times resistance*.

When calculating using this equation, the voltage and ohms (resistance) will result in amperes. Pacing systems use milliamperes, not amperes, so the decimal point has to be moved. There are 1000 mA in 1 A or 1 amp equals 0.001 mA. Thus, if an equation results in a current value of 0.005 A, that converts into 5 mA.

Ohm's law is useful for device clinicians because it explains the relationship between key electrical concepts. Pacemakers are constant-voltage systems; the voltage is programmable and does not vary. What does vary are current and resistance. As the current or flow decreases, resistance increases. Conversely, when current or flow goes up, resistance goes down. *When current changes, resistance changes (in the opposite direction).*

Ohm's law is very useful in helping to troubleshoot lead problems. There are two main ways that pacing leads are compromised: one involves damage to the coil or conductor, often called *fracture*, while the other is insulation failure, sometimes called *breach*. When insulation is breached, resistance to the current flow drops dramatically; that means that impedance (resistance) will increase just as dramatically. An insulation breach typically shows up as a very low resistance or impedance

value. (Insulation damage will drain the pacemaker battery, too.) On the other hand, if the conductor is damaged, then resistance increases sharply and impedance will drop just as sharply. A large and abrupt increase in lead impedance may signal a fractured conductor coil.

Some pacing leads are marketed as *high-resistance leads*. This can only be understood from a knowledge of Ohm's law. If a lead is designed to offer high resistance, this results in a reduced current flow. The reduced current flow spares the battery and can increase device longevity—while keeping voltage delivery constant.

Electrical terms used in pacing

Pacemakers allow programming of the voltage settings as the amplitude or pulse amplitude. These settings are measured in volts, typically from less than 1 V to about 7 or more volts. Amplitude is the term for voltage because it describes how tall the wave appears on an ECG. The other important programmable parameter for the output is the pulse width, sometimes called the pulse duration. Pulse duration is measured in milliseconds (ms) or thousandths of a second and it adjusts how long the device will deliver the voltage. By setting the pulse amplitude (V) and the pulse duration (ms), the clinicians determine the pacemaker's output pulse.

In pacing, the terms impedance and resistance are used interchangeably. Electrical engineers would disagree that these terms are the same thing (they really are not) but for pacing, they are used to describe the same phenomenon, that is, the total opposition to the flow of current. Impedance in pacing is measured in ohms and is not programmable but it is reported by the programmer.

Electromagnetic interference (EMI) can be an important electrical concept in pacing, in that it describes environmental energy that can create noise or even interfere with the proper operation of the pacemaker. An example of EMI occurs when an insulation break occurs that allows electrical signals from within the body but unrelated to the heart to get to the wire and create *noise* for the pacemaker. EMI can also be created in the environment, such as in the presence of large industrial magnets or during arc welding. Pacemaker patients should be cautioned about such environments.

The nuts and bolts of electricity 101

- Electrical energy delivered to the heart causes the myocardial cells to depolarize, and it is this depolarization that results in a cardiac contraction.
- Electricity must travel in a circuit (circular path) and travels from negative to positive pole. The negative pole is called the cathode, while the positive pole is the anode.
- On pacing leads, the tip electrode is the cathode. The anode can be either the ring electrode (bipolar lead) or the pacemaker itself (unipolar lead). The cathode is negative, and the anode is positive.
- In clinical practice today, it is rare to see unipolar leads. This is because bipolar leads today are nearly or as thin as the unipolar leads and bipolar leads offer redundancy. In the event the outer conductor fractures, a bipolar lead can still be viable if it is reprogrammed to unipolar.
- Ohm's law is important to understanding pacemaker energy. It can best be stated as voltage equals current times resistance, abbreviated $V = IR$, where I stands for current.
- In pacing, resistance and impedance are used interchangeably. To electrical engineers, these terms mean slightly different things.

- Current is the flow of electricity. The path along which electricity flows is its conductor (in pacing, this is the lead). Voltage is the *push* that causes the current to flow and can sometimes be called amplitude. Resistance is the force the current must overcome as it flows. In these terms, Ohm's law could be stated as push equals flow times resistance.
- Voltage is measured in volts (V), current is measured in milliamperes or milliamps (mA), and resistance is measured in ohms (Ω).
- One ampere equals 1000 mA. In pacing, resistance is typically measured in mA units.
- Pacemakers are voltage-constant systems. Resistance and current can vary, but voltage is constant. When current changes, resistance changes in the opposite direction, that is, when current goes up, resistance goes down, and vice versa.
- If a lead has a break in insulation, resistance drops; this results in an increase in impedance. If a lead suffers a conductor fracture, resistance goes up and impedance drops. In this way, sudden and large changes in the lead impedance can alert clinicians to possible lead damage.

Test your knowledge

1 In a pacing system, the voltage is 5.0 V and the resistance is 100 Ω. What is the current?
  A 5 mA
  B 0.5 mA
  C 500 Ω
  D 10

2 How many amperes are there in 1 milliamp?
  A 100
  B 1000
  C 19
  D None; they are two totally different things

3 Ohm's law can be stated as $V = IR$. V and R stand for voltage and resistance, respectively. What does the letter I stand for?
  A Impedance
  B Impudence

  C Joules
  D Current

4 In a bipolar pacing system, where is the anode of the system?
  A The tip electrode
  B The ring electrode
  C The pacemaker housing ("can")
  D It doesn't need an anode

5 Which of these is the negative pole?
  A Anode
  B Cathode
  C Diode
  D Electrode

6 When a lead's insulation is damaged, what happens to the impedance?

A It stays the same
B It goes down
C It goes up
D It goes up a little at first and then plateaus

7 When a device clinician notices that the impedance value (resistance) has suddenly gone way down, what is something he or she should suspect?
  A Conductor fracture
  B Insulation breach
  C Battery depletion
  D Nothing; abrupt changes in impedance are normal

8 A unipolar pacing system has a large antenna because:
  A The leads are very large
  B It consumes more electricity

C It uses the can as the pacing anode
D It paces both sides of the heart

9 In the average device clinic, which type of pacing system is seen most often?
  A Unipolar
  B Bipolar
  C Tripolar
  D External

10 In a pacing system, which of the following values is constant?
  A Voltage
  B Resistance
  C Impedance
  D Current

CHAPTER 9

Pacing 101

Learning objectives

- Name the two most basic functions performed by any cardiac pacemaker.
- Define pacing threshold and sensing threshold and explain why these are important for a clinician to know.
- Explain how to create a strength–duration curve and how it can be used in pacing.
- Name the two parameters that define an output pulse and the relative role of each in terms of energy usage.
- State briefly what the pacemaker does when it senses an intrinsic rhythm that differs from the programmed base rate (both faster and slower than base rate).
- Describe the considerations that come into play when setting device sensitivity.
- State why threshold values can vary over time.
- Name and point out the basic components of a pacing lead.
- Explain an easy way to distinguish a bipolar from a unipolar lead just by looking at it.
- Name at least one advantage and one disadvantage, respectively, for silicone and polyurethane lead insulation.
- Briefly explain how and why lead impedance values might relate to lead integrity.

Introduction

Pacemakers really only do two things: they pace and they sense. Pacing means they deliver a small electrical output pulse to depolarize the heart and thus cause a cardiac contraction. Pacemakers also sense, which means they can *see* the patient's intrinsic cardiac activity. A pacemaker has the ability to sense if the patient's heart is beating on its own and how fast it is beating. Sensing allows the pacemaker to *make decisions* as to when to pace and when to withhold or inhibit a pacemaker output pulse. Keep these two basic functions in mind when going through this chapter and do not try to make pacemaker function be more complicated than it is!

There are four components of any pacing system, and this chapter will discuss three of them: the pulse generator, the lead(s), and the programmer. The fourth component that is omitted here should never be forgotten in clinical practice—it's the patient!

Pacing and sensing

Thresholds

A threshold is a minimum value required to accomplish some goal. In pacing, the pacing threshold is the minimum amount of energy required to consistently produce a cardiac contraction. In other words, the pacing threshold defines the minimum output you need to pace the heart reliably. A pacing threshold is a minimum value for the output pulse, which is defined by pulse amplitude (voltage) and pulse width (duration of time). Pacing thresholds are very important values to know, but they can change. A patient does not have a consistent pacing threshold—the pacing threshold varies depending on the device and lead system. Furthermore, during implantation, physicians may find that they get lower (better) thresholds in certain areas of the heart. Over time, thresholds can and do change, with fibrosis of the lead within the heart, advancing

The Nuts and Bolts of Implantable Device Therapy Pacemakers, First Edition. Tom Kenny.
© 2015 John Wiley & Sons, Ltd. Published 2015 by John Wiley & Sons, Ltd.

age, disease progression, and cardiac medications. For that reason, pacing thresholds should be checked often, and clinicians should expect completely new threshold values when a pacemaker system is revised.

The sensing threshold is an entirely different value but equally as important to safe, reliable pacemaker function. The sensing threshold defines how large the minimum intrinsic cardiac signal has to be in order for the pacemaker to be able to reliably detect (sense) it and respond to it. Intrinsic cardiac signals can vary in size (pulse amplitude), and the pacemaker often has to be adjusted so that the pacemaker can *see* the patient's intrinsic signals. An intrinsic signal smaller than the sensing threshold will not be sensed. While clinicians might be tempted to opt for very low sensing thresholds so that nothing gets missed, a very low sensing threshold might see too much and sense noise or extracardiac signals in the body and misinterpret them as cardiac activity.

Sensing is a complex process. First, the lead looks for a difference in electrical potential between two points. In a bipolar lead, those two points are the tip and ring electrodes; in a unipolar lead, those two points are the tip electrode and the pulse generator can. Second, the lead within the heart senses intrinsic cardiac activity in the form of electrical signals at a certain amplitude and frequency range. These signals are carried up the pacing lead and into the pulse generator to a portion of the device known as the *sensing circuit*. The sensing circuit then interprets that signal. If the intrinsic rate being sensed is faster than the programmed rate, the pacemaker inhibits or withholds an output pulse. It might be tempting to think that when the patient's rate is above the programmed base rate, the pacemaker does nothing—but pacemakers never do nothing! They are always observing or sensing the intrinsic rhythm, beat by beat. Based on what is going on intrinsically, the pacemaker will *decide* to pace or inhibit. It is always doing something! By the way, pacemaker can only inhibit the pacing pulse; no pacemaker can inhibit the patient's intrinsic rate. So don't be confused when clinicians talk about a pacemaker's inhibiting activity—*that always means the pacemaker is withholding its output pulse, and it never means the pacemaker is inhibiting the patient's own rate.*

Sensing and pacing work together so that the pacemaker—which watches every single beat of the patient's heart—only paces when the patient requires it. In the early days of pacing, this was called *demand pacing*, a term that you may even still hear today.

To use a simple example, let's take a pacemaker that is programmed to a pacing rate of 60 ppm. If the patient's intrinsic rate is 40 bpm, the pacemaker senses that rate is slower than the programmed pacing rate and then decides to pace so that it can pace the patient's heart at 60 ppm. If the patient's intrinsic rate is 62 bpm, the pacemaker senses that rate and then decides to inhibit its output pulse and allow the heart to beat on its own at 62 bpm. Heart rates vary over the course of the day, sometimes even from moment to moment, so the pacemaker is constantly sensing—beat by beat—and, with each event, deciding to either deliver an output pulse (pace) or withhold an output pulse (inhibit).

Capture

The goal of pacing is not delivery of an electrical output pulse, period. The goal of pacing is to deliver an electrical output pulse that leads the heart to depolarize and thus contract. A pacemaker output pulse or spike that causes depolarization and contraction is said to *capture* the heart. An output pulse that fails to capture the heart does not pace the heart. For that reason, it is extremely important to be sure that the output pulse is sufficient to capture the heart. Capture occurs because the output pulse has sufficient energy to depolarize the heart; if the output pulse does not have enough energy, it will not capture. The output pulse is defined by pulse amplitude (voltage) and pulse width (duration) (see **Figure 9.1**).

Capture can be observed on a paced ECG by finding the pacemaker spike or vertical line that shows the output pulse from the pulse generator and then seeing if it resulted in an immediate depolarization. If a spike appears on the ECG without being followed immediately by depolarization, that spike or output pulse failed to capture the heart. Although the pacing spike looks like a short vertical line on the ECG, if it were slowed down, it would look like Figure 9.1.

The capture threshold is the minimum amount of energy an output pulse must have in order to

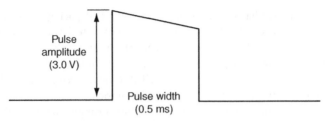

Figure 9.1 The pacemaker output pulse is defined by voltage or pulse amplitude (the height of the waveform) and pulse width or duration of time (the width of the waveform). A typical pacemaker output pulse might be 3 V and 0.5 ms. These values are programmable so clinicians can fine-tune the output pulse for reliable capture. By adjust either pulse amplitude or pulse width or both, the amount of energy carried by the output pulse changes.

reliably and consistently capture the heart. There is not just one single pair of output pulse settings that can capture the heart. The pulse amplitude, for example, can be programmed to 0.5 or 1.0 or 2.0 or 3.0 or even higher voltages. The pulse width can be set to 0.4, 0.5, 0.75, or 1.0 ms or longer. These two values have a relationship to each other, that is, the more voltage you set, the shorter the pulse width has to be to capture the heart. Conversely, the less voltage you apply, the longer the pulse width has to be to capture the heart. At the two extremes, you come to a point where no matter how much voltage you apply to the heart—even 10 or 20 V or more—you plateau in terms of pulse width. Likewise, extending the pulse width beyond about 1.0 ms does not buy us anything in terms of improving capture. A clinician (and nowadays a programmer device) can look at a patient's capture threshold and come up with all of the different pairs of values (pulse amplitude and pulse width) to show a strength–duration curve (strength here means *voltage*). While patients can have quite different capture thresholds, the strength–duration curves always have the same characteristic curved shape that descends sharply from the left and plateaus or flatlines off to the right (see **Figure 9.2**).

Using a strength–duration curve like the one in Figure 9.2, a clinician can determine what pairs of output settings will capture the heart, for example, at a pulse amplitude of 0.4 V, the chart will show that the shortest pulse duration needed for capture is 0.5 ms. The output pulse parameters needed for any device are settings that fall either on the line or in the white portion of the chart (above the curve). Using the example in Figure 9.2, a clinician could easily see that 1.0 V and 0.5 ms would capture the heart, but that 0.25 V and 0.5 ms would not.

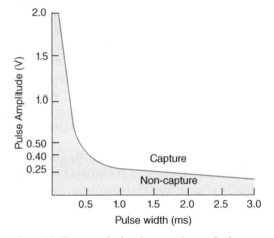

Figure 9.2 The strength–duration curve is actually the pulse amplitude–pulse width chart showing all of the pairs of output pulse parameters (voltage and pulse duration) that will capture the heart. While individual strength–duration curves can vary, they all exhibit the same general curved shape. Note that everything under the curve will not capture the heart, while all values above the curve will.

The center of the curve of the strength–duration curve (sometimes called the *knee of the curve*) is the patient's actual capture threshold. This does not mean it is the only pair of output settings that reliably captures the heart; it just defines *the lowest amount of energy*, which will reliably capture the heart. Obviously, a clinician could reliably capture this patient's heart by programming a 10 V pulse amplitude and a 1.0 ms pulse width, but that is not the most efficient use of energy, and efficient use of energy is very important in an implantable battery-powered device.

Capture thresholds are not static; they change over time and even over the course of a day. Furthermore, capture thresholds can change in unpredictable ways. For that reason, clinicians like to build in a little cushion when programming output parameters. If a patient's capture threshold is exactly 0.5 V at 0.4 ms, it would be risky to program those exact settings because any change upward in the capture threshold will result in loss of capture. And we can't be sure the patient's threshold won't shift upward! Capture threshold is known to be affected by eating, sleeping, electrolyte balance, posture, disease (such as heart failure), and certain medications—all common to pacemaker patients! When choosing the right output pulse parameters for a given patient, the clinician should program an area well above the curve by building in something known as the *safety margin*.

In dealing with strength–duration curves, it is sometimes of academic (more so than clinical) interest to consider the rheobase and chronaxie. All strength–duration curves exhibit the same characteristic curve that plateaus or flatlines off to the right. The rheobase is the lowest voltage value that is still on the strength–duration curve before it flatlines (see **Figure 9.3**). Rheobase is the lowest

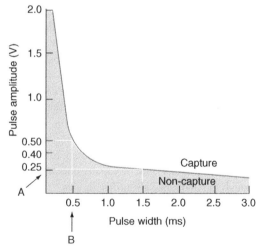

Figure 9.3 The strength–duration curve is characterized by a steep downward slope that eventually flattens out with the capture or stimulation threshold occurring at the inflection of the curve. Rheobase (A) is the lowest pulse amplitude at the longest pulse width that falls on the curve; in this example, rheobase is 0.25 V. Chronaxie (B) is the pulse width at twice rheobase; in this example, that would be the pulse width at 0.5 V (0.25 V × 2 = 0.5 V) or 0.5 ms. Rheobase and chronaxie are largely theoretical values not used directly in clinical practice but may be useful when discussing the strength–duration curve.

voltage that will capture the heart at the longest pulse width; think of rheobase as the lowest voltage at the longest pulse width on the strength–duration curve. In this example, 0.25 V will capture the heart at 1.5, 2.0, or longer pulse widths. Chronaxie is the pulse width at double the rheobase, so if the rheobase is 0.25 V, then 0.25 V × 2 results in 5 volts. Find the point on the strength–duration curve where 5 V captures the heart and that pulse width is the chronaxie value.

The output pulse (pulse amplitude and pulse width or V and ms settings) defines how much energy the pacemaker has to deliver with each pacing pulse. This is a very important setting because the energy the device uses will affect how long the battery lasts. Clinicians who program pacing output parameters balance two very important considerations: how low can these settings be programmed to conserve battery life and how high should these settings be programmed to assure patient safety and reliable capture? The energy that defines how much energy the pacemaker delivers in an output pulse can be described in this equation:

$$\text{Energy (Joules)} = \text{voltage} \times \text{amps} \times \text{time (seconds)}$$

Let's go back and review the old energy equation where *amps* was previous described as I:

$$\text{Amps} = \frac{\text{voltage}}{\text{resistance} (\Omega)}$$

When calculating energy in the pulse generator output pulse, these two equations merge:

$$\text{Energy (Joules)} = \text{voltage} \times \frac{\text{voltage}}{\text{resistance} (\Omega)} \times \text{time (ms)}$$

The purpose of knowing these equations is to better understand safety margin, the extra energy *cushion* programmed to the pulse amplitude and/ or pulse width to allow for variations in the patient's capture threshold. Pacing pulse output is defined by only two parameters: pulse amplitude (V) and pulse width (ms). A clinician can boost the energy in the output pulse by increasing either the pulse amplitude or the pulse width or both. In terms increasing output pulse energy, any of those three methods works. However, clinicians must also think in terms of using the least energy to accomplish the most work. Thus, if a clinician doubles the pulse amplitude or voltage, he or she effectively *quadruples* the energy. By the same token, if the clinic doubles the pulse width (time), he or she *doubles* the energy. Thus, it is *cheaper* to extend the pulse width than to increase the pulse amplitude, but it is not safer. The purpose of the safety margin is inherent in its name: it is there to promote patient safety. So while increasing the pulse amplitude may not be the most energy-saving choice, it is by far the better choice for patient safety. And in this case (like all other cases), patient safety trumps all.

In clinical practice, most safety margins are set using a very simple method. Once the clinician knows the patient's capture threshold—let's say it is 1.0 V at 0.4 ms—the clinician will then double or triple the pulse amplitude and leave the pulse width alone. Using this same example, a patient with a capture threshold of 1.0 V at 0.4 ms will be programmed to 2.0 or 3.0 V at 0.4 ms. This is a *rule of thumb* approach, but it is simple, effective, and widely used.

Remember, *doubling the pulse width doubles the energy but doubling the pulse amplitude quadruples the energy.*

Capture is also affected by the lead. The amount of energy required to capture the heart will change with lead maturation or how long the lead has been in place. When a lead is first implanted, capture thresholds will be much lower than in the coming weeks. As the lead matures, scar tissue forms around the lead and capture thresholds increase, sometimes substantially. Capture threshold depends in part of lead technology; some of the newest leads have porous electrodes that offer lower thresholds than older technologies. Finally, the patient's medications can affect capture threshold as can electrolyte imbalances and other physical conditions.

Output parameters are independently programmable for the atrium and ventricle in dual-chamber pacemakers.

Sensing

Pacemakers sense intrinsic cardiac signals by sensing electrical signals. The body actually generates many different types of electrical signals, including myopotentials or muscle noise. The goal of sensing is to allow the pacemaker to *see* and sense all cardiac signals but not sense smaller extraneous signals like muscle noise. For instance, sensitivity could be set on a pacemaker so that it sensed every possible signal—but that would result in sensing body noise that could inappropriately inhibit pacing. On the other hand, sensitivity could be set so that the pacemaker only saw very large signals—but then it might miss real cardiac signals and pace inappropriately. Ideally, the sensitivity of the pacemaker should be set to a level so that it picks up all cardiac signals and ignores all of the smaller extraneous signals.

Think of sensitivity like a wall in a field. Imagine standing in the field and looking out toward the wall. Anything that is taller than the wall is going to be visible to you. Anything that is shorter than the wall will be hidden. Applying that analogy to sensitivity, imagine setting a pacemaker to a sensitivity of 8 mV. At that sensitivity setting, the pacemaker could only see waveforms that exceeded 8 mV. In practical terms, this pacemaker would *see* or sense nothing at all since waveforms are rarely that big. The pacemaker would sense nothing and would *think* there is no intrinsic cardiac activity and pace. This could be problematic because the patient might have intrinsic activity (just smaller than 8 mV), and the pacing would compete with that intrinsic rate. By the same token, if the sensitivity is set to 1 mV, any waveform larger than 1 mV is visible and this may allow the pacemaker to sense T-waves or myopotentials and inhibit the pacing output inappropriately.

Finding the optimal sensitivity setting involves setting the height of the *wall* tall enough to exclude extraneous signals like myopotentials but low enough to reliably see all cardiac signals.

To make the pacemaker more sensitive, the mV setting is reduced; to make the pacemaker less sensitive, the mV setting is increased. This can sometimes be confusing to new clinicians. Increasing the mV setting decreases sensitivity! A pacemaker programmed to a sensitivity setting of 6 mV is not as sensitive as one programmed to 4 mV.

In a dual-chamber pacemaker, sensitivity is programmed independently for the atrium and ventricle. A typical R-wave is between 5 and 10 mV but should be measured for each patient at regular checkups. A typical P-wave is between 2 and 3 mV and can likewise change over time. Since these so-called sensing thresholds are not static values but fluctuate over the course of the day and with other things such as disease, drugs, posture, and so on, clinicians must rely on a 2:1 safety margin. For example, if a patient's R-wave is measured at 6 mV, sensitivity should be set to 3 mV to allow that 2:1 safety margin so in case the R-wave amplitude decreases, the device will still sense reliably. Likewise, if a P-wave is measured at 2.5 mV, atrial sensitivity should be set to 1.25 mV. In clinical practice, the 2:1 sensitivity safety margin is a rule of thumb and is often rounded to be more generous, so a patient with a 2.5 mV P-wave might be programmed to a sensitivity setting of 1 mV. A good way to think of this is that a sensitivity safety margin is *at least* 2:1. In clinical practice, as long as the measured P-wave and the R-wave amplitudes are acceptable (>2 mV atrial, >5 mV ventricular), most clinicians will leave the device programmed to its nominal parameters (0.5 mV atrial, 2.5 mV ventricular).

The patient's intrinsic signals are measured during implantation to provide intraoperative values and are then measured postoperatively using the sensing test available through the programmer. Regular sensing tests are useful because intracardiac signals can change slightly over time. However, unlike capture thresholds—which exhibit a marked increase after implantation—sensing values will not have a substantial acute-to-chronic change. (They might not even change at all.)

Two of the challenges in pacemaker sensing are undersensing and oversensing. Like the name implies, undersensing means not sensing things that ought to have been sensed, while oversensing means sensing things that should not have been sensed. Since sensing and pacing are linked together in pacemaker function, undersensing results in overpacing, while oversensing results in underpacing. Undersensing and oversensing are common problems in pacing that can be corrected by adjusting sensitivity values.

The pacing system

The pacing system includes the pulse generator, the lead(s), the programmer, and the patient. The patient is the most important single component in the pacing system! The implantable pulse generator (IPG)

is also called the pulse generator, the pacemaker, or even just *the can*. The pulse generator has internal circuitry and an internal battery, an external titanium case, and an epoxy header where the lead(s) plug in.

The programmer is a proprietary laptop-style computer that is used to communicate with the pulse generator, even after it is implanted in the body. Every manufacturer has its own programmer, and they are not interchangeable. This means if you are interrogating a Boston Scientific pacemaker, you must use the Boston Scientific programmer; the Medtronic one will not work. In practice, this means that most pacemaker clinics will have multiple programmers and pacemaker specialists need to be familiar with several different systems. When a clinician is called to interrogate an implanted pacemaker in a new or unfamiliar patient, the first important bit of information needed is the pacemaker manufacturer. This information should be in the patient's medical records, but if records are not available, it can be possible to identify a pacemaker using any of these methods:

- Ask the patient if he or she has a pacemaker ID card. Some patients will have their manufacturer's ID card handy and be able to prove what kind of device they have.
- Some patients may not carry the card but may know the device manufacturer. Ask the patient.
- If the patient does not have the ID card and does not know the manufacturer, you can call the patient registration line of the various pacemaker manufacturers. Using the patient's full name and social security number, you can find out if the patient has a Medtronic, St. Jude Medical, Boston Scientific, Biotronik, or Sorin device. It is required by law that pacemaker manufacturers keep records of patients who have their particular devices implanted. Pacemaker companies all maintain special call-in lines for this that are available around the clock.
- Another method is to perform a chest X-ray to see the implanted pacemaker. Devices have characteristic shapes so a pacing expert may be able to identify the manufacturer of a device just by its silhouette. An X-ray will also reveal a code or numbers that can help identify the device.

The IPG is usually implanted on the left side of the upper chest. Although the pacemaker leads go into the right side of the heart, venous access is usually easier and more direct from the left than the right side. A right-sided implant usually has to make a very sharp bend. While most pacemakers are implanted in the upper-left quadrant of the chest, there are exceptions to this, for instance, if the veins on the left side are damaged or occluded or there are scars or other conditions that would make a left-sided implantation disadvantageous.

Up until about 20 years ago, there were actually right-sided and left-sided pacemakers and the physician had to select the proper device for the implant location. Back then, pacemakers had a coating over the titanium case with a small area in the middle exposed and electrically active. This little exposed window on the front side of the pacemaker (and not the back side) was used for unipolar pacing. The pacemaker had to be implanted with that little electrically active window facing up. Thus, manufacturers created right and left pacemakers. Today, those systems no longer exist. Pacemakers are completely coated and yet can allow for unipolar pacing. Clinicians today may still hear about the old-fashioned *right-sided* and *left-sided* pacemakers, but they are no longer sold. Modern pacemakers from all manufacturers can be implanted in either side, that is, they work just as well right side up and upside down.

The pacemaker casing is titanium (all manufacturers), which is known to be biocompatible and rarely provokes patient allergy. The header or top portion of the pacemaker is made of clear epoxy and has one or more ports where leads plug in. The telemetry coil allows the pacemaker and the programmer to communicate using bidirectional telemetry (communication from and to the pacemaker) (see **Figure 9.4**). The amount of information processed and handled by the pacemaker is phenomenal. In a dual-chamber pacemaker, there are about 20 main parameters but each offers a wide range of settings such that the typical dual-chamber pacemaker offers clinicians about a million parameter combinations.

The *hybrid* is a slang term for a special type of circuit board within the pacemaker. The hybrid contains an integrated circuit, communicating telemetry coil, the reed switch, capacitor(s), resistors, and a sensor, all of which are wire bonded to the hybrid board. Pacemaker manufacturing is not totally automated; a great deal of the work in building the hybrid is done by hand by expert technicians. Even using experienced and highly trained technicians, it takes several days and many people to build one pacemaker. Once the pacemaker is assembled, it takes about 26 more days to run through all of the many quality assurance checks

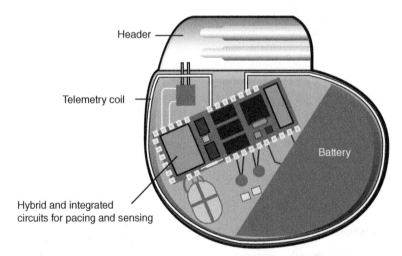

Figure 9.4 About half of the space within the pulse generator is taken up by the battery. The other half is used for the hybrid and integrated circuits necessary for pacing and sensing. Running around the outside circumference of the pulse generator is the telemetry coil that is used by the programmer to communicate with the implanted device. The header typically has one, two, or three ports to accommodate the leads.

necessary to verify that the device works properly. Manufacturers will estimate that it takes roughly 30 days from the start of building a pacemaker until the device is ready to ship out the door.

Pacemakers are composed of numerous components, some of which are very advanced technological parts. Manufacturers do not build all of their own components; manufacturers often rely on vendors to provide specific components for their pacemakers. This allows the manufacturers to be more efficient, but it imposes on them the added burden of checking quality of all incoming parts. Thus, the manufacture of a pacemaker is a labor-intensive and time-consuming process that requires a high degree of skill.

For many years, pacemakers contained a special component called a reed switch, composed of two metal leaflets encased in a tiny glass tube. The reed switch is normally open, that is, the two metal leaflets do not touch each other and form no circuit. Several manufacturers have recently eliminated the reed switch and replaced it with giant magnetoresistors (GMRs), which allow for magnet responses and communication with the implanted device. When a magnet is applied over the implanted pacemaker, it either closes the two metal leaflets on the reed switch or initiates magnet mode via the GMR (see **Figure 9.5**).

Another key component of the pacemaker is the crystal oscillator, which acts as the clock or timing circuit of the device. Since pacemakers constantly measure time in fractions of a second, the crystal oscillator is highly precise. The crystal oscillator is tiny (it would fit entirely on your fingertip) and looks like a miniature metal box.

Probably the most remarkable development in pacemaker technology in the last decades has been battery technology. The early pacemakers from the 1970s and 1980s were literally the size of a hockey puck and often contained several mercury–zinc batteries. The mercury–zinc batteries were heavy, had a large footprint, and lasted just a few months. While these early pacemakers were very large, they offered patients only very limited device longevity. In the 1970s, nuclear technology was considered for pacemakers and, believe it or not, thousands of nuclear-powered pacemakers were implanted. As you can imagine, a nuclear pacemaker created a lot of problems, but it solved one problem—device longevity. A nuclear pacemaker had a longevity of 20 or 25 years! In fact, there may still be a few nuclear pacemakers in patients even today. This approach was soon abandoned for several reasons. First, it is unclear if there was radiation discharge from the devices. Second, patients had to report to federal agencies if they wanted to cross state lines or leave the country because they were traveling with a nuclear device! So the nuclear pacemaker was quickly abandoned.

In the 1980s, a company called Pacesetter developed a rechargeable pacemaker. The idea was that the patient could periodically recharge the

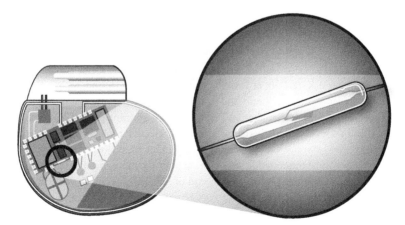

Figure 9.5 In devices with a reed switch, the reed switch closes when a magnet is applied, forcing the device to stop sensing and pace asynchronously. In other devices, magnet mode is achieved through a component known as giant magnetoresistors (GMRs).

pacemaker by sitting with a heating-pad-like device over the implanted device every evening. These devices used a nickel–cadmium battery, and although they could be effectively recharged, many patients did not like having to recharge their devices. Patient compliance became an issue. In addition, even rechargeable batteries eventually wear out. Thousands of rechargeable pacemakers have been implanted, but that idea was also abandoned.

Modern pacemakers rely on a lithium-iodide battery, a very long-lived battery with a reliable discharge curve, that is, they behave in very predictable ways. Most (but not all) pacemaker batteries all use the same battery, a lithium-iodide battery from Wilson Greatbatch. These are small, lightweight batteries that can last a decade or more. Note that one pacemaker manufacturer (Biotronik) manufactures its own batteries. They are the only ones that do not use the Wilson Greatbatch battery. Recently, several manufacturers have changed battery technology in order to accommodate the higher energy drain necessary to provide wireless telemetry. For example, St. Jude Medical has moved to using a Quasar battery from Wilson Greatbatch. More advances in battery technology can be expected in the future.

Batteries are so ubiquitous today that most people have a good understanding of what can impact battery service life. Batteries contain a finite amount of energy, and the rate at which they wear down depends in part on how much they are used (for instance, a dual-chamber pacemaker will consume more battery energy, all things being equal, than a single-chamber pacemaker), the output settings (a pacemaker pacing at 7 V will burn up more energy than a pacemaker set to 1 V), and even resistance within the battery (also called cell impedance). Pacemaker batteries start out at 2.8 V. Over time, the cell impedance increases and the voltage decreases, accordingly; the pacemaker will then decline to 2.4 V and then 2.0 V, usually over a period of 5–10 years.

Patients and clinicians are most interested in specifically how long the pacemaker battery will last because when the battery wears out, the patient needs a new pulse generator. Battery capacity is typically measured in amp-hours. Pacemaker batteries have capacities in the range of 0.4–1.5 amp-hours. As an example, let's take a battery with 1.0 amp-hour

capacity. If the circuit drained 0.5 amps every hour, then the battery would last 2 h ($0.5 \times 2 = 1.0$). If the circuit drained 1.0 amp every hour, then the battery would last 1 h ($1.0 \times 1 = 1.0$). In reality, pacemakers drain much energy than that! Pacemaker battery current drain is measured in microamps, so a 1.0 amp-hour capacity battery actually has 1 000 000 microamps available. If you know how many microamps the pacemaker uses, you could actually calculate how long the battery would last based on the available microamps. The good news is that you don't have to do any math, because the programmer will calculate it for you—and likely more accurately and certainly faster than you can do it.

Still, you might be interested in how battery longevity is calculated. Let's take as an example a fairly typical pacemaker battery of 1.2 amp-hours. We also know that there are 8760 h in a year (365×24). Let's say in this example we knew that this device had a current drain of 20 microamps. The equation would be

$$\text{Longevity in hours} = \frac{\text{battery capacity in hours}}{\text{current drain}}$$

Or in our example,

$$\text{Longevity in hours} = \frac{1\,200\,000 \text{ microamps (h)}}{20 \text{ microamps}}$$

That results in 60 000 h, which is 6.85 years. In clinical practice, nobody calculates battery longevity like this, but it is important to understand how and why programmers arrive at their longevity calculations. Battery longevity may be stated less precisely than that, using a gauge system or perhaps a short description such as *battery life good*. There are three important landmarks in battery life known as beginning of life (BOL) when the battery is fresh, elective replacement indicator or elective replacement time (ERI or ERT) when the battery has about six more months of service life left, and end of life (EOL) when the battery is depleted. No pacemaker should ever hit EOL because at the point, it stops working. When a clinician sees that the pacemaker has reached ERT, replacement surgery should be discussed with the patient and scheduled.

In reality, many pacemakers do reach EOL because some patients are *lost to follow-up*, meaning that for whatever reasons they are no longer being followed by the clinic. There are many reasons for this, including noncompliance, patients' moving, or sometimes patients just feeling so much better with a pacemaker that they stop going to the doctor.

Ideally, when the battery is nearing but has not yet reached EOL, the old pacemaker is explanted and a new one is implanted. The leads are often left in place and just unplugged from the old device and plugged into the new device. This surgery is sometimes called replacement surgery or revision; avoid using the slang term *battery replacement* because it suggests that the battery can be removed and replaced. It cannot. When the battery in a pulse generator wears out, the whole pulse generator is replaced. Patients are often confused about this, so it is better to call it pulse generator or pacemaker replacement.

The decision as to when to replace a pulse generator is made by the physician together with the patient. Once the device hits ERT or ERI, Medicare reimbursement allows for the device to be replaced. Prior to that, the replacement would not be reimbursed. Once the device reaches ERT or ERI, the physician will likely base the decision on when to replace the pulse generator on the patient's degree of dependency on the pacemaker (the more dependent, the sooner the replacement), the patient's condition (a patient who has just undergone surgery may want to postpone generator replacement for a month or two), and the patient's and physician's scheduling preferences.

One might wonder if a pacemaker might reach ERT and the physician decide not to replace it. For example, sometimes a patient gets a pacemaker that ends up never having to pace. After many years of not pacing, the device hits ERT and the physician needs to decide whether or not to replace it. While there are no regulations that would prevent a physician from not replacing the pacemaker, it is rarely handled this way. Most pacemakers are replaced for the simple reason that a physician who opts not to replace a pacemaker puts himself or herself in a position to be legally liable (malpractice) if this turns out to be the wrong decision. The patient got the pacemaker for a reason; if it is removed and the patient turns out to need it, the patient is put at risk and the physician could be held responsible. Most physicians make patient safety paramount and choose conservative options, particularly when they are covered by Medicare or insurance. As a result, in real-world clinical practice, almost all patients who are followed by pacemaker clinics will be offered a device replacement at the proper time. Sometimes, a patient may refuse to have a replacement. In such cases, clinicians have the obligation to make sure the patient is making a fully informed choice, that is, the clinician must explain to the patient clearly why the pacemaker is needed. Some patients may still refuse them, and that is their right.

The pulse generator is hermetically sealed to prevent bodily fluids from entering the device. This creates a problem, because if the pulse generator is hermetically sealed, how does electricity get in and out? Pacemakers rely on tiny wires called feedthroughs, which allow electrical current to flow between the lead(s) and the circuitry encased in the pulse generator.

The header is the clear epoxy connector on top of the pulse generator with one or more ports for leads. The lead must be the proper size to fit into the port of the header. In the early days of pacing, lead connection was a headache because every manufacturer built its own unique header, which only accommodated its own unique leads. The leads from one company did not fit into the pulse generators of another company. What's more, sometimes, a single manufacturer made several different types of headers and leads so they were not even compatible with themselves! In those early days of pacing, many sales representatives carried a wide range of *adapters* aimed at helping make leads fit into incompatible pacemakers. It was very complicated and doctors hated it.

As pacemakers became more prevalent, a standardized system was introduced for pulse generator headers and leads. The idea was that all manufacturers would build pulse generator headers and leads that would work together, even if a doctor crossed manufacturing lines and, for example, tried to use a Medtronic lead in a Boston Scientific pulse generator. The standardization began as Voluntary Standard 1 (VS-1), an industry-led approach to standardizing leads and headers.

VS-1 evolved into International Standard 1 (IS-1). Today, an IS-1 lead from Medtronic will fit perfectly in an IS-1 connector in a Boston Scientific pulse generator.

However, it is not quite as easy as it sounds. The headers of pulse generators actually come in two distinct types. One is IS-1 and the other is called IS-1 Compatible. The difference is the use of sealing rings. When a lead plugs into a pulse generator header port, it relies on something called sealing rings, which help keep fluids from getting into the header. Sealing rings are usually made of silicone. The sealing rings have to be located either on the lead connector pin (the part of the lead that plugs into the header) or the sealing rings have to be located in the connector port. Both methods are effective, but they are incompatible with each other. That is, if you have sealing rings on the lead, that lead will not work well in a port with sealing rings. Also, as the lead is plugged into the connector port, setscrews are tightened to hold the lead in place. When the lead is fully inserted into the port, the implanting physician uses a special torque tool and turns the setscrews until three audible clicks are heard, confirming that the setscrews are tight and, thus, the lead is secured in the port. When inserting a lead in the pulse generator, the implanting physician should look to be sure the lead is fully inserted all the way back into the port (the connector block is clear so this is plainly visible); then the physician tightens the lead by using the torque tool in the setscrews taking care not to overtighten; and finally, the physician should gently tug on the lead after the setscrews are tightened to be sure it is secure.

Leads

Leads carry electrical signals from the heart to the pulse generator and from the pulse generator to the heart. They are one of the most crucial components of any pacing system. All pacing leads have five main components:
- The lead body (i.e., the length of the wire)
- The insulation (the material that protects the wire)
- A fixation mechanism at the tip to secure the lead in place within the heart
- One or more electrodes at the distal end
- A connector at the proximal end (**Figure 9.6**)

There are many different types of leads. Not only can they vary with respect to the above components (for instance, having different kinds of insulation or different fixation mechanisms), they can also vary in polarity (which is a function of the electrodes), whether or not they have steroid medication on the tip (steroid elution), how the conductor coil or wire is designed, and what type of connector pin is in use. In selecting a lead, the implanting physician will consider numerous factors including what is most suitable for the patient, his or her own preferences (some doctors prefer a specific insulation material, for example), and other factors such as the reliability of a given lead type. Leads are the most vulnerable part of the pacing system, and some leads have proven to be more reliable over the long term than others.

Polarity

Pacing systems are either unipolar or bipolar. This term is actually a bit misleading, since all electrical circuits have two poles (positive and negative or anode and cathode). In pacing, polarity refers to how many of those poles are on the distal end of the lead, that is, whether the lead has one electrode (unipolar) or two electrodes (bipolar) at the tip. If the electrode has (or is only using) one electrode at the tip, the pacing system forms its electrical circuit using the generator as the other pole; in other words, the tip electrode on the lead is the cathode and the pulse generator can is the anode. If the lead has (and is using) two electrodes at the tip, the circuit is formed within the heart using the tip

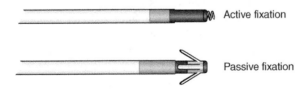

Active fixation

Passive fixation

Figure 9.6 Active and passive-fixation lead mechanisms.

electrode as the cathode and the ring electrode (a little more proximal than the tip electrode) as the anode. Some leads are unipolar right out of the box—they only have one electrode at the tip. Some leads are bipolar out of the box (with both a tip and ring electrode) but can be programmed to function as a bipolar or unipolar lead. Just because a lead has two electrodes does not mean it is functioning as a bipolar lead—although most of the time, that will be the case.

Many physicians today prefer bipolar leads, particularly since modern technology has substantially reduced their size. Many years ago, physicians often hesitated to use bipolar leads because they were very large-diameter leads that did not *fit* well in some patients' veins. That is not the case today. Physicians may select unipolar leads because they are small, handle well, are easier to implant generally, and should be more reliable because there is only one conductor coil (fewer parts). Bipolar leads are more sensitive to intracardiac signals and thus offer better sensing. Bipolar leads eliminate the potential for pocket stimulation, a condition that can occur when a unipolar system transmits signals through the patient's chest that can be perceived. (Pocket stimulation is rare, even in unipolar systems, but it is nonexistent in bipolar systems.) Probably the main advantage of the bipolar lead is that with two leads, it can be

reprogrammed to unipolar if there ever is a problem with one of the electrodes. This happens rarely, but the flexibility may be an important consideration for some implanting physicians. On the other hand, bipolar leads produce smaller pacing spikes on the paced ECG, which can make it harder to read paced tracings. Bipolar leads are usually less flexible than unipolar leads, which can make them more challenging to implant in narrow vessels or in a patient with tortuous veins.

One last consideration in selecting a unipolar versus a bipolar lead is myopotential inhibition. Myopotentials refer to electrical signals generated from the muscles of the body (myo = muscles). *Muscle noise*, a type of extracardiac signal, occurs in everybody, particularly in active people. A unipolar pacemaker—with its wide antenna going from tip electrode to can—is far more sensitive to myopotentials than a bipolar pacemaker. A unipolar pacemaker may sense a myopotential and misinterpret it as a cardiac signal. The pacemaker senses cardiac activity as electrical signals, so it really has no way of knowing whether that electrical signal came from the heart or the pectoral muscle. If the pacemaker senses a myopotential and perceives it as a cardiac signal, it will inappropriately inhibit the pacing output pulse. *Myopotential inhibition* only occurs in unipolar systems (see **Table 9.1**).

Table 9.1 A short overview of unipolar versus bipolar characteristics

	Unipolar	Bipolar
Pacing spike	Large	Small, may even be hard to find
Flexibility of the wire for implant	Very flexible	Not so flexible
Lead diameter	Smaller	Slightly larger
Conductor coils	One	Two
Electrodes	One	Two
Redundant system (can be reprogrammed to the other polarity)	No	Yes
Pocket stimulation	Rare but possible	No
Myopotential inhibition	Rare but possible	No
Sensing	Worse	Better
Reliability	More	Less

Note that leads today are very reliable, but historically, unipolar leads are more reliable than bipolar leads because unipolar leads have only a single conductor coil and a single electrode (fewer parts). The table states that bipolar leads are *less reliable*, which does not mean they are unreliable—they have just historically been more associated with lead problems than unipolar leads. Likewise, sensing characteristics of both types of leads are excellent, but bipolar leads may be considered to offer better sensing than unipolar leads.

In real-world clinical practice, the general preference for most implanting physicians is to use bipolar leads.

Fixation mechanism

The two main types of fixation mechanisms are active and passive. Passive-fixation mechanisms are protrusions at the lead tip, usually tines or fins, which embed themselves into the trabeculae within the heart. The fixation is passive, that is, nothing is attached; the lead is just *snagged* into the dense fiber-like structures inside the heart. Over time, the lead will fibrose itself into place by building up scar tissue around the interface where the lead meets the myocardium. For that reason, passive-fixation leads are usually more difficult to extract, if they ever need to be removed.

An active-fixation lead has a helix or corkscrew at the tip, which is actively twisted into place to affix the lead to the myocardium. When implanting an active-fixation lead, the implanting physician will have to position the lead and, then with some sort of tool or mechanism screw, the lead into the myocardial tissue. (The helix or screw is usually retracted inside the lead as it is maneuvered into place and is then actively fastened to the inside of the heart once it reaches its destination. This kind of lead has an *extendable–retractable helix*.) Active-fixation leads are generally thought to be easier to remove because there is less fibrosis around the lead–tissue interface, and by unscrewing the fixation mechanism, the lead detaches more readily.

Historically, physicians generally used passive-fixation leads in the ventricle and active-fixation leads in the atrium. This made sense in that the ventricles offered the trabeculae that made it easy to implant a passive-fixation lead, while the smooth walls of the atrium required an active-fixation lead. More and more today, the trend is toward using active-fixation leads in both atrium and ventricle. The reason for this migration away from passive-fixation leads is that active-fixation leads are easier to extract. Lead extraction is not common, but it can be necessary if a lead is defective and damaged or the pacing system is infected. In other words, lead extraction is not that common, but when it is necessary, it is usually an urgent matter.

While active-fixation leads offer real advantages, it must be remembered that they have the potential to perforate the heart if they go through the heart wall. In fact, any time an active-fixation lead is fixated in the heart, it injures the tissue. Extendable–retractable leads rely on a delicate mechanism in the lead to allow the helix to extend or withdraw back into the lead body. If the helix is overextended (by turning the lead too many times), it may not retract properly if that is required. Likewise, mechanical problems may occur that prevent the lead from extending the helix properly. While these are rare, they do occur and clinicians need to consider this when choosing a lead. Some implanting physicians will test an extendable–retractable lead before implant by screwing and unscrewing the helix just to confirm proper operation (see **Table 9.2**).

Table 9.2 Summary of active-fixation versus passive-fixation leads

	Active-fixation lead	Passive-fixation lead
Ease of fixation	Easier	Easy
Ease of implant	Easy	Easier
Ease of repositioning	Easier	Easy
Dislodgement	Less common	More common
Acute dislodgement	Less common	More common
Ease of extraction	Less difficult	Difficult
Simplicity of design	Less simple	Simpler
Trauma to patient	More	Less
Risk of cardiac perforation	Greater	Less
Thresholds	Not quite as low	Low
For heart failure patients	May not be the ideal choice	Better choice

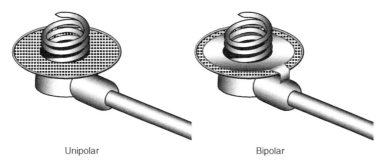

Unipolar   Bipolar

Figure 9.7 Myocardial or epicardial leads attach to the exterior of the heart and are available as unipolar or bipolar leads. The helix is one pole; a bipolar epicardial lead also has a second electrode surrounding the helix.

Myocardial/epicardial leads

Pacing clinicians will mainly deal with transvenous leads, that is, leads that are implanted through (trans) a vein and into the heart. However, there is another type of lead that may be encountered known as the myocardial or epicardial lead (they are the same thing). An epicardial lead is affixed to the exterior of the heart with a helix mechanism (see **Figure 9.7**). An epicardial lead can only be implanted if the heart is exposed, so they are sometimes used if the patient is having a pacemaker implanted along with another surgery, such as valve replacement. Pediatric patients up to about age 10 are paced with epicardial leads because their hearts are still growing and their veins may be too small to accommodate a transvenous lead.

Myocardial or epicardial leads are not frequently used because they require an open-chest surgery or thoracotomy. Another factor to consider is that the pacing thresholds in epicardial leads tend to increase over time.

Steroid-eluting leads

All leads implanted today elute steroids, that is, a small amount of steroid medication on the tip of the lead will dissolve or elute over a matter of a few weeks or months. Steroids decrease inflammation, and the point of adding steroid medication to a lead tip is to reduce inflammation at the point where the lead tip contacts the myocardium.

Before steroid-eluting leads, the lead–tissue interface would become inflamed during implantation, and this inflammation—which often worsened over the first few weeks postimplantation—interfered with the lead's ability to capture the heart. It was not unusual to see a patient's capture threshold at implant increase substantially over the first few weeks after surgery. Implanting physicians were urged to program the device to output settings much higher than the original capture thresholds to accommodate this sudden increase in threshold caused by inflammation. Over time, the inflammation subsided and the capture threshold came back down. At this point, the lead and tissue started to function as one without the inflammatory process; this area of lead electrode(s) and tissue is sometimes called the *virtual electrode*. Pacing experts who have been around for many years remember how pacing output parameters had to be adjusted to accommodate this short increase in capture threshold and then the decrease as the virtual electrode formed.

Steroids made this less of a problem, because the steroid delivered to the lead–tissue interface minimized inflammation. Capture thresholds still increase right after implantation but not as dramatically. Furthermore, steroid-eluting leads decrease capture thresholds overall, and that results in energy savings, which, in turn, increased device longevity. Thus, steroid-eluting leads help pacemakers last longer. This fact is so well accepted in pacing today that no manufacturer even makes a lead without steroid.

Insulation

Lead insulation surrounds and protects the conductor coil(s) of the lead. There are two main types of insulation: silicone rubber and polyurethane. Each of these insulation materials has its own unique attributes; there are pros and cons to using either material. In clinical practice, insulation choice is often a matter of physician preference.

Silicone rubber tends to be sticky, so it can be more challenging to pass a transvenous silicone lead through the vein. When two silicone leads are implanted for a dual-chamber pacemaker, the leads do not always glide over each other easily in the vein. Silicone insulation is biostable and has a track record of about 30 years of safe, reliable use in pacemaker leads.

Polyurethane leads can be maneuvered more easily in the veins, but polyurethane leads have a history of breaking down over time. Polyurethane leads have a slick (rather than sticky) feel to them, but there have been reliability issues over the long term. Most of those issues come from the use of a specific type of polyurethane known as 80A. The industry has moved away from 80A polyurethane to polyurethane 90A and 55D, with the latter being the strongest and toughest version of polyurethane. All polyurethane leads sold today use 55D polyurethane. However, 55D polyurethane is somewhat stiff and rigid and is not as flexible as other types of polyurethane.

Polyurethane insulation offers some important advantages: it does not cut, nick, or tear as easily as silicone. It is a rugged material and resists abrasion. Because it is a smooth material, there is less friction in the bloodstream. If compression strength is applied to the lead in the body, for instance, if it is compressed behind the collarbone, polyurethane holds up to that better than silicone. Polyurethane leads are also thought to be less thrombogenic than silicone leads, that is, there is less risk of a thrombus forming (see **Table 9.3**).

Some bipolar leads may actually use both polyurethane and silicone by using silicone insulation on the inner conductor coil and polyurethane on the outside. Such a lead would handle like a polyurethane lead (slick rather than sticky, stiffer rather than flexible).

While there are two main types of insulation, one company has introduced a new copolymer material that is a combination of silicone and polyurethane (Optim®, St. Jude Medical). The goal of this new material was to combine the advantages of silicone and polyurethane and minimize their respective disadvantages. This material is very new so it does not offer the benefit of long-term reliability data.

Conductor coil

The wire part of the pacing lead is the conductor, sometimes called the conductor coil or just coil. Coils are typically made of a nickel alloy known as MP35N. Sometimes, a nickel alloy wire with a silver core is used, called a Drawn Brazed Strand (DBS). Coils made be unifilar (one wire is coiled) or multifilar (multiple wires form the coil) (see **Figure 9.8**).

Table 9.3 Lead insulation summary. Both silicone and polyurethane 55D are excellent lead insulation materials, but each offers its own unique advantages

	Silicone	Polyurethane
History of good performance	>30 years	Historical reliability issues with 80A
Biostability	Excellent	Good
Flexibility	Very	Not as much
Tear strength	Tears more easily	Resists tears
Cut resistance	Cuts more easily	Resists cuts
Abrasion resistance	Abrades more easily	Resists abrasion
Friction in the bloodstream	More	Less
Easy to pass two leads together in one vein	Less so	More so
Feel	Sticky	Smooth
Thrombogenic	More	Less
Compressive properties	Good	Excellent
Stiffness	Less	More
Environmental stress cracking (ESC)	No	Yes with 80A
Metal ion oxidation	No	Yes
Cautery damage	Less susceptible	More susceptible

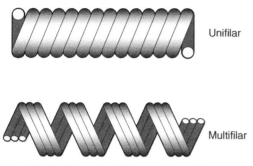

Figure 9.8 Unifilar and multifilar conductor coils.

A unipolar lead has one conductor coil (one wire to one electrode), while a bipolar lead has two conductor coils (one wire to each of two electrodes). Placing two coils into a lead can take up a lot of space, which is why historically bipolar leads had much larger diameters than unipolar leads. New technology now allows for one coil to be placed inside the other to create so-called coaxial leads (leads that share a single axis). This requires insulation on each coil, but it still reduces the overall diameter from the old-fashioned bipolar lead. A bipolar lead may also use coradial technology where the two conductor coils are individually insulated and then wrapped together around the same axis. Coradial bipolar leads are the thinnest bipolar leads, so this design is becoming increasingly common.

Electrodes

A pacing lead has at least one electrode, which is located at the extreme distal tip of the lead. If the lead also has a slightly distal ring electrode, it is bipolar; otherwise, a single-electrode lead is unipolar.

When designing an electrode, the engineer is faced with a contradiction. The ideal electrode has to be small to pace efficiently, but it should be large to sense well. Porous electrodes solve that problem because they can be small (ideal for pacing), but their porosity gives them a relatively large surface area, allowing for good sensing. Porous electrodes also allow for tissue ingrowth, to help hold the lead in place. The porosity of the electrode can only be seen under a microscope. Electrodes are made from many different types of materials such as platinum, platinum alloys (such as titanium-coated platinum–iridium), vitreous carbon, and stainless steel alloys (such as Elgiloy).

When electrical energy is sent from the pacemaker down the conductor coil and through the electrode to the heart muscle, polarization occurs. Polarization occurs because positively charged ions will start to cluster around the electrode as a result of the electrical pulse flowing through it. Polarization is directly proportional to the pulse width (how long the impulse lasts) and inversely proportional to the size of the electrode (i.e., smaller electrodes have higher degrees of polarization). Polarization is inevitable during pacing.

Impedance

Lead impedance is a very important topic that is not always well understood by clinicians. Impedance is the sum of all forces that oppose the flow of current through a circuit, in this case, all of the forces that resist the flow of electricity through the lead. Impedance is measured in ohms (Ω). Every lead, as manufactured, has a specific impedance coming out of the box. The nominal (out-of-the-box) impedance value usually falls between 300 and 1500 Ω.

Impedance values can provide insight into potential lead problems. Some degree of fluctuation in impedance is normal and expected. But when lead impedance values change by more than 20% (either higher or lower), it suggests that there might be a problem with the lead. Thus, when evaluating lead impedance, it is important to consider the trend rather than a specific lead impedance value at one point in time. For instance, knowing lead impedance is 1000 Ω right now does not reveal much about the lead. But knowing that six months ago lead impedance was 600 Ω, that sharp upward trend suggests the possibility that lead integrity is compromised. Likewise, if lead impedance six months ago was 988 Ω and today it is 1000 Ω, this new value suggests the lead is working fine. Pacemakers today automatically measure lead impedance at regular intervals, and programmers present lead impedance trends graphed over time.

When impedance values are very high or are trending sharply upward, this suggests a problem with the conductor coil, such as conductor fracture (broken wire). On the other hand, when impedance values are very low or trend sharply lower, this suggests the problem is with the insulation, such as an insulation breach (broken or torn insulation).

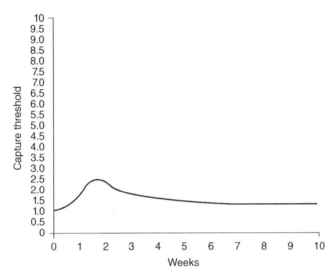

Figure 9.9 Acute-to-chronic threshold increase in a steroid-eluting pacing lead. The intraoperative capture threshold is the lowest value that will ever be achieved in a given patient. A nonsteroid-eluting lead has an even more pronounced acute-to-chronic threshold increase, since the threshold for such a lead can increase as much as fivefold.

Lead problems also show up as capture and sensing problems. For example, when troubleshooting a pacemaker with capture problems and changes in lead impedance, this is good evidence that the lead is the source of the problem.

Leads and thresholds

Earlier, capture thresholds were discussed in terms of what they were and how they worked. The capture threshold for an individual patient is determined by the interaction of that patient's myocardium and the pacing lead. The lowest possible pacing threshold is desired for pacing because it uses up the least battery energy—but the pacing threshold has to be high enough to be consistently able to capture the heart.

When a lead is first implanted, the capture threshold is measured. This intraoperative threshold is the lowest value that will ever be observed for that patient. After implantation, clinicians should expect to see the acute-to-chronic threshold change, which is a marked increase in threshold values attributable to inflammatory processes associated with the new lead. During this acute-to-chronic change, the pacing threshold in a nonsteroid-eluting lead may increase as much as fivefold. Steroid elution has helped to make that acute-to-chronic threshold change less severe, but

it is still a marked increase. As the lead matures over a period of weeks or months, the threshold will decrease and stabilize, but it will never return to the intraoperative level (see **Figure 9.9**). Thus, as long as the acute capture threshold measured intraoperatively is acceptable, the output pulse in a newly implanted device is commonly set at 2.5 V or higher or five times the intraoperative threshold, whichever is greater. However, after 6–8 weeks, thresholds should be reassessed and the chronic pacing output programmed. This will typically be much lower.

Putting it all together

There are four parts to the pacing system: the pulse generator, the lead(s), the programmer, and the patient. Pacemakers can only sense and pace, and these two activities are linked together—the pacemaker will pace based on what it senses or fails to sense. Clinicians concern themselves mostly with patient care and setting the right parameter settings for the pacing system, but understanding these components and how they work together can help. For example, good pacing and sensing depends on good lead integrity, a sound electrode, and appropriate function of the pulse generator.

The nuts and bolts of pacing 101

- The capture or pacing threshold is the minimum amount of energy to consistently depolarize the heart. The capture threshold is used to set the pacemaker's output pulse, which is defined by two settings: pulse amplitude (measured in volts) and pulse width (measured in milliseconds).
- Pacemakers can only do two things: they sense and they pace. Sensing and pacing work together. The pacemaker senses an intrinsic signal or not and *decides* how to respond based on what is sensed. If an intrinsic signal is sensed, most pacemakers will inhibit the output pulse. (No pacemaker can inhibit the patient's intrinsic activity.) If no intrinsic signal is sensed, the pacemaker will pace.
- The strength–duration curve describes the capture threshold and all combinations of pulse amplitude and pulse width that capture the heart. The *knee* of the strength–duration curve is the actual capture threshold. Rheobase is a value on that curve that shows the lowest voltage that will capture the heart at the longest pulse width. Chronaxie is double rheobase.
- Doubling the pulse amplitude quadruples the amount of energy in the output pulse, while doubling the pulse width doubles the amount of energy in the output pulse.
- The typical capture safety margin is 2:1 or 3:1. The typical sensitivity safety margin is at least 2:1.
- Increasing the mV setting of sensitivity lowers the sensitivity (makes the device less sensitive), while decreasing the mV setting increases the sensitivity.
- Oversensing leads to underpacing, while undersensing leads to overpacing.
- Devices are interrogated and followed using programmers, which are unique to each manufacturer. If you must interrogate a pacemaker and do not know the manufacturer, ask the patient to see his ID card, call the pacemaker companies and talk to patient registration to confirm the patient, or take a chest X-ray.
- Pacemakers consist of numerous components, the largest of which is a lithium-iodide battery. Other components include a telemetry coil (to communicate back and forth with the programmer), circuitry, and reed switch. The reed switch can be closed by magnet application and reverts the pacemaker into magnet mode.
- Pacemakers use very precise timing measured in fractions of a second. These timing cycles are controlled by a very tiny part in the pacemaker called the crystal oscillator.
- When a pacemaker battery starts to wear out, it will signal the programmer that it has reached the elective replacement time (ERT, sometimes called the elective replacement indicator or ERI). At that point, the battery will last about six more months.
- The lead is composed of the lead body, insulation, fixation mechanism, electrode(s), and connector. The connector plugs into the header of the pulse generator. Connections today have been standardized and are now IS-1 or IS-1 Compatible. This means that leads from one company will fit and work with any pulse generator, even those from different manufacturers.
- Most physicians today prefer bipolar leads, but unipolar leads are available, too. Bipolar leads have a larger diameter but offer better sensing. Unipolar leads show up on an ECG with a very prominent pacing spike and are thinner, but do not sense as well.
- The clinical trend today is toward more and more active-fixation leads (helix or corkscrew tips), which are often done in an extendable–retractable design. Passive-fixation leads with tines or fins work well in the ventricles but can be more difficult to extract, if removal is ever required.
- Myocardial or epicardial leads (the same thing) are leads that are attached to the outside of the heart rather than fixated inside the heart. They are used in pediatric patients (usually under age 10) and may be implanted when the patient receives a pacemaker during another type of open-chest procedure.
- All leads today are steroid-eluting leads, which decreases the acute-to-chronic threshold rise seen in nonsteroid leads due to the

Continued

Continued

inflammatory process. Nonsteroid-eluting leads could have capture threshold increases up to fivefold in the first few weeks postimplant. Steroid-eluting leads show much less pronounced acute-to-chronic threshold increases.

• Leads today use silicone insulation, polyurethane insulation, or a proprietary material known as Optim, which is a copolymer (St. Jude Medical). Each material offers unique pros and cons. Very often, the choice of lead insulation is based on physician preference in that implanting physicians tend to get used to a particular type of insulation.

• Pacing electrodes tend to have porous surfaces to allow for good sensing characteristics and tissue ingrowth.

• Lead impedance values can provide insight into lead integrity, but it is the trend of impedance values over time that is important. Leads that increase in impedance >20% indicate conductor coil fracture, while leads that decrease >20% suggest an insulation breach.

Test your knowledge

1 What two parameters define the pacemaker's output pulse?
   A Atrial and ventricular channels
   B Pulse amplitude and pulse width
   C Sensitivity and pulse width
   D Impedance and pulse amplitude

2 A clinician follows a pacemaker patient whose ventricular sensitivity is set to 5 mV. The clinician determines that the pacemaker must be made more sensitive because it is missing some cardiac signals (undersensing). How does this clinician program sensitivity to make the device more sensitive?
   A Increase the mV setting (6 mV or more).
   B Decrease the mV setting (4 mV or less).
   C Increase both the mV setting and the pulse amplitude (for larger signals).
   D None of the above.

3 In an emergency situation with a pacemaker patient, why is it crucial to know the manufacturer of the pacemaker?
   A Programmers are manufacturer specific.
   B The pacemaker manufacturer must be notified of all emergencies.
   C To report the problem to the FDA.
   D For potential future litigation.

4 The pacemaker housing or case is usually made of what biocompatible material?
   A Tungsten
   B Stainless steel alloys, such as Elgiloy

   C MP35N
   D Titanium

5 When a magnet is placed over a pacemaker, what action happens that launches magnet mode behavior?
   A It opens the hybrid.
   B It opens the feedthroughs.
   C It closes the reed switch.
   D It activates a small electrically activated window on the front of the pacemaker.

6 Identify the only item below that has *not* been used as a pacemaker battery:
   A Mercury–zinc
   B Nuclear energy
   C Zinc–carbon battery
   D Rechargeable batteries

7 When a pulse generator reaches elective replacement time (ERT), about how much battery life is left?
   A About 6 days.
   B About 6 weeks.
   C About 6 months.
   D None; the battery is depleted.

8 If a lead has two electrodes (one tip and one ring) and two conductor coils, what type of lead is it?
   A Steroid-eluting
   B Bipolar
   C Biphasic
   D Multifilar

9 What are potential advantages of silicone insulation in a lead?

  A History of good reliability

  B Flexibility

  C Biostability

  D All of the above

10 There is a trend in clinical practice toward the increasing use of active-fixation leads. What is causing this shift?

A Active-fixation leads are cheaper.

B Active-fixation leads are easier to remove.

C Active-fixation leads are easier and quicker to implant.

D Active-fixation leads are less likely to have conductor fracture.

CHAPTER 10

Indications for pacing

Learning objectives

- State the primary indications for pacemaker therapy in the setting of sinus node dysfunction.
- State the primary indications for pacemaker therapy in the setting of advanced AV block.
- Briefly explain the differences between class I, class IIa and IIb, and class III indications.
- Explain why and in what situations symptomatic bradycardia as a result of drug therapy might be a pacing indication.
- Define neurocardiogenic syncope and why it occurs.
- Explain what a pacemaker would do that might—as a last resort—help a person with neurocardiogenic syncope.

Introduction

In real-world clinical practice, indications are not always the clear-cut perfectly defined conditions that they can seem to be on paper. Clinicians treat patients and patients are people. Every patient brings with him a unique medical history, personal preferences, possibly a current drug regimen, and risk factors for specific conditions. All of these things factor in to prescribing decisions. Thus, clinicians make prescribing decisions not using a cookie cutter but rather by weighing evidence and exercising judgment. For this reason, clinicians will see that having a certain condition may not necessarily mean getting a pacemaker, or it might mean that patient A gets a pacemaker but patient B does not and patient C is getting a second opinion.

The goal in understanding pacing indications is knowing how to evaluate evidence in reaching a sound but individual patient-centric decision.

Classes and levels of evidence

All of these indications come from the guidelines prepared by the American College of Cardiology (ACC), the American Heart Association (AHA), and the Heart Rhythm Society (HRS) and published in 2008 [1]. This is the definitive guidance for clinicians for pacemaker therapy.

When it comes to indications or in other guidance documents, medical experts weigh evidence based on a class system that attempts to differentiate very solid evidence from more tenuous evidence. This results in categorizing the overall body of evidence into one of five classes (see **Table 10.1**). Class I should be considered as an indication but class III is a contraindication. The evidence that is used to reach these decisions is also weighted using a letter code (see **Table 10.2**). Using these codes, the indications can be better described and appreciated by clinical decision-makers.

When discussing pacing indications, clinicians use terms such as *bradycardia* and *pauses*. For the purposes of the indications, bradycardia should be defined by the cutoff rate of 40 bpm and pauses by 3 s or longer.

The main indications for pacing today can be roughly thought of as sinus node dysfunction, AV block, and *everything else*. Note that the lists made up here are not exhaustive but can be used as good ways to think about pacing indications by grouping certain types of indications together.

The Nuts and Bolts of Implantable Device Therapy Pacemakers, First Edition. Tom Kenny.
© 2015 John Wiley & Sons, Ltd. Published 2015 by John Wiley & Sons, Ltd.

Table 10.1 Classes of evidence describe the body of literature relating to a specific product, device, or therapy

Class	Definition	In other words, implanting a device
Class I	Evidence for and/or general agreement that the procedure is useful/efficacious	Is recommended
Class II	Conflicting evidence and/or a diverge of opinion about the usefulness/efficacy of procedures	
Class IIa	Evidence/opinion is in favor of usefulness/efficacy	Is reasonable
Class IIb	Evidence is less well established	May be considered
Class III	Evidence for and/or general agreement that the procedure is not effective or may be harmful	Is contraindicated

Table 10.2 Levels of evidence describe the relative quality of the individual articles in the literature about a product, device, or therapy

Level of evidence	
A	The strongest evidence, multiple large randomized clinical trials
B	Limited number of trials involving comparatively small numbers of patients and/or well-designed data analysis of nonrandomized studies of observational data registries
C	The weakest evidence, consensus of expert opinion

In evidence-based medicine, the strongest evidence comes from large randomized clinical studies.

Sinus node dysfunction

Today, more than half of pacemaker patients are indicated for pacing because of sinus node dysfunction. This was not the case in the early days of pacing, when AV block was the main pacing indication. The migration toward more pacemakers for sinus node dysfunction occurred not because patients or their conditions changed; it occurred because of our growing understanding of sick sinus syndrome.

Sinus node dysfunction pacing indications: class I

Sinus node dysfunction with documented symptomatic bradycardia, including frequent sinus pauses that produce symptoms, is a class I indication for pacing.

Note that the emphasis is on documented episodes of bradycardia and that these episodes of bradycardia must be associated with symptoms. A form of sinus node dysfunction called chronotropic incompetence is also a pacing indication, providing chronotropic incompetence is associated symptoms; chronotropic incompetence will be discussed in greater detail in the chapter on rate response. For now, a good working definition of chronotropic incompetence is any or all of the following: the inability of the heart to accelerate in response to activity, the inability to maintain a higher rate during activity, and the inability of the heart to decelerate at the conclusion of activity. A healthy heart can ramp up during exercise, maintain an exercise rate during exertion, and then slow down during cool down as the exercise stops. A chronotropically incompetent heart cannot do one or more of those things; when chronotropic incompetence results in symptoms, it is a class I pacing indication.

Another class I pacing indication is a symptomatic sinus bradycardia that occurs as a result of drug therapy necessary to treat a medical condition. For instance, a patient who is prescribed long-term therapy with beta-blockers may experience symptomatic sinus bradycardia as a result. Even though that sinus bradycardia is iatrogenic (literally physician-induced or caused by medical treatment), it is still a pacing indication.

The key to understanding these (and some other) pacing indications is summed up in three words: *symptomatic sinus bradycardia*. Symptomatic sinus bradycardia is associated with depressed cardiac output, which is closely related to the nervous system. For that reason, some of the most frequent symptoms associated with symptomatic sinus bradycardia are neurologic in nature. These symptoms may be described in various ways by various patients but include things like fatigue, tiredness, exhaustion, lethargy, sleepiness, dizziness, vertigo, light-headedness, presyncope, syncope (fainting), wooziness, malaise, and just *not feeling well*.

Note that physicians refer to fainting as syncope or a syncopal spell, while nearly fainting is presyncope; most patients describe presyncopal episodes as *dizziness*. In this connection, clinicians must be careful about this particular symptom in that dizziness can be a symptom of any of a number of conditions, some serious and others benign. Although we are talking about symptomatic sinus bradycardia here, dizziness can also be a symptom of tachyarrhythmias. So while dizziness is a commonly reported symptom in the list of symptoms associated with sinus bradycardia, it may or may not be associated with the sinus bradycardia. Other causes of dizziness include posttachycardic syncope (following an episode of a very fast heart rate), orthostatic hypotension (a drop in blood pressure, which occurs often in older people), neurological syncope, psychogenic syncope (related to psychiatric disturbances), and metabolic syncope (related to blood glucose levels). Causes of syncope are diverse and may relate to hydration, heavy exercise, lack of salt, and other conditions.

Sinus node dysfunction pacing indications: class IIa

With class IIa indication, things are a little less clear-cut.

What if the physician strongly suspects symptomatic sinus bradycardia, but there is *no documentation* of the bradycardia? Let's say a patient has a known sinus node dysfunction and heart rates less than 40 bpm (the patient is measuring his own pulse). The patient is also symptomatic and all of his symptoms are consistent with bradycardia. However, the physician cannot document the bradycardia by, say, being able to produce a surface ECG showing sinus bradycardia. It is not unusual for arrhythmias to be elusive and hard to capture on ECG. In this case, there is a lot of circumstantial evidence for sinus bradycardia—a slow heart rate and symptoms—but no actual documentation. The guidelines make this a class IIa indication, but if documentation were available, it would be class I.

Another class IIa indication for cardiac pacing is syncope of unexplained origin when clinically significant abnormalities of sinus node function are either discovered (for instance, on a surface ECG) or can be provoked in an electrophysiologic (EP) study. In this case, there is no documentation of bradycardia episodes, but there is a symptom (syncope) and clear evidence of some kind of sinus node dysfunction.

Sinus node dysfunction pacing indications: class IIb

A class IIb indication is not necessarily an outright contraindication to pacing, but it suggests that the risk is equal to the benefit.

A class IIb pacing indication is minimally symptomatic patients with chronic heart rates less than 40 bpm. In this case, the slow heart rate has to be chronic; it cannot be a few episodes here and there. The patient also must be symptomatic, although the symptoms can be mild and tolerable. If this kind of patient came to the clinic, should she get a pacemaker? Most experts would say no, but the evidence is not outright against pacing. On the other hand, this is a patient who should definitely be monitored. If the point comes that the symptoms worsen, this changes into a class I indication.

Sinus node dysfunction pacing indications: class III

Class III indications is a bit of a misnomer, since these are actually contraindications. Pacing is contraindicated (or is a class III indication) for patients with sinus node dysfunction (even if it can be documented) if the patient is asymptomatic. Again, this highlights how crucial symptoms are in determining whether pacing is indicated and appropriate for a patient with sinus node dysfunction.

Pacing is also contraindicated in a patient with sinus node dysfunction and symptoms of bradycardia, if there is documented evidence that those symptoms occur in the absence of bradycardia. For instance, a patient with fatigue and light-headedness (both symptoms typical of sinus bradycardia) that occur with or without bradycardia is not indicated for pacing.

Finally, another class III indication relates to an earlier class I indication. If a patient must take essential drug therapy and, as a result, develops documented sinus bradycardia with symptoms, pacing is indicated (class I). However, if the drug therapy in question is not essential, then pacing is not indicated (class III). For example, a patient who takes beta-blockers to treat long QT syndrome (a potentially fatal condition) may develop symptomatic sinus bradycardia and be indicated for a pacemaker; beta-blockers are an essential medical therapy for that patient. A patient who takes beta-blockers to treat occasional migraines (a nonfatal condition that can be treated in many other ways) and develops symptomatic sinus bradycardia is not indicated for a pacemaker. The difference is not the type of medical therapy involved; the distinction is made as to whether or not that treatment can be called *medically essential*.

Sinus node dysfunction pacing indications wrap-up

Clinicians will likely encounter sinus node dysfunction as the most frequent indication for an implantable pacemaker. In this connection, two things stand out. The sinus node dysfunction must always result in symptoms; without symptomatic bradycardia in sinus node dysfunction, there is no pacing indication. The reasons for this are pretty obvious. Many people technically have heart rates that fall below the 40 bpm bradycardia cutoff rate, but they tolerate these rates well and they may even be appropriate for them. Furthermore, some patients do have pathological bradycardia but do not have symptoms or have symptoms so mild that it does not make sense to subject them to device implantation. When symptoms do occur, it is important that they be associated with bradycardia and not present when the patient is not bradycardic.

Another important aspect to sinus node dysfunction is the value of documentation of the sinus bradycardia. Getting evidence on a surface ECG, EP study, or other tracing is very valuable in making the case that a pacemaker is or is not indicated. Of course, the clinical reality is that arrhythmias do not always show up when the ECG monitor is turned on. Sometimes, a *circumstantial case* can be made for pacing even if there is no hard documentation of sinus bradycardia.

AV block

In the first decades after pacemakers were invented, AV block was the most common indication for cardiac pacing. AV block had been well known for many years before the pacemaker was invented and resisted treatment. The pacemaker was a very welcome option for individuals who otherwise had little hope of having a normal heart rhythm. Today, sinus node dysfunction has surpassed AV block as a pacing indication. This is not because AV block is rarer today than it was back then. It is because our growing understanding of the SA node and its function has expanded our awareness about symptomatic sinus bradycardia.

AV block: class I

There are nine main class I indications in the setting of AV block. The first six to be discussed all relate to third-degree AV block or advanced second-degree AV block (second-degree AV block type II). Third-degree AV block, also known as complete heart block, is the most severe form of AV block. Third-degree AV block refers to a heart rhythm in which the atrial rate and the ventricular rate are independent or dissociated from each other. The indications group third-degree AV block together with advanced second-degree AV block (second-degree AV block type II); these two rhythm disorders are sometimes collectively called *high-grade AV block*. All of these high-grade AV block class I indications refer to AV block *at any anatomic level*, meaning that it is not of importance for the pacing indication as to exactly where the AV block originates. Most first-degree and second-degree type I AV blocks originate at the AV node; most second-degree type II AV block and third-degree AV block originate below the AV node or in the bundle of His. However, for these first six class I indications, the anatomical point of origin of the AV block is not important.

There are six main class I indications for patients with advanced AV block:

1 Third-degree or advanced second-degree AV block at any anatomic level with symptomatic bradycardia is a class I indication. The key here is symptomatic bradycardia. Note that the AV block can be at any *anatomic level*, meaning that the block may be in or around or near the AV node; the actual anatomical location of the block is not important for this indication.

2 Another class I indication for pacing is third-degree or advanced second-degree AV block at any anatomic level associated with arrhythmias and other medical conditions that require drug therapy that results in symptomatic bradycardia.

This would refer to a patient on drug therapy with resulting symptomatic bradycardia. The drug therapy must be *required* and essential.

3 The third class I indication for pacing associated with AV block is third-degree or advanced second-degree AB block at any anatomic level in awake, asymptomatic patients in sinus rhythm who experience documented periods of asystole greater than or equal to 3 s or escape rates less than 40 bpm or with an escape rate that originates anatomically below the AV node. In this class I indication, the patient need not have symptoms (although he or she might very well have symptoms, even severe symptoms!). In these patients, there is documented evidence of third-degree or advanced second-degree AV block plus at least one of the following: pauses, bradycardia, or an escape rate originating below the AV node. The clinician needs to find only one of these to make this a class I pacing indication, but more than one may very well be present. This type of rhythm disorder is considered so severe that symptoms are not part of the requirements. In this case, bradycardia is defined as a rate less than 40 bpm, and pauses have to be at least 3 s or longer.

4 The fourth class I indication for third-degree or advanced second-degree AV block is AV block at any anatomic level following catheter ablation of the AV junction. AV ablations may be carried out in patients with persistent atrial fibrillation and rapid ventricular response; in this case, the AV node is ablated (small areas of tissue destroyed) so that it cannot conduct electricity. This effectively and permanently dissociates atria from ventricles. Following an AV ablation, a pacemaker is often implanted; in fact, these procedures are sometimes nicknamed *ablate-and-pace* operations.

5 Number five on the list of class I indications is third-degree or advanced second-degree AV block at any anatomic level that is associated with postoperative AV block and is not expected to resolve after cardiac surgery. Cardiac surgery patients may sometimes experience advanced AV block after surgery. If this block is deemed temporary, no pacemaker is required, but if it is not expected to resolve on its own or if it fails to resolve on its own, it is a class I pacing indication.

6 Finally, the sixth class I indication for pacing is third-degree or advanced second-degree AV block at any anatomic level associated with neuromuscular diseases such as Kearns–Sayre syndrome, Erb dystrophy, and peroneal muscular atrophy.

Other class I indications for AV block include more detail about the type of block:

1 Second-degree AV block associated with symptomatic bradycardia, regardless of the type of site of the block. The key to this important indication is that the patient must have symptomatic bradycardia.

2 Asymptomatic persistent third-degree AV block at any anatomic site with an average awake ventricular rate of 40 bpm or higher if one or more of the following are present: cardiomegaly or left ventricular dysfunction or the block site is below the AV node. In this case, the patient has third-degree AV block but no symptoms and must have cardiomegaly (enlarged heart), some type of pump compromise (left ventricular dysfunction), or an AV block site below the AV node. AV block sites below the AV node are more common in advanced AV block.

3 Second-degree or third-degree AV block during exercise in the absence of myocardial infarction. In acute myocardial infarction, symptomatic bradycardia can be transient, that is, it may go away on its own. For such patients, temporary pacing may be a preferable option.

4 Asymptomatic second-degree type II AV block with a wide QRS is a class I indication; if the QRS in this case is narrow, it is a class IIa recommendation.

AV block: class IIa

There are four main class IIa indications for pacing in the setting of some form of AV block. The class IIa indications for pacing are:

1 Persistent third-degree AV block with an escape rate greater than 40 bpm in asymptomatic patients with cardiomegaly (enlarged heart).

2 Asymptomatic second-degree AV block at intra- or infra-His levels as determined by an EP study. In this case, the AV block need not be advanced and symptoms need not be present, but there must be documented evidence from an EP study that the AV block is below the AV node. This anatomical location for AV block is more associated with advanced forms of AV block.

3 First- or second-degree AV block with symptoms similar to those of pacemaker syndrome or hemodynamic compromise. Normally, first-degree

AV block is not an indication for pacing, but in this case, it is (along with second-degree AV block), provided that a specific type of symptom occurs, namely, pacemaker syndrome. Pacemaker syndrome is an older term that relates to symptoms specifically associated with the loss of AV synchrony (today, clinicians might describe it as symptoms associated with AV dyssynchrony). This includes hypotension, retrograde conduction (from ventricles to atrium, backward through the heart), fatigue, light-headedness, and lack of rate support to meet physiologic need (leading to the possibility of syncope). Since these symptoms are typical of advanced AV block, it is easy to understand why they should be considered for potential pacemaker implantation.

4 Asymptomatic second-degree type II AV block with a narrow QRS; note that if the QRS is wide, the indication becomes class I.

AV block: class IIb

There are two important class IIb indications to be considered for pacing in the setting of AV block. Remember that a class IIb indication is not well named; it is actually a case where pacing is not recommended but not outright contraindicated.

Cardiac pacing may be considered for patients with certain neuromuscular diseases, such as myotonic muscular dystrophy, Erb dystrophy, or peroneal muscular atrophy with any degree of AV block or without symptoms, because there may be unpredictable progression of AV conduction. The concept of pacing in these patients is to prevent the patient from experiencing the symptoms associated with AV dyssynchrony, which may occur in patients with these neuromuscular conditions. However, the idea of pacing such patients even without symptoms and first-degree AV block is not generally endorsed.

AV block is known to occur with the use of certain drugs or drug toxicity. In some cases, AV block may be transient and resolve on its own or when the drug is discontinued. If the AV block is temporary, pacing is contraindicated. But if it is expected that AV block will recur even after drug use is discontinued, it is a class IIb indication. Again, this means that pacing is not generally advocated in such cases but could still be considered.

AV block: class III

Class III indications are actually the contraindications to pacing for patients with AV block. Cardiac pacing is contraindicated (class III) in patients with asymptomatic first-degree AV block. This condition may be more prevalent than we realize, and if the patient tolerates first-degree AV block well, there is no need to implant a pacemaker.

Pacing is contraindicated (class III) for asymptomatic second-degree AV block type I at the anatomic level of the AV node (so-called supra-Hisian or above the bundle of His) or for asymptomatic second-degree AV block not known to be intra-Hisian or infra-Hisian. Thus, for second-degree AV block type I with no symptoms and an anatomic block at or around the AV node, pacing is contraindicated.

Finally, pacing is not indicated in patients who have AV block that is expected to resolve on its own or is unlikely to recur. This may occur in patients with poisoning or Lyme disease or in transient episodes associated with sleep apnea or other conditions. The idea is that if AV block occurred because of a specific situation and it is not likely to continue or come back, pacing is not necessary or appropriate.

AV block pacing indications wrap-up

When thinking through the pacing indications for AV block, it is important to differentiate advanced AV block (third-degree and second-degree type II AV block) from other types as more pacing indications are associated with advanced AV block than lesser forms of AV block. In fact, first-degree AV block is almost never an indication for pacing (pacing is only indicated for first-degree AV block if the patient has symptoms of pacemaker syndrome, that is, AV dyssynchrony, which suggest a more severe AV block is actually going on). As with sinus node dysfunction, pacing indications often require the patient to be symptomatic. However, some indications for AV block pacing may allow for asymptomatic patients if the location of the AV block is below the AV node, which again is suggestive of more severe forms of AV block.

An interesting and frequent situation comes up with a patient with first-degree AV block and a very long but stable PR interval of 400 ms with heart failure or, to be more specific, left ventricular dysfunction. Is pacing indicated? Clearly, if the patient had normal left ventricular function (no heart failure), pacing would be contraindicated. In particular, if the patient had no symptoms or only very mild symptoms, there would be no reason to consider pacing. However, sometimes, heart failure patients can be paced in a way that optimizes their AV delay (PR interval); in this case, pacing can help to remodel the heart and improve their left ventricular function. In such cases, dual-chamber pacing may be indicated. The indication is based on the fact that forced AV pacing can restore ventricular function.

Other indications for pacing

There are some indications for pacing that do not fit neatly in the two main categories described above (sinus node dysfunction and AV block). Indeed, these are less frequently encountered indications but are still important. Hypersensitive carotid sinus syndrome and neurocardiogenic syncope (NCS) are both encountered by pacing clinicians. These are completely different and unrelated conditions that should not be confused.

Hypersensitive carotid sinus syndrome

Hypersensitive carotid sinus syndrome occurs because the carotid vessels, located in the neck, can affect the heart rate. During carotid massage, patients can experience a lowered heart rate. In some individuals, the carotid is hypersensitive so that even light pressure—such as a shirt collar or a gentle touch—can cause bradyarrhythmias or even asystole.

Neurocardiogenic syncope

NCS is not an arrhythmia at all but a disorder of the autonomic nervous system. In fact, NCS occurs when there is a miscommunication between the autonomic nervous system and the heart. NCS is also known as vasovagal syncope or neurally mediated syncope (these terms mean the same thing). NCS typically occurs with postural changes, such as when a person is lying down and suddenly stands up and faints. When you go from lying down or sitting to standing, about 40% of your circulating blood volume is suddenly dumped into the periphery. In the healthy individual, the heart's

baroreceptors will signal the brain that there is a shift in blood volume and the brain orders adrenaline. As discussed earlier, adrenaline increases conduction, heart rate, contractility, and vasoconstriction. For healthy people, this is the reason that we can go from lying down to standing up without passing out! In people with NCS, the system does not function. As blood volume shifts abruptly to the periphery, the brain turns off the adrenaline—with the result that conduction slows, heart rate drops, contractility decreases, and vasodilation occurs. The patient suffers from hypoxia (lack of oxygen) in the brain. This results in the patient's feeling woozy and dizzy and can cause fainting.

About 25–40% of fainting disorders can be attributed to NCS, and it often occurs in young otherwise healthy individuals with no history of any type of structural heart disease and no neurological disorders. Some adolescent patients with NCS may suffer multiple episodes every day. However, many pediatric and young patients outgrow NCS, typically in the mid-20s. NCS is the most common cause of fainting in adolescents. Since it often resolves on its own without therapy, NCS in adolescent patients may not be treated at all.

In some NCS patients, the heart raises the blood pressure by increasing the rate and vigor of the cardiac contractions, but this actually makes the problem worse. When heart rate and contractility increase, the message is sent to the heart's receptors that the ventricles are full (which they are not). This, in turn, sends a message to the neurological receptors that the blood pressure is too high (which it is not—it is actually too low). This causes the brain to slow the heart rate and dilate the blood vessel, resulting in a drop in blood pressure. Less blood is pumped to the brain and the patient's risk of fainting increases.

NCS has been associated with the body's *fight-or-flight* reflex, and it has been observed to occur when a person is suddenly confronted with something frightening or a very stressful situation.

NCS seems to occur in two main types of population differentiated mainly by age. In younger patients, NCS tends to be more related to heart rate, while in older individuals, NCS seems to relate more to blood pressure. Geriatric patients are more likely to have vasodepressor NCS, while younger patients are more likely to have cardioinhibitory

Table 10.3 A short description of the various types of NCS

Type	Description	What happens	Rate/asystole	Sequence
1	Mixed	Heart rate drops at time of asystole but no long pauses; blood pressure drops before heart rate	Not under 40 bpm (or under 40 bpm < 10 s) and no asystole or pauses < 3 s	Blood pressure drops before heart rate
2A	Cardioinhibitory without asystole	Heart rate drops below 40 bpm >10 s and pauses may occur but are never >3 s	Under 40 bpm >10 s and no asystole >3 s	Blood pressure drops before heart rate
2B	Cardioinhibitory with asystole	Heart rate drops and asystole >3 s	Under 40 bpm >10 s and asystole >3 s	Blood pressure drop coincides with or slightly precedes drop in heart rate
3	Vasodepressor	Blood pressure drops but heart rate does not decrease	Heart rate does not drop more than 10% from its peak	Blood pressure drops but the heart rate does not (or drops only slightly)

types of NCS (see **Table 10.3**). Note that NCS is very rare; only about 1% of the population has any form of NCS.

Mixed NCS is by far the largest category with perhaps 50% or more of NCS patients. Diagnosis of NCS depends on taking a thorough patient history and may involve echocardiography, stress testing, carotid massage, Holter monitoring, the use of an event recorder or an implantable loop recorder, or an EP study. By far the best diagnostic tool is the tilt table in that it will provoke NCS episodes. Tilt-table testing involves having a patient lying down and then tilting the table so that the patient is in an upright position; the patient may remain upright for as long as 60 min because the NCS response may not occur at once but may only be observed after about 20 or 30 min of being upright. Note that tilt- table testing is considered somewhat controversial among physicians who are concerned that the test can result in false-negatives (somebody who has NCS but the test does not show it) and false-positives (somebody who does not have NCS but the test shows it). While it may be true that tilt-table testing (like many other diagnostic tools) can have false-negative and false-positive results, tilt-table testing is still very useful in diagnosing NCS, particularly when long pauses are observed.

There are many treatment options for NCS, most of which do not involve a pacemaker. The appropriate treatment of NCS may depend on the age of the patient and the type of NCS. For example, it has been observed that in young people, NCS is often related to dehydration and low sodium levels. Some NCS patients (but not all) can sense when a fainting spell is approaching; with counseling, they can learn to anticipate episodes and sit or lie down. With prompt and proper response, NCS patients may avoid passing out but might still experience a so-called brownout. For that reason, *psychological counseling* is probably the best first line of treatment for NCS in that patients should be taught to anticipate these episodes as much as possible so that they can prepare for them. Since a typical NCS episode lasts about 2–5 min, the patient may be able to avoid fainting and come back to normal in a reasonably short period of time. If these approaches are not successful, drug therapy may be tried. Typical drugs used to treat NCS include beta-blockers, Florinef, Norpace, Prozac, Zoloft, and theophylline. Beta-blockers may seem counterintuitive since beta-blockers are known to slow the heart rate and slow heart conduction, but it appears that the beta-blockade can block the autonomic nervous system from lowering blood pressure and heart rate. It is unclear how antidepressants affect NCS, but there is clearly an emotional component to the disorder. Thus, physicians who deal with NCS patients have a long list of potential drugs to consider for use in these patients. If—and only if—no drug therapy works, the physician may consider pacing. Cardiac pacing must be considered as a therapy of last resort for NCS.

If an NCS patient is treated with an implantable pacemaker, the clinician must realize that pacing does not cure NCS. At best, cardiac pacing can decrease symptoms, but even then, pacing will not eliminate symptoms. Paced NCS patients should get specific patient education that pacing will not reduce their episodes or cure them of the condition—it will only make their symptoms more tolerable. Managing patient expectations can be an important part of achieving good pacing outcomes. As the name suggests, pacing works best in patients with *cardioinhibitory forms* of NCS. Since cardioinhibitory NCS tends to occur more in younger than older patients, this makes pacing even less appealing because most physicians do not want to implant a permanent pacemaker in a young and otherwise healthy person who very well may outgrow NCS.

Paced NCS patients require special programming since they are not *typical* pacemaker patients and usually do not need any pacing the vast majority of the time. Pacemakers may offer special features that are useful for NCS patients. Since pacing for NCS is uncommon, it is important to know about these important (but rarely used) features:

- *Rate drop response* (Medtronic) will start dual-chamber pacing at an elevated rate when an abrupt drop in atrial rate is sensed. The elevated dual-chamber pacing (usually around 80–100 ppm and for a programmable duration of time) is intended to boost cardiac output.
- *Sudden brady response* (Boston Scientific) likewise offers elevated dual-chamber pacing for a programmable duration when a sudden drop in atrial rate is sensed.
- *Advanced hysteresis* (St. Jude Medical) offers elevated dual-chamber pacing for a programmable rate and duration when there is a sudden drop in the patient's atrial rate.
- *Closed-loop stimulation* or CLS (Biotronik) may be requested by some prescribers for treating NCS. Unlike the other three features, which are triggered by an abrupt rate drop, CLS is closed-loop physiologic pacing. It has been shown that changes in myocardial contractility occur right before a syncopal episode occurs, and since CLS allows those changes to trigger pacing before the rate drops, it may benefit the NCS patient by pacing before the *episode* occurs, potentially preventing the episode.

Other indications for pacing: class I

Pacing is indicated in patients with recurrent syncope caused by spontaneously occurring carotid sinus stimulation and carotid sinus pressure that induced ventricular asystole of greater than 3 s. Remember, hypersensitive carotid sinus syndrome is *not* NCS, although it is often grouped together with NCS as a sort of *miscellaneous* category of pacing indications. The fact is that there is no class I pacing indication for NCS. There is a class I indication for hypersensitive carotid sinus syndrome.

Other indications for pacing: class IIa

Pacing is reasonable for patients with syncope without a clear, provocative event or with a hypersensitive cardioinhibitory response of greater than 3 s. Pacing is indicated in the presence of known hypersensitive carotid syndrome and is reasonable if the patient has hypersensitive cardioinhibitory response (suggestive of the syndrome). Again, pauses must be 3 s or more in duration. This is not NCS!

Pacing is considered reasonable in patients with significant symptomatic and recurrent NCS associated with bradycardia documented spontaneously or at the time of tilt-table testing. This is a clear NCS pacing indication (class IIa), but it requires three things: significant symptoms, recurrence, and documentation. In this class IIa indication, pacing is *reasonable* but only after other treatment options, including drug therapy, have been tried.

Other indications for pacing: class IIb

Pacing may be considered for significantly symptomatic NCS associated with bradycardia, documented spontaneously or at the time of tilt-table testing. NCS has, as the name implies, some pretty significant symptoms in that patients with this condition are at risk of passing out. It is rare for patients to present with documented spontaneous NCS, so the clinician must rely on a patient history and interview and a tilt-table test to recreate the symptoms.

Other indications for pacing: class III

Pacing is contraindicated (class III indication) for patients with hypersensitive cardioinhibitory response to carotid sinus stimulation with symptoms or vague symptoms. For pacing to be considered, cardioinhibition must occur spontaneously (without stimulation). Pacing is also not indicated (class III) for situational vasovagal syncope (also known as situational NCS), which refers to vasovagal syncopal syndromes that occur based on specific behaviors. Instead of pacing, patients are advised to avoid those behaviors.

Conclusion

The indications for pacing are based on medical evidence but applied to real-world situations and real people, which is to say that things are not always as neat as the guidelines might suggest. Pacing indications are grouped by classes, with class I what we might call an indication and class III a contraindication. Between them are classes IIa and IIb where pacing may be reasonable (IIa) or may not be reasonable (IIb), but there is some conflicting evidence. As a general rule, the two main indications for cardiac pacing are sinus node dysfunction and AV block, but the class of indication depends on the severity of the symptoms, documented evidence, and the degree of AV block. Pacing can also be used for hypersensitive carotid sinus syndrome and NCS, but these conditions are rarer. Although the indications tend to group hypersensitive carotid syndrome and NCS together, they are different conditions. Hypersensitive carotid syndrome is a cardiac condition, while NCS is technically a neurologic condition that affects the heart.

The nuts and bolts of indications for pacing

- There are three main classes of indications: class I (indication), class II (conflicting evidence or divergence of opinion), and class III (contraindication).
- Class II indications can be divided into classes IIa and IIb, where the difference of opinion either favors the intervention (class IIa) or does not favor it (class IIb).
- When evidence is evaluated, it is grouped as level A, B, or C. Level A evidence is the strongest and is based on large randomized clinical trials.
- The two main indications for pacing involve sinus node dysfunction and AV block, with more patients getting a pacemaker for sinus node dysfunction.
- As a rule of thumb, the cutoff rate for bradycardia is less than 40 bpm; for pauses, the cutoff duration is 3 s.
- Sinus node dysfunction with symptoms and documented bradycardia is a class I pacing indication. Pacing is contraindicated in patients with sinus node dysfunction if the patient has no symptoms.
- Symptomatic sinus bradycardia without documented bradycardia is a class IIa indication.
- Patients who have pacing indications as a result of medically necessary drug therapy or a medical procedure (such as AV nodal ablation) may be indicated for permanent pacing. If the drug therapy is not medically necessary, pacing is not indicated.
- If the patient has syncopal spells and there is evidence of sinus node dysfunction, pacing is a class IIa indication even if there is no documented bradycardia.
- A class IIb indication is sinus node dysfunction for patients with chronic heart rates less than 40 bpm but mild to no symptoms.
- Pacing is contraindicated in patients with sinus node dysfunction and symptomatic bradycardia if there is evidence that those symptoms also occur in the absence of bradycardia.
- Typical symptoms of bradycardia include fatigue, dizziness, light-headedness, wooziness, a sense of malaise, and tiredness. These symptoms can be mild to severe. Syncope (fainting) is a symptom of bradycardia as is its predecessor, presyncope (feeling like one might faint).
- Most pacing indications related to high-grade (also called advanced) AV block, which can be defined as third-degree AV block (the most severe form where atria and ventricles are dissociated from each other) and second-degree

Continued

Continued

AV block type II. There are several indications for patients with high-grade AV block.

- In some AV block indications, it may be important to know at what anatomic level the AV block occurs; in general, higher blocks (sometimes called supra-Hisian or *above the bundle of His*) are more dangerous than lower blocks (at the AV node itself).
- Advanced AV block with symptomatic bradycardia is a class I pacing indication. The anatomic level of the AV block does not matter for this indication. Moreover, second-degree AV block type I with symptomatic bradycardia is also a class I indication for pacing.
- AV block may sometimes occur postoperatively, in the immediate period after a myocardial infarction, or as the result of short-term drug therapy. In such cases, pacing is contraindicated if the AV block might resolve on its own or after treatment is discontinued.
- Second-degree type II AV block with a wide QRS complex (>120 ms) is a class I pacing indication, while second-degree type II AV block with a narrow or normal-duration QRS complex is a class IIa indication.
- Pacing is only ever indicated for first-degree AV block (class IIa) in the case where the patient has symptoms indicative of hemodynamic compromise, such as hypotension, retrograde conduction, fatigue, presyncope, syncope, and lack of rate support to meet physiologic requirements.
- Certain neuromuscular diseases (such as Erb dystrophy, myotonic dystrophy, and others) and drug therapy/toxicity can result in AV block, but pacing in this setting is contraindicated (class III) unless the patients meet specific pacing indications.
- Hypersensitive carotid syndrome and neurocardiogenic syncope (NCS) often are listed together in pacing indications, but these are totally different conditions. Hypersensitive carotid syndrome is a heart condition, while NCS is a neurologic disorder that affects the heart.
- Patients with hypersensitive carotid sinus syndrome with spontaneously occurring episodes of ventricular asystole greater than 3 s have a class I pacing indication. If the patient has hypersensitive cardioinhibitory response (which is suggestive of the syndrome) and pauses greater than 3 s occur without a clear provocative event, the patient has a class IIa indication.
- Note that there are no class I or IIa indications for pacing for NCS. About 1% of the population has NCS, which is a disorder based on miscommunication between the brain (the autonomic nervous system) and the heart. For NCS patients, permanent pacing should be considered a therapy of last resort to be tried when all else fails.
- There are four types of NCS. The largest group of NCS patients have the mixed syndrome, and younger patients tend to have cardioinhibitory forms of NCS (types 2A and 2B), while geriatric patients are more likely to have vasodepressor NCS (type 3).
- Other names for NCS are vasovagal syncope and neurally mediated syncope.
- Young people who get NCS (typically the cardioinhibitory type) may outgrow it; pacing is not recommended for them. They may respond well to learning how to manage their condition (such as how to anticipate syncopal spells) and improve hydration and salt replacement.
- NCS is not a common disorder and pacing therapy is not a common therapy. However, the major pacemaker manufacturers offer features for NCS patients. These may be elevated pacing in response to a sudden rate drop (Medtronic, St. Jude Medical, and Boston Scientific) or closed-loop stimulation (Biotronik). Closed-loop stimulation is physiologic pacing, which is thought to anticipate changes in contractility and start pacing, which in theory might prevent an NCS episode.
- In the event that a patient with NCS receives a pacemaker, patient education is crucial. Pacing does not cure NCS; episodes will still occur. Pacing, at best, can help reduce symptoms.

Test your knowledge

1 If a patient has a clear class III indication for pacing, what is the best course of action?
   A A pacemaker should be implanted at once.
   B It might be reasonable to implant a pacemaker and this should be discussed with the patient.
   C The patient should be put on a Holter monitor.
   D A pacemaker should not be implanted (it is contraindicated).

2 A patient has third-degree AV block at the supra-Hisian level and symptomatic bradycardia. What is the pacing indication?
   A Class I
   B Class IIa
   C Class IIb
   D Class III

3 A patient has sinus node dysfunction and has symptomatic bradycardia, but the clinic cannot get documentation of the bradycardia on an ECG. The patient has measured his own pulse during these episodes, and his heart rate appears to be around 30 or 40 bpm. What is the pacing indication?
   A Class I
   B Class IIa
   C Class IIb
   D Class III

4 A patient has undergone AV nodal ablation and as a result now has permanent third-degree AV block. What is the pacing indication?
   A Class I
   B Class IIa
   C Class IIb
   D Class III

5 A patient has second-degree AV block type I but has no symptoms. The clinic can determine that the AV block is at the AV node. What is the pacing indication?
   A Class I
   B Class IIa
   C Class IIb
   D Class III

6 When discussing pacing indications, what is the minimum duration for a pause?

A 10 s
B 5 s
C 3 s
D Anything >1 s

7 A patient is hospitalized for digitalis toxicity and has documented evidence of third-degree AV block; she reports severe symptoms. What is the pacing indication?
   A Class I
   B Class IIa
   C Class IIb
   D Class III

8 If a patient has hypersensitive carotid sinus syndrome and has spontaneous episodes of ventricular asystole for more than 3 s, what is the best therapy?
   A Pacing, class I
   B Hydration
   C Drug therapy
   D Psychological counseling so he can learn to anticipate syncopal episodes

9 There are different types of neurocardiogenic syncope. Which main type responds best to pacing?
   A Mixed
   B Cardioinhibitory
   C Vasodepressor
   D Hypersensitive carotid syndrome

10 Below are some pacemaker features that could potentially be used to help a patient with neurocardiogenic syncope with one exception. Which is the only feature below *that would not be helpful* in dealing with neurocardiogenic syncope?
   A Rate drop response
   B Mode switching
   C Sudden brady response
   D Closed-loop stimulation

Reference

1 Epstein, A.E., DiMarco, J.P., Ellenbogen, K.A. *et al.* (2008) ACA/AHA/HRS 2008 guidelines for device-based therapy of cardiac rhythm abnormalities. *Journal of American College of Cardiology*, **51 (21)**, e1–62.

CHAPTER 11

Pacemaker implantation

Learning objectives

- Name and briefly describe the main steps in pacemaker implant.
- Name the two main sites of venous access.
- Identify the pieces in an introducer kit and state the function of each tool.
- Explain the retained guidewire technique.
- Name a situation in which a physician might opt for the double-wire technique.
- Describe the function of the PSA and how it is used during implantation.
- State appropriate emergency ventricular pacing settings for the PSA and why these should be set up prior to the implantation.
- Name two or three different measurements obtained from the pacemaker at implant.
- Name three or four potential complications associated with pacemaker implantation.
- Describe the current of injury and how clinicians should treat it.
- Name at least two potential complications from pacemaker surgery.

Introduction

Pacemaker implantation is considered a fairly simple routine procedure, but just because this is a minimally invasive surgery, it does not mean that there are not some very important techniques and technical tools that implanters must learn. While many pacing clinicians are not routinely involved in device implant, it is essential to understand the key steps involved in an implant procedure along with potential complications.

The basic steps of device implant are deceptively simple:
- The patient is prepped and a pocket is created in the upper chest and drenched in antibiotics.
- The implanting physician selects a vein and gains access using an introducer kit. There are different veins and access techniques possible.
- The lead is maneuvered under fluoroscopy through the vein and into the heart where it is fixated in place.
- Intraoperative values are obtained and the lead is repositioned if necessary to get optimal values.
- The leads are plugged into the device and the device is placed into the pocket. The pocket is sewn closed.

In reality, there are potential pitfalls at each step and specific strategies to facilitate implantation and make the procedure as safe as possible for the patient.

The pacemaker implantation procedure: prepping the patient

Pacemaker implantation must be done in a sterile environment, but its exact location depends on the facility and the physician. Some pacemakers are implanted in an operating room (OR); others can be implanted in a cardiac catheterization lab (cath lab) or an electrophysiology (EP) lab. The typical setup will include the pacemaker tray (the boxes with the sterile pacemaker and leads), a tray of surgical instruments including a scalpel, drapes to cover the patient, cautery equipment, and sterile basins. The exact equipment and room may vary somewhat depending on whether the implanting physician is an electrophysiologist, a cardiologist, a cardiac surgeon, or a general surgeon.

The Nuts and Bolts of Implantable Device Therapy Pacemakers, First Edition. Tom Kenny.
© 2015 John Wiley & Sons, Ltd. Published 2015 by John Wiley & Sons, Ltd.

A large C-arm fluoroscope will be available to help observe the lead during its transvenous passage.

The patient will be brought into the room awake. ECG, oxygen saturation, and blood pressure monitoring equipment will be attached to the patient and gentle restraints applied to keep the patient's arms out of the surgical field. The skin area around the implant site (typically the left upper chest) is shaved and prepped. Finally, the surgical area is cordoned off with sterile towels and the patient's body is draped. In many cases, the patient is awake during the procedure; drapes may be set up so that the patient cannot see the implant site.

The implant side is numbed with a medication, such as lidocaine or xylocaine. In most cases, the patient is lightly sedated to help relieve anxiety. An introducer kit will be used to help gain venous access (discussed more in detail in the following text). Every manufacturer offers an introducer kit, and there are other kits from manufacturers who do not make pacemakers (e.g., Pressure Products). The selection of the introducer kit depends on physician and facility preference.

Selecting a vein

In order to pass a transvenous lead into the heart, the implanting physician must access a vein. Venous access can be one of the most challenging aspects of pacemaker implantation. Any number of veins is technically available for venous access, but most implanting physicians will select either the cephalic or the subclavian vein, and more rarely, the axillary vein. However, in some cases, the internal or external jugular veins could be used (see **Figure 11.1**). The selection of the most appropriate vein depends first and foremost on the patient's anatomy and also on physician preference.

In selecting the appropriate site of venous access, the implanting physician should consider a condition known as clavicular crush, which occurs when a pacing lead is exposed to compressive pressures exerted by the clavicle. In subclavian access, the insertion point or *stick* site is very close to the intersection of a joint, ligaments, and a muscle.

Venous access

When the cephalic vein is used, the physician typically exposes the vein and makes a small incision with a scalpel. This is called a *cutdown*. Since the veins are low-pressure systems, there will not be a large outflow of blood under pressure. The physician can then insert the guidewire (described in the next section) after the incision. There are important advantages to a cephalic cutdown:
• There is relatively low stress in this area so it does not put undue stress on the lead.

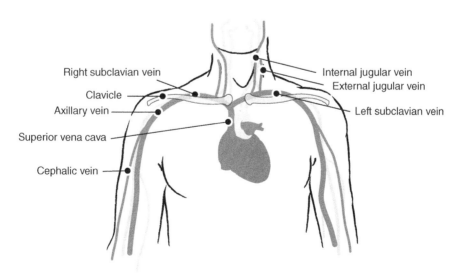

Figure 11.1 The three main veins used for transvenous leads in cardiac pacing are the subclavian vein, the cephalic vein, and the axillary vein. The subclavian and cephalic veins are the most frequently used.

- There is no risk of pneumothorax with this approach.
- It has a lower rate of complications than subclavian access.
- It is commonly used for pacing and defibrillation leads as well as chronic indwelling catheters.

It is also possible to access a vein without a surgical incision using a needle and the Seldinger technique [1]. A needle is advanced into the vein through which the sheath (introducer) and guidewire can then be inserted. This method requires some technical expertise, but when properly done, it allows for safe, rapid, and easy venous access. This *stick* method can be used in any vein, but it is often used for subclavian venous access in what might be called a *blind stick*. In this method, the implanting physician palpates the upper chest from the sternal notch to the medial third of the collarbone; the needle is inserted about 1 cm below and lateral with respect to the medial third of the clavicle.

Subclavian access is very frequently used for pacemaker lead implantation and offers the advantage of a large-diameter vessel (the subclavian vein can be about the size of the patient's pinkie finger).

The introducer kit

Regardless of how venous access is achieved or which vein is selected, the implanting physician will require an introducer kit for lead placement. Introducer kits may be roughly grouped into *hemostatic* or *nonhemostatic* types. Hemostatic introducer kits offer a hemostatic introducer that helps manage blood flow and prevent bleed-back during the procedure. The components of the introducer kit generally include the introducer (which may or may not have a hemostatic valve), a dilator, a syringe, a needle, and a guidewire (see **Figure 11.2**).

The kit includes a *syringe* and a *needle* contained in a protective plastic tube for safety. Prior to the implantation, a clinician will assemble the syringe by putting the needle into the syringe barrel. This will be set on the operating table and saved for use later in the procedure. The *dilatator* (sometimes called dilator) is a thin plastic cylinder with a blunt tip that helps to open up the vein and facilitates passage of the introducer through the vein. The dilatator is inserted into the *introducer* so that

the introducer/dilatator is one single tool. The *guidewire* is typically described as a 0.035 wire, which is the diameter of the wire in inches. The guidewire is a very thin metal wire that is provided in a hoop-type holder to facilitate handling. Guidewires have soft, blunt tips (atraumatic tips) so they do not damage the vessel as they pass through it. Some guidewires are straight, while others may have a J shape. All of these tools will be laid out on a tray prior to implantation.

There are different introducer kits available; all of the pacemaker manufacturers have their own introducer kits and some other companies make them as well. The selection of a specific introducer kit will likely be a decision based on the preferences of the implanting physician or the institution or what is available. It is possible to use an introducer kit from one manufacturer and the lead from another.

Introducer kits come in different sizes, stated in French (Fr), which is a diameter measurement. The size of the introducer depends on the size of the lead to be implanted. A pacing lead will state on its box label and in its instructions for use the *minimum introducer size*, which is the smallest introducer size that will work. In some cases, it might be wise to opt for a slightly larger French size, for example, if a pacing lead requires a *minimum 7 French introducer*, the use of an 8 French introducer may be smart.

Introducing the lead into the vein

Once the needle with the syringe is inserted into the vein, the implanting physician will draw back on the syringe to see if blood enters the barrel (confirming that a vessel was accessed) and to confirm that this blood is dark in color (from the venous system) rather than bright red (which would suggest that it came from the arterial system). The venous system is a low-pressure system, so when the implanting physician removes the syringe barrel gently from the hub of the needle, only a slow drip of blood occurs, which can be temporarily stopped by placing a finger over the opening. The physician will now take the 0.035 guidewire. The guidewire is then threaded through the needle and into the vein. Fluoroscopy is used to confirm visually that the wire is entering the vein and traveling through the vein toward the heart.

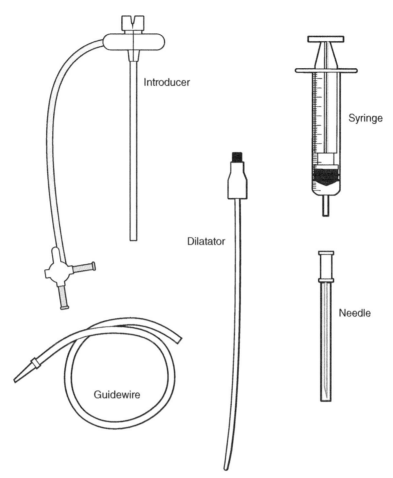

Figure 11.2 The basic components of a hemostatic introducer kit. These kits are manufactured by several different device manufacturers and the brand of introducer kit is usually a matter of hospital or physician preference. Physicians may request introducer kits with and without hemostatic valves on the introducer, by French sizes (such as 7 or 8 Fr), and introducer length (standard vs. long).

Using gentle, careful motions, the physician passes the guidewire through the vein, through the superior vena cava (SVC), and into the heart. When the guidewire is inside the right atrium, venous access has been achieved, and the guidewire now serves as a *placeholder* for the introducer, also known as the sheath. Note that the guidewire is never passed over the tricuspid valve; its destination is the right atrium. At this point, the needle and syringe are removed and discarded.

If the patient's vein is narrow, the physician may insert the dilatator by itself to help stretch or dilate the vein. (This step may be omitted.) The dilatator is inserted into the introducer and—as one unit—the introducer/dilator is put over the tip of the guidewire. Using the guidewire, the introducer/dilatator now *slides* into place. As the name implies, the purpose of the guidewire is to help *guide* the introducer into position.

From the patient's perspective, this point of the procedure may be associated with some discomfort and sensations of pressure and even pain. The clinical team may advise the patient of this and reassure the patient during this particular phase of the implant.

Once the introducer/dilator unit is in place—inserted into the vein—the physician will carefully remove the dilatator. Most physicians leave the guidewire in place, but it is possible that in some procedures the guidewire will be removed after the

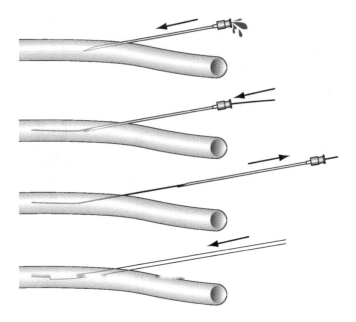

Figure 11.3 The Seldinger technique involves insertion of the needle into the vein (the *stick*) shown in the top illustration. The backflow of blood at low pressure confirms that a vein has been accessed. The guidewire is then inserted into the needle and into the vein in the second illustration. The guidewire is a very thin wire with a blunt tip. Once the guidewire is in place, the needle is removed (as shown in the third drawing) and the introducer/dilatator assembly is inserted over the guidewire (bottom drawing).

dilatator. (When the guidewire is retained in position, it is called the *retained guidewire technique*.) The implanting physician uses the introducer or sheath to pass the transvenous lead (see **Figure 11.3**).

Ventricular lead

In a dual-chamber pacemaker implantation, the ventricular lead is almost always implanted first. Safety is the main reason for this: the ventricular lead should be in place as soon as possible in the rare event that the patient requires emergency pacing support.

The lead is passed through the introducer, which is why the French size of the introducer must be large enough to accommodate the French size of the desired lead. The ventricular lead may have a passive-fixation mechanism (tines or fins) or it may have an active-fixation mechanism (helix or corkscrew). Active-fixation leads will have the mechanism protected in some way during venous passage. In an extendable–retractable

active-fixation lead, the screw-in tip will be retracted into the lead (it can then be extended when it reaches its destination). Some leads may have the active-fixation mechanism encased in a material that dissolves during venous passage; this protects the vessels from being nicked or torn by the screw-in helix.

In order to implant a lead through the introducer, the physician or the clinician helping to prepare for the implant will insert a thin wire into the lead. This thin wire, called a *stylet*, stiffens the lead enough to make it maneuverable. First, a straight stylet is inserted into the lead. Once the stylet is in place, the distal end of the lead is inserted into the introducer and then passed carefully under fluoroscopy to the venous system into the heart. Note that in some cases, the physician may experience a little resistance when the lead is first inserted into the introducer in that some introducers have a sort of diaphragm system near the opening to control bleed-back.

The ventricular lead is carefully advanced through the vein, into the SVC, and into the right atrium. When it reaches the right atrium, the straight stylet is withdrawn and replaced with a J stylet. A J stylet is a stylet that has been formed into a J shape at the tip. A J stylet allows the physician to pass the lead tip in a prolapsed position over the tricuspid valve and into the right ventricle. If the straight stylet were used, it is possible that the lead tip (active or passive) could snag and possibly damage the tricuspid valve.

Once the lead is safely across the tricuspid valve and in the right ventricle, the physician will remove the J stylet and replace it with a straight stylet. At this point, the implanting physician must select the desired fixation site for the lead. Most implanters will select either the right ventricular apex (the tip of the heart or the most distal point in the right ventricle) or the right ventricular outflow tract (RVOT). The ventricular lead can also be fixated in the ventricular septum, but this is usually not the implanting physician's first choice. The decision as to where the right ventricular lead should be fixated is based on the patient's anatomy, the type of lead used, and the physician's preference.

Once the lead is in place, the implanting physician will secure or fixate it in place. If a passive-fixation lead is used, it is lodged or snagged into the dense trabeculae of the ventricles that hold it in place; eventually, it will fibrose in place. If an active-fixation lead is used, the physician will extend the helix and then turn or twist it into position. A variety of different active-fixation leads are available and most rely on a simple plastic tool that twists or turns the proximal end of the lead in a certain way to extend the helix and screw it into the myocardium.

This portion of the implantation sounds relatively straightforward, but it can be slow work because the lead has to be advanced very gently and with great care. Most of the clinical team will be watching the progress of the lead on the fluoroscope monitors in the room. When the lead is in proper position, intraoperative testing is conducted (see next section). If the implanting physician is happy with the intraoperative test values, the lead is left in place and the atrial lead is implanted.

It is not unusual for the implanting physician to reject the intraoperative values of a particular lead position. This would happen, for example, if the lead interfaced with diseased or damaged myocardial tissue. Since finding healthy myocardial tissue is a matter of trial and error (it cannot be identified using fluoroscopy!), the implanting physician may decide to move the lead and try again. Repositioning the lead is not uncommon during pacemaker implantation and may happen several times before the implanting physician is convinced that he or she has found optimal intraoperative values. Sometimes, even slightly repositioning the lead by a matter of millimeters can improve its performance.

When the physician is happy with lead position, the introducer is removed by breaking it apart. Grasping the two wings on the introducer, the introducer is pulled back and apart, taking care that the lead is not dislodged with it. The introducer is designed to break away neatly in this manner; it is then discarded. If another lead is implanted, a new introducer is needed.

Atrial lead

In a dual-chamber system, the atrial lead is typically implanted once the ventricular lead is in place. The implanting physician can do this using *one stick* by means of the retained guidewire technique. In this case, the guidewire is left in place but a second introducer sheath is required. The implanting physician places the new introducer sheath over the guidewire. Once the introducer is in place, the retained guidewire is removed and the atrial lead is inserted into the introducer and passed through the vein.

The physician now inserts a J stylet into the atrial lead. When the stylet is fully inserted into the lead, it takes on a straight shape to facilitate lead passage, but when the stylet is pulled back slightly, the stylet takes on its distal J shape. The stiffened atrial lead is inserted into the introducer and is passed through the vein under fluoroscopy until it reached the mid-right atrium. Most atrial leads use an extendable–retractable helix so the active-fixation mechanism is retracted within the lead at this point. The most frequently used implant site for the atrial lead is the right atrial appendage (RAA). Patients who have undergone a coronary artery bypass graft (CABG) or valve replacement procedure may not have an intact RAA; in such cases, the alternate position for the atrial lead is the lateral wall.

Once the lead is in the proper position, the implanting physician retracts the stylet slightly and the lead assumes its J shape, which *pops* it into the RAA or desired implant site. (Alternately, some physicians opt to implant the atrial lead with a straight stylet and switch it for a J stylet right before fixation.)

The physician now activates the active-fixation mechanism to screw the helix or corkscrew into the atrium.

Atrial leads are available in J shapes or straight. The atrial J lead is particularly useful for an RAA implantation and accounts for the lead's popularity. However, a straight atrial lead can be advantageous if the lead is to be fixated in the atrial lateral wall.

Active versus passive fixation

Pacing leads must be secured in the inside of the heart. Ventricular leads often use passive fixation mechanisms, such as fins or tines, which lodge in the trabeculae lining the interior of the ventricle. The fins or tines *snag* the lead into position, and over time, fibrosis grows over the interface between lead and tissue such that the lead is firmly in place in the heart. In fact, chronic leads are so securely fixated by fibrosis that they can be difficult to extract if that is ever necessary.

Atrial leads typically use active-fixation mechanisms because the interior of the atria tends to be smooth walled and possesses no trabeculae. Of course, active-fixation leads can also be used in the ventricles, if the implanting physician chooses. An active-fixation lead has a corkscrew or helix or another mechanism that is deployed and twisted or screwed into the heart. There are a number of active-fixation leads on the market and most usually involve a small tool to twist or turn to deploy the active-fixation mechanism. These leads are securely fixated right at implant and can be easier to remove, if necessary.

Implanting physicians may have ideas as to where they want the leads to be fixated, such as the right ventricular outflow tract, but finding the optimal lead location can involve some trial and error. Once a lead is secured in the heart, it has to be tested to be sure that the electrical characteristics are acceptable. A lead can be properly placed mechanically but yield suboptimal electrical results. In such cases, the physician moves the lead to a new spot and tests it again. It is not at all unusual during implant for a

physician to move the leads a few times to achieve the desired electrical performance.

Intraoperative testing

The electrical performance of the implanted leads is tested intraoperatively using a special peripheral device known as a pacing system analyzer (PSA). A PSA works like an external pacemaker and is used together with a programmer. As with other pacing equipment, there are different types and manufacturers, so that pacing experts need to be familiar with several systems. For our purposes, our descriptions will be somewhat generic with the caveat that the precise instructions for each device may vary.

A PSA is an external pacemaker that is used during the implant procedure to test the electrical performance and patient response of the implanted leads. While that is the main function of the PSA and the one that will occupy the most time for pacing experts, the PSA also should always be ready—at a moment's notice—to pace the ventricle. In an emergency situation, the clinical team counts on the PSA to deliver ventricular pacing support. Thus, the PSA should be set up well in advance of the procedure and the person operating the PSA must be mindful of its emergency pacing function. Most PSAs have an emergency or other red button for this purpose.

As each lead is implanted, a series of measurements are taken to confirm proper placement and optimal function of the lead at that particular location in the myocardium. In a dual-chamber system, the first lead implanted (almost always the ventricular lead) is tested before the second lead is implanted. In general, intraoperative measurements and tests might include:

- Sensing threshold
- Pacing impedance
- Stimulation threshold
- Slew rate
- Retrograde conduction time (not all patients have this)

These intraoperative measurements are taken primarily to assess that the lead is fixated in contact with healthy myocardial tissue and can function appropriately. Desired values appear in **Table 11.1**. These intraoperative values may differ from chronic desired values. For instance, *chronic* stimulation thresholds should be less than or equal to 3 V for atrial and ventricular leads, but intraoperative (acute) values are much lower. Stimulation thresholds can be expected to rise substantially from intraoperative values, so care must be taken to find appropriately low values at implant in order to provide good long-term results.

During implant, the implanting team will measure the patient's intrinsic R-waves (ventricular lead sensing) with the goal of finding an intrinsic R-wave of 5 mV or larger. During this test, no pacing is performed. An R-wave of this amplitude is suggestive of healthy myocardial tissue. There may be situations where despite numerous placements, the implant team cannot find a sufficiently large R-wave. In such cases, a second measurement may be taken; the slew rate provides the voltage over time, defined as volts per second (or millivolts per milliseconds). Another way to think of this is that slew rate is the *slope* of a signal, that is, how steep it is. Slew rate can be another measure of myocardial tissue health. Ideal values are at least 0.5 V/s. However, slew rates can change over time by as much as 25%. Not all implanting physicians will

measure slew rate, but it may be used to confirm viable myocardial tissue. If a slew rate value is desired, it is available as a one-button option on most PSAs.

Most PSAs measure intrinsic signals *peak to peak*, that is, from the highest point to the lowest point (see **Figure 11.4**). However, Boston Scientific pulse generators measure intrinsic signals from baseline to peak. There are two key take-away measures: the bigger the intrinsic R-wave, the better, and clinicians should not be surprised if the PSA measurement of an intrinsic signal differs— even substantially—from the implanted pulse generator's measurement of the intrinsic signal.

Pacing impedance is often measured at implant to evaluate lead integrity, that is, the proper function of the lead. Lead impedance values can only be measured during pacing, so the pacing function must be activated. In general, pacing impedance values are not particularly sensitive to lead location; lead impedance values will be similar whether the pacing lead is connected to healthy myocardial tissue or is free floating in the ventricular blood. The main point in measuring pacing lead impedance intraoperatively is to confirm that the lead is fully functional. The impedance value should fall within the ranges specified on the lead label or in the lead package insert; values are typically stated in broad ranges and can vary from lead to lead (for instance, 200 Ω may be an appropriate value for one type of lead but out of range for another). If pacing impedance values jump all around during intraoperative assessment, for instance, from 200 to 600 to 100 to 800 to 500 Ω and so on, that suggests that there is poor contact with the myocardial tissue and the lead should be repositioned. Because proper lead function is essential to stimulation thresholds, pacing impedance should be measured prior to stimulation threshold testing.

Table 11.1 Target value ranges for intraoperative for pacemaker implantation

	Atrial	Ventricular
Acute sensing threshold	≥2 mV	≥5 mV
Pacing impedance	Per specifications	Per specifications
Stimulation threshold at 0.5 ms	≤1.5 V	≤1.0 V
Slew rate	≥0.5 V/s (mV/ms)	≥0.5 V/s (mV/ms)
Retrograde conduction time (VDD/DDD)	100–400 ms (stable value, if present)	

Note that atrial and ventricular values are different.

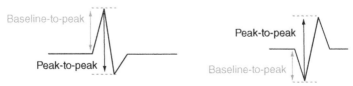

Figure 11.4 Pulse generators and PSAs may measure intrinsic signals in different ways, depending on whether they use a peak-to-peak measure or a baseline-to-peak measure.

Capture or stimulation threshold assessment is an important consideration because the patient's threshold determines how much energy the pacemaker will use to pace the heart. Thresholds that are initially high (and thresholds will increase somewhat over the next several weeks) can end up costing a lot of pacemaker energy and shortening the device's service life. Thresholds have been known to vary—sometimes considerably—by lead location. For this reason, the physician may ask that multiple threshold assessments at different locations be taken until an appropriate one is found. Threshold measurement is facilitated by annotations and markers, so that capture can be confirmed. The key point to remember in intraoperative threshold assessment is that the goal is to find the lowest possible threshold values.

The reason that stimulation threshold assessments are so crucial at implant is a process known as the acute-to-chronic threshold transition. This process describes how thresholds can change from the acute (implant) phase to the chronic phase (long-term use). The acute-to-chronic transition occurs in three main steps. At implant, the electrode of the lead touches myocardial tissue; this is the point at which the lowest possible capture thresholds are observed. In the first 4 weeks after implant, an inflammatory reaction occurs all around the electrode and changes the nature of the electrode/myocardial interface. At this point, there is a marked increase in stimulation threshold. Steroid-eluting leads attempt to minimize this inflammatory reaction, but it still occurs to some extent along with the threshold rise. (With older leads, the transition increased threshold values by a factor of 5; today with steroid-eluting leads, one can expect thresholds to roughly double at 1–4 weeks after implantation.) At about 6–12 weeks after implant, the inflammation subsides and a small bit of scar tissue (the *fibrotic capsule*) forms around the lead. Thresholds decrease to levels only slightly above the intraoperative stimulation threshold and stabilize (with a steroid-eluting lead, one can expect chronic thresholds to be about 1.5 times the intraoperative stimulation threshold) (see **Figure 11.5**). The fibrotic capsule around a chronically implanted lead is sometimes called the *virtual electrode*.

Retrograde conduction refers to the patient's ability to conduct an electrical impulse backward through the heart. Not all patients even have the ability to conduct in retrograde fashion. Retrograde conduction tests may be conducted intraoperatively or postoperatively, and many physicians do not do this sort of test unless it appears that the patient is having a problem with retrograde conduction. However, it is included in this list because some implanting physicians may opt to test for retrograde conduction at implant, which may be available as an automated or a semiautomated test. If retrograde conduction is found, the PVARP should be programmed to a value about 25 ms longer than the measured retrograde conduction time.

Diaphragmatic or phrenic nerve stimulation occurs when the pacing output pulse stimulates the diaphragm or phrenic nerve that can result in pocket twitching or hiccups in the patient. To test

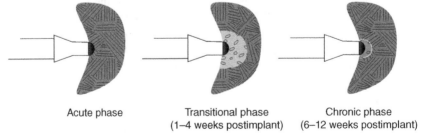

Acute phase   Transitional phase   Chronic phase
(1–4 weeks postimplant)   (6–12 weeks postimplant)

Figure 11.5 The acute-to-chronic transition is a physiologic process that is reflected in changing threshold values from the acute phase (at implant) to the chronic phase. The stimulation threshold is lowest in the acute phase when the pacing electrode makes direct contact with myocardial tissue. At 1–4 weeks after implant, inflammation around the lead/tissue interface causes a marked stimulation increase. As time passes, the inflammation subsides and a fibrotic capsule forms around the lead/tissue interface. At this point, around 6–12 weeks after implant, the pacing threshold decreases (but never again as low as acute values) and stabilizes to provide a chronic threshold value.

for diaphragmatic/phrenic nerve stimulation, a high output setting must be selected (typically 10 V) to pace each chamber as the clinical team checks for any possible inappropriate stimulation. The best way to assess this is to pace the heart while the clinician holds his or her hand over the patient's diaphragm to see if any twitching or stimulation is perceptible. If inappropriate stimulation occurs, the clinicians may try to find the voltage at which it occurs and make sure the pacemaker is programmed to values lower than that (for instance, stimulation occurs at ≥ 8 V but not below that). Better yet, the pacemaker leads should be repositioned to a spot where inappropriate stimulation does not occur even at 10 V.

Current of injury

The current of injury differs from the acute-to-chronic threshold transition described earlier.

An active-fixation lead is affixed with a corkscrew or helix into the heart muscle, causing an injury. While this is a temporary injury, it results in something called the *current of injury* that appears as an ST elevation on the electrogram. From an electrical standpoint, the current of injury represents that tiny area of the endocardium that was damaged and is now being irritated by the presence of an electrode. Current of injury is a temporary phenomenon and may only last 5 or 10 min. While current of injury is not generally a cause for alarm—it is transient—it can affect pacing and sensing thresholds when an active-fixation lead is secured in place and thresholds are tested immediately.

Closure

Once the implanting physician has obtained proper lead placement, the leads are plugged into the actual pulse generator that is placed in the pocket and sewn closed. The pocket is drenched in antibiotics and, ideally, offers a snug fit for the pacemaker that does not allow too much *wiggle room*.

In most pacemaker implant procedures, the patient is consciously sedated and the implant site numbed, but the patient is awake and responds to the clinical team. The clinical team is wise to address the patient occasionally and to find out if there is any discomfort. Be aware that the patient

does not really understand what is going on, so clinicians should avoid making remarks that could be misinterpreted. I once observed an implant procedure where a lead was being tested by the pacing thresholds that were very high in that particular location. One of the clinical team called out, "We're losing him!" The patient immediately panicked and required nitroglycerin, probably because he thought he was in danger, when in reality all the clinician meant was that capture was being lost at a specific location.

Complications

All surgery is associated with some degree of risk, including minimally invasive pacemaker implantation. Clinicians should think about complications as being acute, that is, associated with the implant procedure or the immediate postoperative period, and delayed. Delayed complications are those that become apparent or occur only after the passage of time.

The three most common general categories of acute complications involve venous access, lead placement, and pulse generator insertion (see **Table 11.2**). Pneumothorax can be thought of as air in the pleural cavity around the lungs. This can occur with and without symptoms; it is possible to find evidence of pneumothorax in an asymptomatic patient on a chest X-ray. If symptoms occur, they are typically going to be pleuritic or chest pain, difficulty breathing, and coughing. In some emergency situations, a chest tube may have to be inserted to help draw air out of the pleural cavity so that the lungs can reexpand. More minor cases of pneumothorax can often be treated with supplemental oxygen. As a general rule, symptoms tend to occur and be worse with more severe pneumothorax. Pneumothorax is, unfortunately, one of the more common pacemaker surgery complications.

Hemothorax involves the entry of blood into the thoracic cavity and occurs when the subclavian artery or vein (or some other vessels) is injured. Such injuries can often be managed by applying gentle pressure to the injury site, but severe cases may require drainage and surgical repair. Hemothorax is not a common complication and, when it does occur, can usually be treated effectively.

Table 11.2 It can help clinicians to understand the main types of complications as related to the aspect of implantation as well as whether the complications are likely to occur in the acute or delayed phase

	Acute complications	Delayed complications
Venous access	Pneumothorax	Lead perforation
	Hemothorax	
	Air or foreign body embolism	
	Perforation of the heart	
	Perforation of a central vein or artery	
	Entry into an artery	
Lead placement	Brady–tachy arrhythmias	Intravascular thrombosis
	Perforation of the heart	Intravascular constriction
	Perforation of central vein	Macrodislodgement of lead
	Damage to heart valve	Microdislodgement of lead
	Lead damage	Fibrosis at electrode/myocardial interface
	Improper lead connection	Infection
		Lead failure (insulation breach or conductor fracture)
		Retention wire fracture
		Chronic perforation
		Pericarditis
Pulse generator insertion	Wound pain	Pain
	Hematoma	Erosion
		Pocket infection
		Migration
		Premature failure
		Damage due to external energy
Patient condition	Unique to the patient	Twiddler syndrome
		Pacemaker extrusion
		Lead erosion

This list is by no means exhaustive, but it does capture the most frequently encountered complications.

Air embolism is usually obvious when it occurs, because the clinical team will hear a hissing sound as air is taken into the catheter. Fortunately, this complication has been drastically reduced by catheters today, which have one-way valves that do not allow for air to be sucked into the catheter. However, a deep inspiration by the patient may draw air into the system, which is one reason many implanting physicians do not want a pacemaker patient to be heavily sedated. Heavily sedated patients can start to snore and the deep inspirations in snoring can put a patient at risk for an air embolism. Symptoms include respiratory distress, chest pain, hypotension, and arterial oxygen desaturation. Treatment depends on the extent of the problem: supplemental oxygen may suffice for mild cases, while catheter aspiration or inotropic cardiac support

(e.g., with dobutamine) may be required in more severe cases.

Acute lead problems include arrhythmias. For example, passing a ventricular pacing lead into the right ventricle could brush up against the right bundle branches and trigger a ventricular tachyarrhythmia, tachy–brady syndrome, or asystole. It usually relates to an unexpected vagal reaction, excessive anesthesia, a bruise to the right bundle branch in a patient with left bundle branch block, or *ticklish* or hypersensitive ventricular tissue.

The lead can also perforate the heart and the perforation may be internal (from one chamber to another chamber) or external (from the heart into the pericardium). Lead perforations are probably far more common than we realize because the heart is often able to seal itself very quickly and effectively and the problem is never noticed. However, larger perforations may provoke symptoms such as chest pain and tamponade. Signs of perforation include an extremely distal lead position, an ECG pattern with right bundle branch block, poor sensing characteristics, and poor or very high threshold values. The population at highest risk for lead perforation is small-framed women with heart failure. If severe lead perforation occurs, pericardiocentesis drainage may be needed.

The ventricular pacing lead may also damage the tricuspid valve as it passes over it.

Lead connection problems should also be considered a potential implant complication. This may involve loose or improperly tightened setscrews on the header or putting the leads into the wrong ports (such as an atrial lead in the ventricular port and vice versa). Loose setscrews may show up on an ECG or electrogram as noise.

Delayed complications can be grouped into three main categories: those related to the patient's condition, those related to lead placement, and finally those related to generator insertion.

One of the most unusual (and not infrequent) late complications of pacemaker implantation is Twiddler syndrome, which is caused by the patient manipulating the implant site to the point that the generator is moved and leads are dislodged or loosened. Twiddler syndrome is usually not diagnosed until sensing problems or lead complications occur. When diagnosed and confirmed on X-ray, it usually requires surgical revision.

Infection remains the most common complication of device implantation and is delayed but can be defined as early (within 60 days of implant) and late (any point after 60 days). The most common pathogen involved is *Staphylococcus aureus*. When infection occurs, the pacemaker and lead(s) must be removed and antimicrobial therapy begun. A new device and lead system can be implanted at a later date. Because of the patient's risk for morbidity and mortality, *the entire system* must be removed. Note that delayed pain is often a sign of possible infection.

Some complications such as a mild pocket hematoma or a small degree of wound pain often resolve on their own with conservative management. Wound pain and tenderness may occur right after surgery but should diminish over time; pain that persists or worsens days after implant suggests infection. The best treatment for hematoma is observation; unless the patient is decompensating or there is evidence to support an intervention, avoid inserting anything into the wound site. Hematomas are not uncommon and most resolve on their own with time.

Patient education

The physician and his or her clinical team officially provide patient education for the pacemaker recipient and the family, but this does not mean that other people are not asked questions. Providing clear *nonmedical* answers can be very helpful and reassuring, particularly about the pacemaker implant procedure.

First, patients should be encouraged to discuss their particular surgery with the physician because there are many factors that can vary by individual. For instance, many people stay overnight in the hospital when they get a pacemaker—but sometimes patients get pacemakers as outpatients and other patients may need to be hospitalized for a few days. Most patients receive conscious sedation during implantation, but others will be under general anesthesia. Patients should be informed that even if they are awake, they will be given numbing medicine for the surgery and a medicine to relax them. They should not experience pain, although it is possible during the procedure that they may feel some sensations and pressure.

Most device manufacturers publish patient manuals and other materials specifically aimed at helping people understand their pacemakers and pacemaker surgery. Physicians should be encouraged to request such free materials to provide to their patients.

Conclusion

Pacemaker implantation is a minimally invasive procedure in which one or more leads are implanted and connected to a pulse generator implanted in a pocket in the upper chest. Leads are implanted by venous access using an introducer kit. The two most commonly used veins are the subclavian vein (subclavian stick) or the cephalic vein (cephalic cutdown). An introducer kit is used with a guidewire and introducer to facilitate introduction of the transvenous lead into the vein; the lead is maneuvered under fluoroscopy through the vein and into the heart, where it is attached to the endocardium (inside of the heart). In a dual-chamber system, the ventricular lead is placed first. Different implant techniques may allow for one guidewire to be used for implanting two leads (*retained guidewire technique*). Once in place, leads are tested using a PSA, which will measure the acute sensing threshold(s), pacing lead impedance, and stimulation threshold(s). For sensing thresholds, the larger the intrinsic signal, the better. If an optimal intrinsic signal cannot be found, the physician may decide to reposition the lead and test again. Stimulation thresholds are measured and also should be as low as possible, since they should increase in the acute-to-chronic transition (about double in 1–4 weeks postimplant and then about 1.5 times the acute threshold at about 6–12 weeks for the chronic value). Pacing impedance evaluates lead integrity (not lead location) and values should fall within the manufacturer's specified range. It is possible to evaluate slew rate (the slope of the signal) and retrograde conduction at implant, but these measurements are less frequently taken. An active-fixation lead will produce an ST-segment elevation on the electrogram known as the *current of injury* for about 10 min after implant; this is a transient phenomenon. Although pacemaker surgery is minimally invasive and is often performed under conscious sedation, all surgery is associated with a risk of complications. Patient education prior to implantation can help manage patient anxiety and expectations.

The nuts and bolts of pacemaker implantation

- Pacemaker implantation is considered minimally invasive surgery and is often performed under conscious sedation on an outpatient basis or with an overnight hospital stay. Pacemaker surgery is often performed in an EP lab or a cath lab, but can also be performed in an operating room.
- The implant site is typically numbed with lidocaine or xylocaine and the patient is given a light sedative but is awake during the procedure.
- The two main venous access sites are the subclavian vein (subclavian stick) or the cephalic vein (cephalic cutdown). Less frequently, the axillary vein is used.
- An introducer kit is used for lead implantation. The two main types are those with and without a hemostatic valve to help manage blood flow and prevent bleed-back.
- A syringe and needle are needed for subclavian stick. The biggest drawback to subclavian stick is the risk of subclavian crush. Proper lead insertion can minimize the risk of subclavian crush.
- A guidewire is a thin wire (0.035 in. in diameter) that is used to *guide* the passage of the lead. The guidewire is inserted into the vein first and passed into the superior vena cava (SVC) of the heart. Once in place, the guidewire becomes the *placeholder* for the introducer.
- The introducer kit contains a dilatator (or dilator) for optional dilation or stretching of the vein.
- A stylet (thin wire) is inserted into the pacing lead to temporarily stiffen it; the stylet and lead are inserted through the introducer and passed under fluoroscopy through the vein. Once in place, the stylet is withdrawn from the lead and discarded.
- Dual-chamber pacemakers require two leads: one in the right atrium and one in the right ventricle. In most cases, the right ventricular lead is implanted first. In an emergency situation, a patient may require ventricular pacing support.
- The diameter of leads and introducers is stated in French (abbreviated Fr). Typical lead and introducer sizes might be 7, 8, or 9 Fr.
- Leads are fixated to the endocardium using active-fixation (helix, corkscrew) or passive-fixation (tines, fins) mechanisms.
- Once the lead is in place, it must be tested to be sure it is making contact with healthy myocardial tissue. This testing is done with a pacing system analyzer (PSA).

- During implant, the clinical team will want to measure the intraoperative sensing threshold (the size of the intrinsic signal), the intraoperative stimulation or capture threshold, and the pacing lead impedance. Pacing lead impedance assesses the integrity of the pacing lead. Other tests that might be performed during implant include the slew rate (the slope of the signal) and retrograde conduction, but this type of testing is less common. Many physicians will also test for diaphragmatic and phrenic nerve stimulation at implant.
- The acute sensing threshold test measures the patient's native P-wave (atrial lead) and R-wave (ventricular lead). A good rule of thumb with the intraoperative sensing threshold is *the bigger, the better*. Atrial signals should ideally be 2 mV or larger, while ventricular signals should be 5 mV or larger. If such signals cannot be found, the implanting physician may reposition the lead.
- No pacing should be going on during sensing threshold testing.
- During pacing impedance testing, the PSA must pace the heart. The lead impedance value is taken and compared to the manufacturer's stated specification (in the package labeling). Pacing lead impedance verifies proper function of the lead, not its proper position in the heart.
- An intraoperative capture or stimulation threshold test is performed using the PSA. The acute capture threshold is the lowest it will ever be. The acute-to-chronic transition defines an increase in capture at 1–4 weeks after implantation and then a decrease at 6–12 weeks. Although the chronic threshold decreases from the maximum, it will be about 1.5 times the acute value for a steroid-eluting lead.
- The purpose of slew rate testing is to confirm that the myocardial tissue where the lead is affixed is healthy. This test may be omitted, particularly when good sensing values are obtained.
- Clinicians may notice that signal measurements differ between a PSA and a device. Actually, devices and pulse generators may measure signals peak to peak or baseline to peak.
- Retrograde conduction may also be measured at implant as an automatic PSA test but not all implanting physicians will do this. Not all patients even have retrograde conduction, which is the heart's ability to conduct an electrical pulse backward along the conduction pathways.
- The PSA offers emergency ventricular pacing in the form of a one-button function. This is rarely necessary, but the clinical team should be familiar with how to initiate emergency ventricular pacing via the PSA during intraoperative testing.
- Current of injury refers to a transient ST-segment elevation of the electrogram following implantation of an active-fixation lead. This phenomenon typically lasts about 10 min and resolves on its own.
- Pacemaker surgery is considered minimally invasive, but there is always a risk for complications. Although rare, complications of pacemaker implantation surgery include pneumothorax, hemothorax, lead perforation, cardiac tamponade, hematoma of the pocket, wound pain, and infection. Early infection (within 60 days of implant) is usually easier to detect than late infection. If a pacemaker system is infected, all of its components must be extracted and antimicrobial therapy must be conducted.
- Patient education is recommended before implantation to help the patient know what to expect during surgery, to reduce anxiety, and to help manage patient expectations and improve patient satisfaction.

Test your knowledge

1 Which of these veins is *never used* for pacemaker implantation?
  A Axillary vein
  B Subclavian vein
  C Carotid vein
  D Cephalic vein

2 In some implants, the implanting physician will use the needle to make a *stick* and then examine the blood that is drawn back into the syringe. What is the physician looking for?
  A Bright red blood.
  B Blood under high pressure.

C Dark blood.

D No blood at all should be in the syringe.

3 All of the following are typical components of an introducer kit except for which item?

A Surgical markers

B Guidewire

C Needle

D Syringe

4 What is the main advantage of the *retained guidewire technique*?

A You can reuse the guidewire in multiple patients, saving money.

B You can use one guidewire to insert two leads for a dual-chamber pacemaker.

C You keep the guidewire in place, eliminating the need for fluoroscopy.

D No stylet is needed in the lead.

5 In a dual-chamber pacing system, which statement is *not true* about the atrial lead?

A It might be straight or J shaped.

B It is almost always implanted after the ventricular lead.

C It is usually a passive-fixation lead.

D It is often implanted in the right atrial appendage.

6 If emergency ventricular pacing were ever required during an implant, how would this most likely be carried out?

A External defibrillator.

B The physician would hurry and hook up the pacemaker to the external leads.

C The emergency button on the PSA.

D The clinical team would perform CPR.

7 The intraoperative sensing threshold value for a ventricular lead should be:

A At least 10 mV

B ≥5 mV

C ≥2 mV

D 1 V

8 The intraoperative stimulation threshold is:

A The lowest value it will ever be

B Measured in volts at 0.5 ms

C Will be lower than 1.5 or 1.0 V, depending on the chamber

D All of the above

9 What is the current of injury?

A It describes the inflammatory process that occurs about 1–4 weeks after lead implant.

B It is one of the most common pacing complications and requires removal of the entire pacing system.

C It is responsible for threshold increases of up to five times the intraoperative value.

D It describes a transient ST-segment elevation on the electrogram that lasts about 10 min.

10 If it is determined that a pacemaker is infected, what step is the most appropriate course of action?

A Remove all of the components of the system and begin antimicrobial therapy.

B Remove only the infected part(s) of the system and begin antimicrobial therapy.

C Leave the pacemaker system in place but begin antimicrobial therapy.

D Call the manufacturer and determine the appropriate course of action.

Reference

1 Seldinger, S.I. (1953) Catheter replacement of the needle in percutaneous arteriography: a new technique. *Acta Radiologica*, **39** (5), 368–376.

CHAPTER 12

Connecting the leads to the pulse generator

Learning objectives

- Briefly walk through the main steps in connecting a lead to a pulse generator.
- Explain the difference between an IS-1 and an IS-1 Compatible lead and IPG.
- Know confidently the proper ports for atrial and ventricular leads in all IPGs.
- Describe the proper use of the torque tool and some common pitfalls.
- State what a single-pass lead is and why it might be used.

Introduction

The implantable pulse generator (IPG) relies on the proper connection of one or more leads for its operation. This seemingly straightforward step was not always easy. Historically, the earliest pacemakers had unique headers and lead connectors, making it difficult to use leads from one manufacturer with another manufacturer's IPG—in fact, sometimes, leads from a manufacturer did not fit even in all of the IPGs from that manufacturer! Today, standardized connectors make this much simpler and leads and IPGs from different companies work well together. However, attaching leads to the pulse generator is not necessarily a simple process; it must be done with care. Clinicians will find the greatest challenges not with new device implantations but when replacing an IPG and using an indwelling lead system. Leads typically have long service lives, so it is not unusual to see older types of leads during replacements. Clinicians should do their homework prior to a generator replacement to know what lead(s) the clinical team is going to encounter to make sure that the replacement IPG is compatible.

Implantable pulse generator

The IPG is hermetically sealed to prevent the intrusion of bodily fluids into the circuitry and battery of the device. A feedthrough wire in the header of the IPG allows electrical current to flow between the circuitry (encased in the IPG) and the leads. The feedthrough connects to the IPG's internal circuitry. When the lead is properly in plugged into the port, the lead is connected by way of the feedthrough wire to the internal circuitry of the IPG.

The leads plug into the clear epoxy header (also called the connector) of the IPG. In order to achieve the proper fit, the lead must be the right size for the header. When the lead is properly plugged into the port, sealing rings help create a seal so that bodily fluids do not infiltrate the lead port. These sealing rings can be located on the lead or in the port (or both). When selecting leads for a particular device, the clinician must look at lead size and sealing ring configuration.

Today, we use International Standard-1 (IS-1) and IS-1 Compatible lead and header configurations. This configuration will be stated prominently on the lead and IPG product labels. It is possible to use leads from one manufacturer with an IPG from

The Nuts and Bolts of Implantable Device Therapy Pacemakers, First Edition. Tom Kenny.
© 2015 John Wiley & Sons, Ltd. Published 2015 by John Wiley & Sons, Ltd.

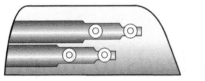 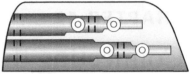

IS-1   IS-1 compatible

Figure 12.1 IS-1 and IS-1 Compatible leads and headers differ in terms of length of the lead receptacle and the location of sealing rings. The IS-1 header has no sealing rings, while the IS-1 Compatible header has sealing rings.

another manufacturer, provided that both are either IS-1 or IS-1 Compatible (see **Figure 12.1**).

IS-1 leads are 3.2 mm in diameter, have sealing rings on the lead itself, and have a relatively short terminal pin. IS-1 leads are available in unipolar and bipolar configurations. The IS-1 IPG has a port that accommodates such a lead; there will not be sealing rings in the IPG port. Since leads generally have a very long service life, clinicians will often encounter older leads. In fact, clinicians may often encounter the old VS-1 leads (no longer manufactured but still indwelling in many patients), which have a short terminal pin and sealing rings—they are in many ways similar to the modern IS-1 lead.

Leads

The extreme proximal end of the lead plugs into the connector block (or header) of the IPG. This end of the lead is sometimes called the terminal pin. The terminal pin itself acts as an electrode; in a bipolar lead, there will also be a ring electrode. Pacing leads can be visually inspected at either proximal or distal ends to determine whether or not they are unipolar (one electrode) or bipolar (two electrodes, best visualized as the presence of a ring electrode). To establish a good connection and prevent the intrusion of bodily fluids, there must be sealing rings. Sealing rings may be present on the lead (see **Figure 12.2**) or in the IPG port.

However, you may also encounter some historical oddities. The *low-profile* or LP lead has a 3.2 mm diameter but differs from the IS-1/VS-1 leads in that it has a long terminal pin and no sealing rings on the lead. The *LP* name comes from the fact that the lead does not have sealing rings and has a smaller profile; some clinicians use the LP name as a mnemonic device to remember that LP leads have a *long pin*. A 3.2 mm LP lead must be plugged into an IPG with sealing rings in the IPG port. LP leads are no longer manufactured, but it may occur in clinical practice that a clinician will want to plug an indwelling and still viable LP lead into a new IPG during generator replacement. To accommodate this kind of revision, an IS-1 Compatible IPG can be used. An IS-1 Compatible IPG was designed specifically to accommodate this kind of older lead (see **Figure 12.3**). Even older leads are the 5 and 6 mm leads; these are becoming very rare in clinical practice and have not been manufactured in years.

An IS-1 lead can be connected to an IPG with an IS-1 header or an IS-1 Compatible header. In the event that an IS-1 lead (with sealing rings) is plugged into an IS-1 Compatible IPG, sealing rings will be present on both the lead and the IPG receptacle. This is not a problem. As long as sealing rings are present (either on the lead, in the receptacle, or both), the lead can work. In the event that an IS-1 lead is plugged into an IS-1 Compatible receptacle, some resistance might be felt as the lead is pushed into place because of the sealing rings on both lead and receptacle. In the box with the IPG are several accessories, including a small vial of sterile silicone oil. When plugging an IS-1 lead into an IS-1 Compatible port, a drop or two of silicone oil can facilitate lead insertion.

Lead insertion

By far, the most common clinical scenario will be the insertion of an IS-1 lead into an IS-1 pulse generator; this will undoubtedly be the case for new implants and is very common for pulse generator replacements. The IS-1 lead has a short terminal pin and sealing rings on the lead; it is inserted into the IS-1 header port with a short receptacle and two connector blocks for setscrews. For proper lead function, the lead pin must be fully inserted into the lead receptacle, that is, the tip of the terminal

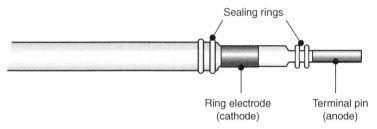

Sealing rings

Ring electrode
(cathode)

Terminal pin
(anode)

Figure 12.2 The terminal pin of a bipolar IS-1 lead. Note the sealing rings on the lead body. Sealing rings may be located on the lead, in the IPG receptacle, or both, but there must be sealing rings to assure a tight seal and prevent fluid intrusion.

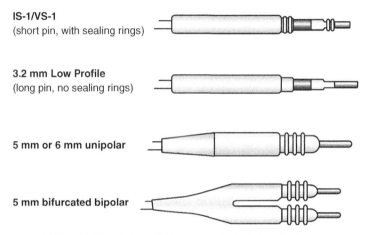

IS-1/VS-1
(short pin, with sealing rings)

3.2 mm Low Profile
(long pin, no sealing rings)

5 mm or 6 mm unipolar

5 mm bifurcated bipolar

Figure 12.3 While the top lead (IS-1) is the only type of lead manufactured today, clinicians may encounter some older leads during IPG revision. These include the VS-1 (similar to IS-1, top), the low-profile lead with its characteristic long pin and no sealing rings, and the wider 5 and 6mm leads. These last two leads are rarely, if ever, encountered in clinical practice today.

pin must be fully inserted into the port. The best way to check for proper insertion is to look through the clear header and make sure that the distal pin is visible beyond the second setscrew and is fully inserted to the end of the port (see **Figure 12.4**).

In a dual-chamber pacemaker, the atrial lead plugs into the top receptacle, while the ventricular lead plugs into the bottom receptacle. There are no dual-chamber devices that do it differently: atrial is on top and ventricular is on the bottom (similar to cardiac anatomy, the atria are the upper chambers and the ventricles are the lower chambers). The ventricular lead is nearly always placed first in the patient. The implanting physician will plug the ventricular lead into the lower receptacle, make sure it is fully inserted, and then tighten the setscrew. Once the lead is securely in position, the clinical team

should observe the surface ECG to confirm the presence of ventricular pacing. Ventricular pacing is a good confirmation that the ventricular lead is in the right port! Another good way to double-check this is to look at the model numbers of the leads, which should be visible from both the lead labels on the packages and on the lead itself, near the point at which the lead plugs into the header. A team member can call out the lead model number and state whether it is in the top or bottom port while another clinician checks the lead labels to confirm that it is the appropriate (atrial or ventricular) lead.

Once the lead is fully inserted into the lead receptacle, the implanting physician uses a small tool (included in the IPG box with the accessories) and tightens each of the two setscrews. This tool is called a torque wrench or wrench; it is sterile and

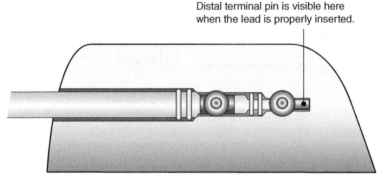

Distal terminal pin is visible here
when the lead is properly inserted.

Figure 12.4 An IS-1 lead inserted into an IS-1 connector must be fully inserted for proper function. The distal end of the terminal pin will be visible through the clear epoxy header and should extend completely to the end of the lead receptacle.

included in the IPG box with the pacemaker accessories. The pointed end of the tool is inserted through a self-sealing rubber septum to engage the setscrew and tighten it. The tool is specifically designed and calibrated to apply just the right amount of torque to tighten the setscrew firmly, but there is a bit of technique to learn. The wrench should be held perpendicular (straight) with respect to the header. Each turn will produce an audible click. Turning the tool too much (beyond three clicks) or not enough (less than three clicks) may result in an improper lead connection. The purpose of the setscrews is to hold the lead securely in place. If they are not properly tightened, the lead may be too loose (and wiggle out of place or have only intermittent electrical connection), or the setscrews may be damaged by overtightening, which can also result in a loose lead. Most experienced implanters have developed good technique with tightening the setscrews, but one potential problem can occur when the implanting physician removes the torque wrench somewhat laterally—which can lead to a loose lead. As soon as the three clicks occur, the tool should be removed by pulling it straight upward (not sideways) (see **Figure 12.5**).

After the setscrews are properly tightened, the implanting physician will tug lightly on the lead to confirm that it is securely held in place by the setscrews.

Troubleshooting lead connections

Lead connection problems are largely preventable with the right techniques. However, clinicians will encounter situations where there are device prob-

lems that can be traced back to a faulty lead connection. When a lead connection problem is suspected, an X-ray of the pulse generator can help. With an X-ray, you may be able to confirm:

- Leads are in proper ports (atrial on top, ventricular on the bottom).
- Leads are fully inserted (tip of terminal pin visible at end of receptacle).

Poor lead connection will manifest as very high impedance values along with intermittent or constant problems with capture and sensing. These problems tend to get worse with time. The only way to fix a problem with an improperly connected lead is to take the patient back to surgery. This is an extreme solution to a problem that is often preventable!

The single-pass lead (VDD)

A single-pass lead (also called a VDD lead) has a unique design that gives it two terminal pins but only a single distal end. Designed for use with VDD(R) pulse generators, the lead actually has two sets of electrodes: a far distal set (for use in the ventricle) and a more proximal pair of ring electrodes, which are located in the atrium and are able to pace through the atrial blood pool. While relatively unusual in the USA, these leads are more frequently used in Europe and other locations. The concept of a VDD pacemaker is pace and sense in the ventricle and sense in the atrium, making it a kind of *single-chamber dual-chamber* pacemaker. This type of lead is sometimes called a *single-pass* lead because one single lead offers dual-chamber sensing along with single-chamber pacing. The main advantage to a single-pass lead is its simplicity; it offers atrial

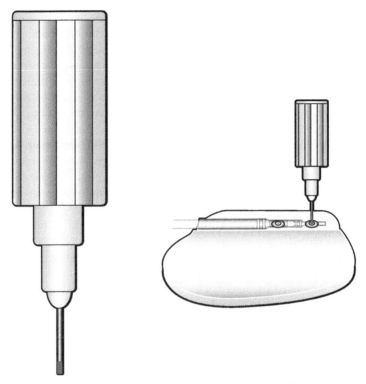

Figure 12.5 The physician uses a special tool called a torque wrench included in the IPG accessories to insert into the self-sealing rubber septum and tighten the setscrews (shown left, much enlarged). The implanting physician uses the tip of the torque wrench to pierce the septum over the setscrew; the tip engages the setscrew. Still holding the tool straight up, the setscrew is tightened with three audible clicks. The tool is removed by pulling it straight up and away (not laterally); the septum closes back over the setscrew and prevents fluids from entering the lead receptacle and connector block.

sensing (and atrial tracking) in what is essentially a single-chamber design (see **Figure 12.6**).

Characteristics of the ideal lead

The pacing lead is a vitally important component of the pacing system. When there are device problems or voluntary recalls, they often involve the pacing lead. While the perfect pacing lead has not been invented yet, pacing specialists agree on their ideal characteristics:

- Long-lasting
- Durable
- Stable
- Flexible
- Biocompatible
- Corrosion resistant
- Easy to pass through the vein
- Easy to fixate in the heart
- Efficient in delivering energy

- Low stimulation thresholds
- Excellent sensing characteristics

Leads have to be designed to work reliably in one of the harshest environments on earth—inside the human body. Considering that leads in the heart have to flex with every beat of the heart, it is clear that this is a *high-stress* environment. Imagine how a power cord to a lamp, for example, might function if it were flexed once a second for 10 or 20 years. Modern leads are extraordinary products of advanced engineering, but they can be vulnerable to problems associated with their design, implantation, or long-term wear.

Lead extraction

It sometimes becomes necessary to remove an indwelling pacing lead. In fact, clinicians are facing lead extractions more and more often for several reasons:

- More leads are being implanted (1.2 million new leads are implanted every year).
- Today's more complex devices may require more leads (an advanced CRT system of today requires three leads compared to the single-lead pacemaker of not so long ago).
- People are living longer—which means they may have pacemakers for 20, 30, 40, or more years.
- When devices get upgraded, sometimes, the old leads become redundant.
- Leads can break, tear, or suffer other malfunctions.
- Infection.
- Over time, veins can become overcrowded or become blocked or weakened.

When an indwelling lead is no longer to be used, the physician has two options. The first is that the lead can be capped and abandoned, meaning that it is unplugged from the pulse generator, capped so that it is electrically inactive, and left in place.

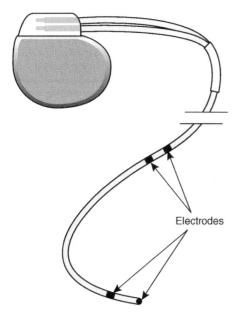

Figure 12.6 A single-pass lead is a specially designed lead for use with a VDD pacemaker. A VDD pacemaker, as the name implies, paces and senses in the ventricle and senses in the atrium. A lead is bifurcated at the proximal end and plugs into two pulse generator receptacles (atrial and ventricular). The bifurcations merge and form a single-lead body with just one pair of distal electrodes (this is a bipolar system) to be affixed in the ventricle for pacing and sensing. Two ring electrodes on the lead *float* in the right atrium and can provide sensing (the electrodes can sense through the atrial blood pool).

Capping an indwelling lead is usually a relatively simple process during a pulse generator revision, but the downside of abandoning a lead in place is that it leaves unnecessary hardware in the body. In the future, it may be more difficult or even impossible to insert a new lead because the vein is too crowded. Furthermore, leaving an abandoned lead in the body may be associated with elevated risks of venous thrombosis, infection, and endocarditis. The other option involves removing or extracting the lead. This offers the clear advantage that the patient is rid of the unnecessary hardware and that the lead cannot damage the body or *clog up* the veins. However, lead extraction is a surgical procedure that historically has been associated with morbidity and mortality risks. New tools and techniques, specifically in the field of laser-assisted lead removal, have reduced these risks but require special training on the part of the physician. There are physicians and centers that specialize in lead extraction, and when possible, patients requiring lead removal should be referred to these specialists. As with many procedures, higher-volume centers statistically show higher success rates. However, even with the newest tools in the hands of experts, lead extraction carries with it a risk of procedural mortality (<1%) and patients should be made aware of the risks and benefits of a lead extraction procedure.

There are many factors to consider when a patient has a redundant lead. Extracting a lead becomes increasingly more difficult the longer the lead is in place; thus, if a lead is to be removed surgically, the sooner the better. Another factor is the patient's age and health; leaving such a lead in place with a *wait-and-see* attitude may cause the patient to face lead extraction at an older age or with a comorbidity. On the other hand, some pacemaker patients with redundant leads may simply not be good candidates for surgery, on account of frailty, advanced age, or other conditions.

Methods of lead extraction

In the early days of pacing, the only way to remove a lead was simple traction. If the lead had not been in the body very long, this method was reasonably efficient. Active-fixation leads could be unscrewed from position and pulled. Ventricular passive-fixation leads were much more challenging because they fibrosed into place in the dense network of trabeculae in the ventricle. A chronic ventricular passive-fixation lead was literally fibrosed into the heart—making it very stable but also very hard to remove. Soon, more advanced traction devices were developed to ease this type of procedure, but lead extraction at that time carried significant morbidity and mortality risks to the patient.

New equipment includes mechanical sheaths, laser sheaths, electrosurgical sheaths, rotating threaded-tip sheaths, and telescoping sheaths, all of which surround and *cut out* the lead. The idea is that the sheath is advanced over the lead until it comes to a place where the lead is attached to the interior of the heart. Once it hits one of these so-called binding sites, the laser or other tool is activated so that the binding site can be ablated. Once the binding site is cleared, the sheath advanced forward, to the next binding site. Eventually, all of the tissue holding the lead in place is removed and the lead can be extracted with gentle traction.

These devices and techniques can be highly effective, but the procedures still have a complication rate of around 2%. Typical complications for lead extraction include death, cardiac avulsion, pulmonary embolism, pericardial effusion, hemothorax, hematoma, migration of lead fragments, tearing of surrounding blood vessels, perforation of the heart, blood clots, and stroke.

The nuts and bolts of connecting the lead to the pulse generator

- The IPG is hermetically sealed to prevent fluid intrusion. When a lead is plugged into the receptacle on the header, a feedthrough wire allows for the electrical connection of the lead to the IPG circuitry.
- Today, leads and pulse generators are standardized (IS-1) and leads from any manufacturer can be plugged into IPGs from any manufacturer.
- The two main connector standards that clinicians will encounter today are IS-1 (this is the one being manufactured today) and IS-1 Compatible. IS-1 Compatible is older but may be seen during IPG replacement surgery.
- An IS-1 or IS-1 Compatible lead has a 3.2 mm diameter. IS-1 leads have a short terminal pin and sealing rings on the lead itself. IS-1 Compatible leads have a longer terminal pin and no sealing rings.
- Sealing rings must be present on the lead, in the IPG receptacle, or both.
- The low-profile (LP) 3.2 mm lead is no longer manufactured but may be indwelling in some patients. It has no sealing rings (which is why it is called *low profile*) and a long terminal pin.
- Historically, 5 and 6 mm diameter leads were manufactured but are almost never encountered in clinical practice today.
- In the event that a clinician wants to insert an IS-1 lead (with sealing rings on the lead) into an IS-1 Compatible header (with sealing rings in the receptacle), a drop or two of sterile silicone oil may be needed to facilitate lead insertion.
- The lead should be inserted so that the terminal pin is pushed all the way into the lead receptacle; this can be visually confirmed by looking through the header to see the tip of the terminal pin.
- In a dual-chamber system, the atrial lead port is always on top and the ventricular lead port is always on the bottom. Plugging the leads into the wrong ports will result in system malfunction and necessitate revision surgery. Unfortunately, this is not an unheard-of complication!
- Once the lead is in the header receptacle and pushed all the way in, a torque wrench is used to tighten the setscrew through a self-sealing septum. The torque wrench should be inserted and pulled out straight (not laterally). It should be pushed through the self-sealing septum to engage with the setscrew and then turned until three audible clicks are heard.
- Once the two setscrews are tightened, the implanting physician will tug lightly on the lead to confirm that the setscrews are holding the lead securely in place.
- When troubleshooting lead problems, it may be necessary to use a chest X-ray. A chest X-ray can show if the leads are in the proper ports and fully inserted into the receptacles.

Continued

Continued

> • Leads are designed to be robust and flexible, have good electrical performance, and be easy to implant. If there is a breakdown in a pacemaker system, the lead is often involved. In fact, in terms of product recalls, leads are recalled more often than IPGs or programmers.
> • A single-pass lead senses and paces in the ventricle and senses in the atrium (VDD function) as a single lead. It has two terminal pins but only one distal end. Atrial sensing is performed by two ring electrodes that float in the atrial blood pool and can sense (but not pace).
>
> Although not very common in the USA, single-pass leads are used more extensively in some parts of the world. They offer a good and simple solution for single-chamber pacing with the added benefit of atrial tracking.
> • Lead extraction or removal can be necessary for any number of reasons, including to remove a damaged or broken lead. In the early days of pacing, lead extraction was associated with a risk of morbidity and mortality. Today, lead extraction using laser sheath technology has made the procedure much safer.

Test your knowledge

1 What is the diameter of pacing leads today?
  A 3.2 mm
  B 5 mm
  C 5/6 mm
  D They vary

2 Please select the newest lead and pulse generator standard.
  A VNS-1
  B VAS-1
  C IS-1
  D IS-1 Compatible

3 When selecting an IPG for a generator replacement that will use indwelling leads, what is an important consideration in choosing the IPG?
  A Leads and generator must be compatible (IS-1, IS-1 Compatible).
  B Leads and generator must be from the same manufacturer.
  C Leads must always have sealing rings or an adapter is needed.
  D All of the above.

4 Pick the true statement.
  A Sealing rings are always located on the lead.
  B Sealing rings can be on the lead or in the IPG receptacle but never both.

C Sealing rings are the same as wire feedthroughs.
  D Sealing rings can be on the lead, in the IPG receptacle, or both.

5 The IPG box contains some sterile accessories including:
  A Lead adapters
  B A torque wrench and silicone oil
  C An extra lead
  D Sealing rings

6 When implanting a dual-chamber pacemaker, which receptacle in the header is used for the ventricular lead?
  A The top one.
  B The bottom one.
  C It does not matter; they both work with either lead.
  D It does matter, but it varies by manufacturer and device model.

7 When inserting a lead into the IPG receptacle, what should the implanting physician do to confirm that the lead is fully inserted?
  A Visually confirm that he or she can see the lead tip all the way at the end of the receptacle.
  B Visually confirm proper insertion on a chest X-ray.

C Listen for audible clicks.

D Tug on the lead.

8 When using the torque wrench, how does the implanting physician know when the setscrew is properly tightened?

A It will not turn anymore.

B An indicator light will blink.

C Three audible clicks are heard.

D It is a matter of *feel* and experience.

9 After implantation of a single-chamber system, the physician observes off-the-chart impedance values and intermittent capture and sensing problems. What does this suggest and what should he or she do?

A It suggests an infection and the entire system should be removed at once.

B It suggests that the lead is loose; an X-ray should be taken and, if necessary, surgery must be performed to tighten it.

C It suggests that the lead has broken; an X-ray should be taken and, if necessary, the entire lead ought to be replaced.

D The system can most likely be fixed by reprogramming lead impedance settings.

10 Which of the following is an approved and well-known technology used to extract indwelling pacemaker leads?

A Neurolysis

B Cryosurgical ablation

C Lithotripsy

D Laser sheath ablation

CHAPTER 13

Pacemaker modes and codes

Introduction

In the early days of pacing, several manufacturers had devices on the market. While these devices had similar functions, each manufacturer employed its own unique terminology to describe device function. In some cases, three different companies might use three different terms to describe the very same thing. The result was a lot of confused clinicians! The Inter-Society Commission for Heart Disease (ICHD) was formed by a group of concerned physicians to help standardize the ways pacemakers were being described. The original ICHD code was published in 1974. Since that time, the code has evolved with pacemaker technology.

This chapter discusses the current rather than the historical code, although we should be aware of why and how pacemaker codes got started in the first place.

Among other things, the code differentiates single-chamber from dual-chamber devices. This chapter will not only discuss how the codes work and explain these differences, but it will also go into reasons why a physician might select a single-chamber versus a dual-chamber device. There are not only specific indications for single-chamber and dual-chamber pacemakers, but there may be other factors that enter into consideration as well. After all, pacemakers can last 10 years or more, so selecting the right pacemaker is sort of like planning for the patient's therapeutic needs for the next decade!

Pacemaker modes may help preserve AV synchrony, that is, the rhythm in which there is one atrial beat for each and every ventricular beat. This is the normal pattern of the healthy heart, and to the extent possible, pacemaker modes should try to imitate this healthy rhythm by allowing for maximal AV synchrony. Understanding AV synchrony will help to explain why certain device and mode choices are made.

NBG code

The pacemaker code used today is often called the NBG code, which is actually shorthand for the North American Society for Pacing and Electrophysiology (NASPE) and British Pacing and Electrophysiology Group (BPEG) code. NASPE may be known to some veterans of pacing in that it

The Nuts and Bolts of Implantable Device Therapy Pacemakers, First Edition. Tom Kenny.
© 2015 John Wiley & Sons, Ltd. Published 2015 by John Wiley & Sons, Ltd.

Table 13.1 The current NBG code as we have it today. A device may be described using three, four, or five positions

Position	I	II	III	IV	V
Category	Chamber(s)	Chamber(s)	Response to	Rate modulation	Multisite pacing
Letters used	O=none	O=none	O=none	O=none	O=none
	A=atrium	A=atrium	T=triggered	R=rate modulation	A=atrium
	V=ventricle	V=ventricle	I=inhibited		V=ventricle
	D=dual (A+V)	D=dual (A+V)	D=dual (T+I)		D=dual (A+V)
Manufacturers' designation only	S=single (A or V)	S=single (A or V)			

Note that *manufacturers' designation only* refers to letter codes that might be seen in the field or on product labeling but which are not technically part of the official NBG code.

was the original name of the specialty society known to us today as the Heart Rhythm Society (HRS). Originally, NASPE and BPEG joined forces to create a code that would allow for descriptions of pacemaker, ICDs, and cardiac resynchronization therapy devices. The NBG code has actually been updated three separate times to the code we have today. It consists of three to five letters (see **Table 13.1**). While five letters may be used in mode descriptions, most commonly, these codes are expressed in three or four letters only.

First and second positions

The first letter in the mode code refers to where the pacemaker is pacing the heart. This is most often stated as D, meaning dual (both atrial and ventricular pacing). However, in single-chamber systems, this may be V, such as would be used in a pacemaker that paces the ventricle only.

The next letter refers to where the pacemaker senses intrinsic signals from the heart. This will most often be D because most pacemakers in the USA are dual-chamber systems that sense in both atrium and ventricle.

This mode code may seem counterintuitive to clinicians, because pacemakers sense first and then—based on whether or not the heart beats intrinsically—paces or withholds the pacing output pulse. Thus, clinicians may think of pacing as sensing first then pacing second. However, the code states this the other way around: the first position is pacing, the second sensing!

Third position

The third position can be somewhat confusing, particularly to clinicians new to pacing. The purpose of the third letter in the code is to explain what the pacemaker will do when it senses an intrinsic beat, that is, when the patient's heart beats fast enough spontaneously on its own. When the patient's heart beats on its own, the pacemaker may trigger (or initiate) an output pulse, it may inhibit (or withhold) an output pulse, or it may do both of those (dual), inhibiting in the same chamber when an intrinsic beat is sensed or triggering a ventricular output pulse when an atrial event is sensed. The dual response is only possible in a dual-chamber system.

The two most common pacemaker modes in clinical practice are DDD (paces and senses in both atrium and ventricle and triggers/inhibits in response to an intrinsic activity) and VVI (paces and senses in the ventricle only and inhibits an output pulse when an intrinsic activity occurs). Note that inhibition does not refer to the patient's rhythm; it refers to inhibition of the *pacemaker*. A common confusion in pacing might occur when a patient has a VVI pacemaker programmed to 70 ppm. The patient has atrial fibrillation at 90 bpm. The clinician notices the patient's rhythm is right around 90 bpm and wonders why the pacemaker is not *inhibiting*. The pacemaker is inhibiting—it is inhibiting itself from delivering a pacing output pulse. It does not inhibit the patient's rhythm; pacemakers cannot slow down a heart rate.

Some pacemakers have no response to an intrinsic event, that is, they use an O code in the third position. This does not mean that they inhibit (that's I)—they have zero response to a sensed event, which means they keep right on pacing. A pacemaker in the VVO mode just paces at the programmed setting without any regard at all to the patient's own heart rate. VVO mode is something that clinicians may encounter when a magnet is placed over an implanted device. Magnet mode is typically characterized by pacing and sensing at programmed settings but with no consideration of the patient's intrinsic cardiac activity. VVO is not a therapeutic mode, but it may be used in device testing for short periods of time or in certain specific settings.

The triggered response (T) can confuse even experienced clinician. A triggered response means that the pacemaker will fire an output pulse in response to an intrinsic beat. Today, there is no reason to ever want to pace the same chamber when a patient's heart beats, but back in the early days of pacing, triggered pacing was actually a testing mode. Modern pacemakers allow clinicians to evaluate intracardiac electrograms or activity from within the heart itself. The earliest pacemakers did not offer anything even remotely like this, so to be sure that a pacemaker was sensing properly, the triggered mode was used. A VVT test strip would prove that the device was sensing the ventricle if every time the ventricle beat on its own, a confirmatory triggered ventricular pacing spike appeared. If the pacing spike appeared on top of a T-wave, this suggested a sensing problem, that is, the pacemaker was sensing T-waves as ventricular activity. Thus, originally, VVT and AAT were modes that had a genuine utility for testing and troubleshooting but served no therapeutic purpose. Over time, electrograms and annotations and other features make this type of VVT or AAT testing unnecessary.

Today, the term triggered refers to what is also called tracking, that is, if a dual-chamber pacemaker senses an intrinsic beat in the atrium, it will respond by triggering or initiating a ventricular pacing output pulse. Today, the letter T always involves two chambers—sensing in one chamber (the atrium) will trigger in the other chamber (the ventricle). The point of this type of *triggering* is to preserve AV synchrony, that is, to try to match atrial activity to ventricular activity.

In the early days of pacing, triggering was always in the same chamber—wherever you sensed, you also triggered. Today, triggering is better described as tracking and always means sensing in the atrium and pacing in the ventricle in response.

A dual-response system allows for tracking but it also inhibits. Inhibition of the output pulse occurs whenever an intrinsic event is sensed *in that same chamber*. For instance, if the pacemaker senses a natural atrial beat, it inhibits the atrial output pulse. If it senses an intrinsic ventricular beat, it inhibits the ventricular output pulse.

Fourth position
Rate modulation is also called rate response or rate adaptation and is described by the fourth position. Typically, when a device is described by only three letters, it has no rate modulation; the fourth position is mostly used only when the device is rate modulated. Thus, DDD has no rate response but DDDR does. (It is rare to see the designation written as DDDO although that is technically correct.)

Rate modulation relies on a sensor within the pacemaker. Do not confuse the sensor with sensing—they are two different things. The sensor helps to gauge the patient's level of activity and increase the patient's pacing rate in response.

Today, every pacemaker manufactured has rate response (i.e., a sensor is built into every device), but this feature is not always activated or programmed on.

Fifth position
The fifth position is almost never used in actual practice, but it would make sense if multisite pacing were common.

Manufacturers' designation only
After the code was developed, manufacturers adapted it for their own labeling by adding the letter S to mean *single*, that is, single chamber. An SSI device can be a VVI or AAI device, depending on where the lead is located. Likewise, an SSIR device can be VVIR or AAIR once it is implanted. Although not official code lingo, these designations were practical for device companies since a single-chamber pacemaker can function as an AAI or VVI device, depending on where the lead was positioned. Labeling such single-chamber devices

as SSI made sense for devices still in the box, and clinicians may see such designations on cans or in product literature.

Putting It together

Codes are used for devices (the highest possible mode is described in product labeling) or for the currently programmed mode. Using the code, you can tell a lot about how the pacemaker paces and functions. By far the most common devices in the USA are DDD, DDDR, VVI, and VVIR systems.

Single-chamber pacing

A single-chamber pacemaker is—as the name implies—a pacemaker that works in one chamber of the heart. In order for the pacemaker to pace and sense, it requires a lead. A single-chamber atrial pacemaker has one lead in the right atrium. A single-chamber ventricular pacemaker has one lead in the right ventricle. The same single-chamber device can function as an atrial single-chamber or ventricular single-chamber pacemaker, which is why manufacturers prefer to describe them as SSI devices.

Single-chamber atrial pacing

An atrial single-chamber pacemaker can be programmed to main single-chamber atrial modes, of which the most common is AAI. To use the code, AAI means that the pacemaker paces in the atrium (first letter) and senses in the atrium (second letter), and when it senses an intrinsic activity in the atrium, it inhibits or withholds the atrial output pulse (third letter). On the other hand, if the pacemaker senses no activity in the atrium, it will pace the atrium. The pacing output in the atrium should result in atrial

depolarization, leading to an atrial contraction, which would conduct to the ventricle.

Although far less common, one might also encounter AOO. This device paces the atrium (first letter) but senses nowhere (second letter), and its response to nothing is to do nothing (third letter). An AOO device paces the atrium constantly at the programmed rate. This type of pacing—constant pacing with no regard to intrinsic activity—is called asynchronous pacing because it is not timed to the heart's intrinsic events (see **Figure 13.1**). Asynchronous pacing will go on regardless of whether the patient's own heart is beating; it may even compete with the native rate. Most clinicians will encounter AOO pacing when a magnet is placed over an implanted single-chamber atrial pacemaker; magnet mode (the way a pacemaker will respond upon magnet application) is typically asynchronous pacing at a specified rate.

Single-chamber atrial pacemakers are not very common in clinical practice; in fact, most of the time, the term *single-chamber pacing* refers to single-chamber *ventricular* pacing. Atrial pacing is effective only in patients who have reliable AV conduction, that is, the atrial beat conducts consistently and reliably across the AV node to depolarize the ventricles. Patients with sick sinus syndrome (dysfunctional SA node) may be indicated for an AAI pacemaker provided that they have normal AV conduction—and most of them do. However, if a patient with sick sinus syndrome has high-degree AV block (Mobitz II or third-degree AV block), AAI pacing will no longer provide adequate pacing support. Sick sinus syndrome is a collective term that refers to five different rhythm disorders: sinus bradycardia, sinus arrest, SA exit block, atrial

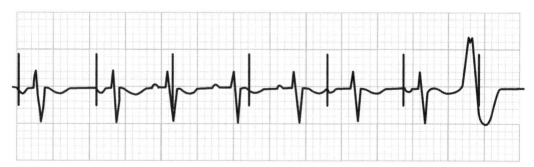

Figure 13.1 AOO pacing. Note that atrial pacing spikes occur before atrial depolarization, indicating atrial capture. An intrinsic atrial activity is not sensed and pacing is asynchronous at the programmed (or magnet) rate.

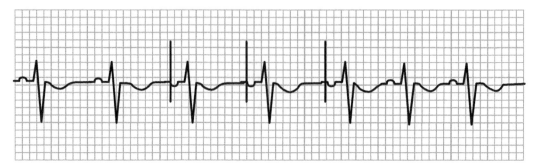

Figure 13.2 AAI pacing with atrial pacing (atrial spikes result in atrial depolarizations). Note that intrinsic atrial events are sensed, resulting in the inhibition of the atrial output pulse.

fibrillation with a slow ventricular response, and tachy–brady syndrome (see **Figure 13.2**).

While AAI devices work well in most sick sinus syndrome patients, the problem is that pacemakers can last 5, 7, even 10 years, or more. In that time, a sick sinus syndrome patient could potentially develop AV block and require a new pacemaker. For that reason, many physicians opt for different devices for their sick sinus syndrome patients. In the USA, most physicians will opt for a dual-chamber system instead; interestingly, in Europe and other less litigious parts of the world, AAI pacing is far more common.

Some physicians prefer to use AAI pacing whenever possible because they believe there are good reasons to try to preserve AV conduction and a normal physiologic ventricular rate as long as possible. AAI pacing is safe in patients with sick sinus syndrome provided that they have good AV conduction, and this is a risk factor that a physician can evaluate in the electrophysiology (EP) lab. In this test, the patient's atrium is paced at normal ranges (60, 70, and 80 ppm) and then progressively faster. Everybody—even people with healthy hearts—will develop physiological Wenckebach at rates around 150 or higher. Wenckebach rhythms are characterized by the progressive lengthening of the PR interval until a QRS drops out. At high enough atrial rates, even people with healthy hearts will experience physiological Wenckebach. The risk assessment for the sick sinus syndrome patient determines at what point the patient develops Wenckebach rhythms. If Wenckebach rhythms develop at or around 150 ppm, this is normal and physiologic. The patient is not at any particular risk for

conduction abnormalities. On the other hand, if Wenckebach commences around 70 or 80 ppm (or at any rate <100 bpm), this is pathological Wenckebach and it indicates a risk for future conduction abnormalities.

It may seem curious that physicians would bother with single-chamber atrial pacing at all, given the risks (however slight) and the hassles of EP testing. There is a reason that some physicians favor atrial pacing whenever possible: the reason is that ventricular pacing creates a degree of dyssynchrony in the heart. In a ventricular pacemaker, the ventricular pacing lead is placed somewhere inside the right ventricle, most often in the right ventricular apex but, on occasion, in the septum or perhaps the right ventricular outflow tract (RVOT). The electrical output that depolarizes the ventricle is not coming from the AV node outward and downward—as would occur in a healthy beat—but comes from the bottom or middle of the right side and goes outward. This causes the right side to conduct before the left side—which is not how the healthy heart contracts. It also uses different conduction pathways. The risks of right ventricular pacing are not entirely clear. Right ventricular pacing may worsen heart failure. Many pacing experts try to limit right ventricular pacing as much as they can—that is why some physicians will opt for AAI pacing whenever they feel it can be safely used. Another method to offer a patient the benefits of AAI pacing with the safety of ventricular support is to implant a DDD pacemaker, which will automatically switch between functional AAI and DDD, depending on the patient's conduction status. This type of pacing behavior will be discussed more in detail later.

Single-chamber ventricular pacing

A single-chamber device with one lead in the right ventricle, typically at the right ventricular apex or septum, is a single-chamber ventricular pacemaker that might function in VVI or VOO mode. VOO mode is magnet mode (asynchronous ventricular pacing) (see **Figure 13.3**).

VVI pacing paces in the ventricle (first letter) and senses in the ventricle (second letter), and when it senses an intrinsic event in the ventricle, it responds by inhibiting the output pulse to the ventricle. Thus, if the pacemaker senses intrinsic ventricular activity, it withholds the ventricular output pulses. If it senses no intrinsic ventricular activity, it will pace the ventricle (see **Figure 13.4**).

VVI pacing is more common than AAI pacing in part because ventricular pacing support is more urgently required by patients. Note that a VVI pacemaker does not sense any atrial activity so it will not be able to synchronize atrial activity to ventricular pacing. The big advantage of VVI pacing is that ventricular pacing support can be crucially important. The potential drawback, as mentioned earlier, is that many experts are raising concerns about right ventricular pacing, particularly about unnecessary right ventricular pacing.

Dual-chamber pacing

A dual-chamber pacemaker has two leads: one in the right atrium and other in the right ventricle. Dual-chamber devices not only can be programmed to pace and sense in both upper and lower chambers, the activity in each chamber leads to adjust-ments in the timing cycles of the other chamber. Dual-chamber pacing is more complex than single-chamber pacing, but it often provides patients with a higher degree of therapy.

Asynchronous dual-chamber pacing

The magnet mode of dual-chamber pacemakers is DOO; DOO may also be used as a temporary mode in other situations. Like AOO and VOO, the DOO mode is asynchronous. The D in the first position means that the pacemaker will pace both atrium and ventricle at the programmed (or magnet) rates. The other positions state that there is no sensing and, thus, no response to information sensed (see **Figure 13.5**).

Tracking

A DDD pacemaker paces in both atrium and ventricle (first letter), senses in both atrium and ventricle (second letter), and has a dual response to sensed intrinsic activity (third letter). This dual response includes *tracking* (sometimes called triggering) and inhibiting. This section looks at tracking, which means that an intrinsic activity sensed in the atrium will cause the pacemaker to try to time ventricular activity so that 1:1 AV synchrony is preserved, that is, the pacemaker will try to match intrinsic atrial beats to ventricular activity as much as possible, even if it means pacing the ventricle at rates above the programmed rate.

All pacemakers rely on internal *clocks* or timing cycles to know when to pace. Dual-chamber pacemakers have about 20 of these internal clocks, but two are of primary importance to us. The first is the

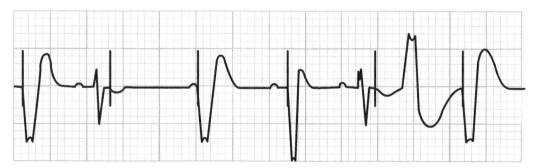

Figure 13.3 VOO pacing paces in the ventricle but does not sense. When the ventricular output pulse results in a ventricular depolarization, capture is confirmed. Note that QRS complexes associated with ventricular pacing are wider and look different than intrinsic QRS complexes. The reason for this is that right ventricular pacing stimulates the right ventricle and the depolarization goes outward and around, slower than an intrinsic depolarization. It is possible that VOO pacing may result in a pacing spike hitting the T-wave, which can potentially result in an arrhythmia.

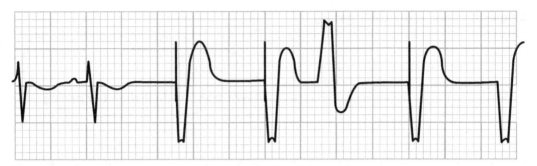

Figure 13.4 VVI pacing senses in the ventricle so intrinsic ventricular beats will inhibit the output pulse. Note that there is a PVC, which is an intrinsic beat. It resets the timing; note the next output pulse is timed to the PVC.

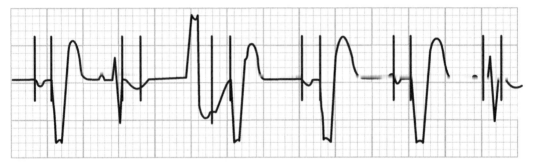

Figure 13.5 DOO pacing with atrial and ventricular pacing occurring with no regard for the patient's intrinsic activity. Note that the third pacing spike occurred during the vulnerable period of the T-wave. However, this third spike is an atrial pacing spike (notice the timing). An atrial spike on the T-wave poses no risk of arrhythmia.

clock that times the programmed rate (sometimes called the base rate or the lower rate limit). For example, if you have a dual-chamber pacemaker programmed to 60 ppm, the 60 ppm clock is the programmed rate clock. *In a DDD pacemaker, the programmed rate is based on the atrium.* As the pacemaker times out one beat to the next, it is synching the internal clock continually back to the atrium. This mimics the natural physiology of the healthy heart. Thus, with a DDD pacemaker at a programmed rate of 60 ppm, the atrium will never be allowed to go slower than 60 ppm (if no intrinsic atrial activity occurred, the pacemaker would fill in the missing beat and pace it so it went at 60 ppm). This first dual-chamber clock is observing the atrium; if the programmed rate is set to 60 ppm, the first clock makes sure that the atrial rate never falls below 60 ppm, and if an intrinsic atrial activity is faster than 60 bpm, the first clock inhibits atrial output pulses.

If the atrial event, whether intrinsic or sensed, does not conduct over the AV node to depolarize

the ventricle, the DDD pacemaker will pace the ventricle in an effort to maintain 1:1 AV synchrony so that each atrial event matches up to a corresponding ventricular event in a 1:1 ratio. The second most important clock in a DDD pacemaker is the AV interval (sometimes called the AV delay). This timing cycle actually spans both chambers. The AV interval clock starts with an atrial event, and if it expires before an intrinsic ventricular event occurs, then a ventricular output pulse is delivered. The AV interval clock searches for the next ventricular event; if an intrinsic ventricular event occurs before the clock times out, the AV interval clock inhibits or withholds the ventricular output pulse. This stops the clock, which resumes again with the next atrial event.

The programmed rate clock of a pacemaker set to 60 ppm is going to be 1000 ms, that is, the pacing interval associated with 60 ppm or one beat per second. The AV interval timing clock mimics the PR interval, which, in a healthy individual, is about 200 ms. A typical AV interval is programmed around 200 ms to allow the ventricles ample opportunity to depolarize spontaneously and contract. Programming the AV interval too short may result in unnecessary right ventricular pacing, because it does not allow the ventricles chance to beat intrinsically.

Tracking (also called atrial tracking or P-wave tracking) occurs when the pacemaker senses an intrinsic atrial activity and paces the ventricle in response. Tracking is possible in DDD pacemakers, but it can only occur if the patient has an intrinsic atrial activity (see **Figure 13.6**).

The goal of tracking is to maintain 1:1 AV synchrony as much as possible, since this is the rhythm of a healthy heart and provides for optimal hemodynamics. When the atrial rate hovers around the programmed rate, it is easy to see how tracking works. But what about a DDD pacemaker patient with a pacemaker programmed to a base rate of 60 ppm but who has an intrinsic atrial rate of 70 beats a minute? In this case, the atrial output pulse would be inhibited. In order to provide 1:1 AV synchrony, *the tracking function will allow the ventricle to be based faster than the base rate*. That is, the patient's native atrial rate will be 70 bpm, and the pacemaker will make sure that the ventricles keep up or *track* to the atrial rate and also beat at 70 ppm.

Tracking will continue at rates above the base rate. Using the same example, the DDD pacemaker will keep tracking the patient's atrial rate, even at rates of 80 or 90 or 100 bpm. In fact, the DDD pacemaker will keep tracking up to its *speed limit*, which is a programmable rate sometimes called the maximum or max tracking rate (sometimes abbreviated MTR or also known as the upper rate limit). In a patient with a DDD pacemaker and an MTR of 120, the DDD device will track an intrinsic activity from right above the base rate (61 bpm) all the way up to the MTR (120 ppm). This means that in a DDD device and a patient with an intrinsic atrial activity, it is possible to see ventricular pacing at rates far above the programmed base rate. Thus, as the DDD patient's intrinsic atrial rate increases, the ventricular pacing rate *keeps track*!

In a DDD pacemaker, you should see atrial pacing only at the programmed base rate, but ventricular pacing can occur at rates up to and including the MTR. Ventricular pacing in a DDD pacemaker is driven by the base rate or patient's intrinsic atrial rate, whichever is faster.

Types of dual-chamber events

There are really only four main types of things that can occur with a DDD pacemaker, as described in **Table 13.2**.

Nontracking dual-chamber modes

There may be situations where a clinician does not want tracking during dual-chamber pacing. The most common nontracking dual-chamber mode is DDI. The third position of the code says that in response to sensed activity, a pacing output pulse is inhibited or withheld. DDI pacing does not track, that is, the atrial rate will never drive the ventricular

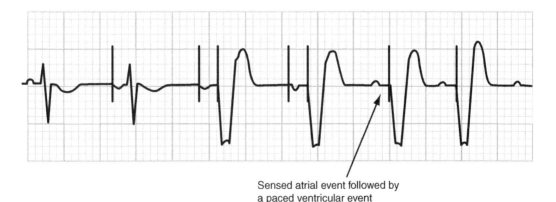

Sensed atrial event followed by
a paced ventricular event

Figure 13.6 Tracking in DDD mode occurs when a sensed atrial event is followed by a paced ventricular event. The sensed atrial event launches the AV delay timing clock, but if no ventricular activity occurs when that clock times out, the pacemaker paces the ventricle to promote 1:1 AV synchrony or one atrial beat matching up to one ventricular beat.

Table 13.2 While DDD pacing can seem complicated, it breaks down to only four types of events

What is going on	What the paced ECG shows	Nickname
The patient's atrial rate and ventricular rate will both be above the base rate, so the pacemaker inhibits in both chambers	Sensed atrial event, sensed ventricular event	AsVs
The patient's atrial rate is above the base rate, but there is no conduction over the AV node. The pacemaker inhibits in the atrium but paces the ventricle	Sensed atrial event, paced ventricular event	AsVp
The patient's atrial rate is below the base rate, but there is good conduction over the AV node. The pacemaker paces the atrium but inhibits in the ventricle	Paced atrial event, sensed ventricular event	ApVs
The patient's atrial and ventricular rates are both below the base rate. The pacemaker paces in both atrium and ventricle.	Paced atrial event, paced ventricular event	ApVp

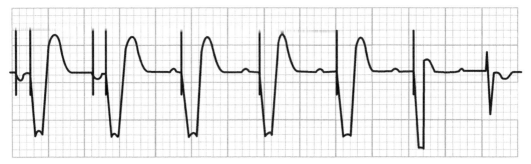

Figure 13.7 DDI or nontracking dual-chamber pacing will not allow the ventricle to track an intrinsic atrial activity, which can be useful in patients with atrial fibrillation.

rate. This kind of mode might be used effectively in a patient with a very high intrinsic atrial rate or atrial fibrillation. The drawback to DDI pacing is that you lose 1:1 AV synchrony because the pacemaker will not try to marry an intrinsic atrial event to a ventricular event (see **Figure 13.7**).

Rate response

Rate-responsive pacemakers have an R in the fourth position of the code, such as VVIR or DDDR. Rate response is covered in detail in a subsequent chapter, but for now, it is important to know that in a rate-responsive pacing, the pacing rate may be under the control of a sensor and exceed the programmed base rate. The goal of rate-responsive (also known as rate-adaptive or rate-modulated) pacing is to provide adequate pacing support during activity so that the pacemaker can pace faster when the patient is exercising, for example, than when he is sitting in a chair. The types of sensors and their various algorithms vary by manufacturer and even by models from a single manufacturer. However, in general, it is important to know that in rate-responsive pacemakers, under certain conditions, the sensor can take control of the rate and the clinician will see faster-than-base-rate pacing.

The sensor has a *speed limit* in the form of a programmable parameter known as the maximum sensor rate (also called max sensor rate or MSR). For example, if a patient has a DDDR pacemaker with an MSR of 120 ppm, the pacemaker might pace as fast as 120 ppm, but it will never go above that rate in response to sensor input. DDDR pacemakers thus have two important speed limits: the MTR and the MSR. Usually, these are set to the same value, which is often 120 or 130. However, they are independently programmable. A short summary appears in **Table 13.3**.

Table 13.3 Atrial and ventricular pacing in DDD and DDDR modes

	Atrial pacing	Ventricular pacing
DDD	Atrial pacing will only ever occur at the base rate	Ventricular pacing is driven by the AV interval and will be in the range of base rate to MTR, but if it is faster than the base rate, it will be tracking the atrium
DDDR	Atrial pacing will occur within the range of base rate to MSR	Ventricular pacing is driven by the AV interval and will track to the atrium up to the MTR or MSR

Thus, AV pacing (paced atrial event followed by a paced ventricular event) occurs in DDD at the base rate but in DDDR may occur at any rate from the base rate to the MSR, for example, from 60 to 120 ppm.

In single-chamber pacemakers, the rate response affects only the paced chamber, for example, VVIR pacing offers rate response only to the ventricle. VVIR pacemakers are often employed in patients with atrial fibrillation with a slow ventricular response.

Mode Selection

While there are numerous choices available to clinicians today in terms of pacemaker mode, clinicians will see two predominate modes in practice: VVIR pacing for patients with atrial fibrillation with a slow ventricular response and DDDR pacing for everybody else. In Europe and other parts of the world, there tends to be more single-chamber pacing than in the USA. While rate-responsive devices are common (all devices today have a built-in sensor), clinicians should be aware that rate response is activated in only about half of all devices. Just because a patient has a DDDR device, it should not be assumed that rate response is turned on. This is something that should be checked on the programmer or may be evident on a paced ECG.

AAI or AAIR pacemakers may be implanted in patients with sick sinus syndrome, a healthy AV node, and low risk for developing high-degree AV block. Those with sinus node dysfunction or AV block should be paced with dual-chamber pacemakers, DDD or DDDR modes.

Some of the more obscure modes like VOO or DDI actually do show up in clinical practice but in specific circumstances, such as testing or magnet mode or as a response mode for a mode switch algorithm.

Conclusion

The pacemaker mode code may seem simple, but it is inextricably linked to pacing and sensing behaviors of the device, which, in turn, related to pacemaker timing cycles. The code describes where the pacemaker paces, where it senses, how it responds when it senses an intrinsic event, and whether or not it has rate response. Generally, if a mode code is stated as three letters only, there is no rate response (DDD vs. DDDR rather than DDDO vs. DDDR). The fifth position on the code is almost never used. Single-chamber modes are AAI(R) and VVI(R) and pace and sense only in one chamber and inhibit an output pulse when they sense an intrinsic activity.

Dual-chamber pacemakers on the other hand have two timing clocks. First, they have a base rate clock that is timed to the atrium. Second, they have an AV interval clock that times an atrial event to the next ventricular event. DDD(R) devices may also track in that they time ventricular paced events to intrinsic atrial events. Tracking occurs when the patient's intrinsic atrial rate exceeds the base rate; the pacemaker will pace the ventricular to *keep track* with the higher atrial rate up to the programmable MTR (usually around 120 ppm). The goal of tracking is to maintain 1:1 AV synchrony.

All pacemakers today contain a sensor but these sensors are not always activated; when they are, the pacemakers offer rate response that paces above the base rate in response to patient activity. It is possible to see faster-than-base-rate pacing in rate-responsive devices! The sensor takes control of the pacemaker only when it detects patient activity increasing. The sensor-driven rate is governed by a second *speed limit* known as the MSR. The MTR and MSR are independent of each other but are often programmed to the same value of around 120 ppm.

In a dual-chamber pacemaker, only four types of events are possible, which can be described as AV (atrial paced event, ventricular paced event), AR (atrial paced event, ventricular sensed event), PV (atrial sensed event, ventricular paced event), and PR (atrial sensed event, ventricular sensed event).

The most frequently observed pacemakers are VVI(R) and DDD(R). VOO, AOO, and DOO are magnet modes that are sometimes used for a short period of time for test purposes. DDI mode may be used in dual-chamber patients when tracking has to be turned off, that is, in the presence of high intrinsic rates.

The nuts and bolts of pacemaker modes and codes

- The pacemaker code is a simple series of letters that helps clinicians understand the type of device or its mode. The first standardized code was the Inter-Society Commission for Heart Disease (ICHD) code published in 1974. Today, the code has evolved with pacemaker technology.
- The code used today is often called the NBG code but it is really the code from the North American Society for Pacing and Electrophysiology (NASPE, today known as the Heart Rhythm Society or HRS) and the British Pacing and Electrophysiology Group (BPEG).
- The NBG code has five positions, but for all practical purposes, only the first three or four positions are used. The first and second positions describe the chamber paced and sensed, respectively; the code shows an A, V, or D for atrial, ventricular, or dual (both), respectively. Thus, a VVI pacemaker paces and senses in the ventricle, while a DDD pacemaker paces and senses in both atrium and ventricle (dual).
- Manufacturers sometimes use an S for the first or second position but this is not officially part of the code. Clinicians sometimes see products labeled or discussed as SSI. The S stands for *single chamber* and it means that the device can be used in either the atrium or ventricle. An SSI pacemaker is only SSI while it is in the box. Once it is implanted in a patient, it can become an AAI pacemaker (if it is attached to an atrial lead) or a VVI pacemaker (if it is attached to a ventricular lead).
- The third position in the code refers to what the device does in response to a sensed signal, in other words, what the pacemaker does if it senses that the heart has beat appropriately on its own. The main letter codes here are I for inhibit (meaning the pacemaker inhibits or holds back a pacing output pulse) or T for triggered.
- Triggered is actually an outdated term. In the early days of pacing, sometimes, a pacemaker could be programmed so that for testing purposes, it delivered an output pulse whenever it sensed native cardiac activity. That is not done today. However, sometimes, a pacemaker will *track*. Tracking means that the pacemaker may make decisions about how to pace the ventricle based on what it senses in the atrium. A dual-chamber pacemaker can track the atrium so that the ventricle beats in 1:1 synchrony with the atrium. Thus, the term *triggered* today really means *tracking*.
- The third position can also be D for dual or both inhibition and triggering (which is really tracking). In this case, the pacemaker inhibits an output pulse when it senses activity in the same chamber (sensed atrial event results in inhibited atrial output; sensed ventricular event results in inhibited ventricular output) but it tracks activity by pacing the ventricle to keep up with the patient's intrinsic atrial rate.
- The fourth position is R for rate modulation, also known as rate response. If a device does not have rate response, it may use the O for none in the code. However, it is more common to see a device just use a three-letter code if it does not have rate response. Thus, DDDR is a dual-chamber rate-responsive pacemaker, while a dual-chamber pacemaker without rate response would describe itself as DDD.
- The fifth position stands for multisite pacing, but this is not used in ordinary clinical practice.
- All of the codes have the option of O for none. Thus, a VOO pacemaker paces the ventricle but does not sense or respond to sensed activity. Such modes do occur in clinical practice but are typically used only for very short periods of time under clinical supervision for testing purposes.

- Single-chamber atrial pacing is not very commonly used in the USA but does exist. A good reason to implant an AAI or AAIR device is to preserve natural AV conduction and a normal physiologic ventricular rate as long as possible. Furthermore, ventricular pacing is known to promote mechanical dyssynchrony of the heart. Single-chamber atrial pacing is safe for patients with sick sinus syndrome provided that they have good and reliable AV conduction.
- Ventricular single-chamber pacing is the more common single-chamber mode but it does not take into account the patient's atrial activity. Thus, VVI and VVIR pacing are associated with a loss of 1:1 AV synchrony.
- In the USA and many other parts of the world, DDD and DDDR pacing are the most common modes.
- In dual-chamber pacing, there are only four possible cardiac events. These are a sensed atrial event followed by a sensed ventricular event (nicknamed an AsVs event), a sensed atrial event followed by a paced ventricular event (AsVp), a paced atrial event followed by a sensed ventricular event (ApVs), and a paced atrial event followed by a paced ventricular event (ApVp). Most dual-chamber paced rhythms tend to have a dominant type of event, that is, some patients have mostly AV events, others mostly AR, and so on.

- During tracking or rate response, the pacemaker might pace faster than the programmed base rate.
- In order to provide some limits, most devices have a maximum tracking limit (max tracking rate) and a maximum sensor-driven rate limit (max sensor rate), which define the fastest rate the device will pace in response to an intrinsic atrial activity or a sensor input, respectively. The max tracking and max sensor rates are often the same (they are independently programmable) and tend to be about 120 or 130 ppm for most patients.
- All devices manufactured today have a built-in sensor for offering rate-responsive pacing but only about half of devices have rate response turned on. There may be many reasons for this, including that rate response is not necessary or appropriate for that particular patient.
- There are two predominant modes for pacemaker patients in real-world clinical practice: VVIR pacing for patients with atrial fibrillation and a slow ventricular response and DDDR for everybody else.
- When a magnet is placed over an implanted device, it reverts to magnet mode. These are usually modes like DOO, VOO, or AOO in which the device paces asynchronously (i.e., without regard to any sensed activity). Magnet mode is useful for testing purposes.
- In dual-chamber devices, the programmed rate is always timed using an atrial clock.

Test your knowledge

1 The pacemaker code in use today is called:
 A ICHD code.
 B NASPE code.
 C NBG code.
 D All manufacturers use their own individual code systems.

2 If a pacemaker is a VVIR device, what can be said about it?
 A It paces and senses in the atrium.
 B It does not have rate response.
 C It will pace the ventricle by tracking intrinsic atrial activity.

 D It paces and senses in the ventricle and has rate response.

3 What does it mean when the code says the device responds to a sensed event by *inhibiting*?
 A The pacemaker inhibits or holds back the pacing output pulse.
 B The pacemaker inhibits the patient's intrinsic rate.
 C The pacemaker inhibits the sensor so rate response is disabled.
 D The pacemaker will deliver an output pulse when it senses an event.

4 Why would a manufacturer want to label a pacemaker SSI?
  A Because a single-chamber pacemaker can work in the atrium or ventricle; you don't know if it will be an AAI or a VVI device until it is implanted.
  B This is a holdover from the old ICHD code and is still seen on product labeling.
  C Manufacturers are required by the FDA to use this designation.
  D None of the above.

5 Which of the following modes might be used as a magnet mode?
  A VDD
  B DDI
  C DDDR
  D VOO

6 When a dual-chamber pacemaker tracks, what does it do?
  A It paces the ventricle to keep up with the intrinsic atrial rate as much as possible.
  B It inhibits ventricular pacing whenever it senses intrinsic atrial activity.
  C It slows the base rate to allow for intrinsic activity as much as possible.
  D It allows the pacemaker to pace as fast as the patient's activity level requires.

7 Why is dual-chamber tracking a good thing?
  A It preserves battery life.
  B It reduces cardiac output.

  C It preserves 1:1 AV synchrony as much as possible.
  D It encourages physiologic intrinsic ventricular activity as possible.

8 What is the max sensor rate?
  A It defines the pulse amplitude of the sensed cardiac signal.
  B It sets how fast the pacemaker will pace in response to sensor input.
  C It is the fastest rate the ventricle can be paced in response to sensed atrial activity.
  D It's another word for max tracking rate.

9 Pick the one reason below why a correctly functioning DDDR pacemaker might pace the patient faster than the patient's programmed base rate;
  A Magnet mode.
  B Inhibition.
  C The sensor shows the patient is very inactive and likely asleep.
  D The sensor shows the patient is active and needs a faster rate.

10 Pacemaker timing cycles can be described as internal *clocks*. In a dual-chamber pacemaker, how is the base rate timed?
  A By the atrial clock
  B By the ventricular clock
  C By the average or the atrial and ventricular clocks
  D By a T-wave clock used only in dual-chamber systems

CHAPTER 14

Single-chamber timing cycles

Learning objectives

- Describe what magnet mode is, why it might be useful, and what type of pacing behavior occurs.
- Explain what sensing means and when a device will inhibit an output pulse.
- Define capture and explain why this function is essential to pacemaker therapy.
- Briefly explain how a clinician would determine if a pacemaker patient is pacemaker dependent.
- Calculate the ms interval for pacing at a rate of 80 ppm and explain the formula for this conversion.
- In brief terms, explain the difference between fusion and pseudofusion and their relationship to capture.
- Name the two components of a pacemaker refractory period and the key difference between them.
- Describe how a clinician might change the alert period of a pacemaker.
- Define and differentiate the automatic interval from the escape interval in single-chamber pacing.
- Describe rate hysteresis and the type of pacemaker patient that might benefit from it.

Introduction

Single-chamber timing cycles are without doubt one of the most crucial topics for the pacing clinician, because virtually all understanding of timing cycles, device function, troubleshooting, paced rhythms, and device features builds on this foundation. Dual-chamber pacing is essentially two single-chamber pacemakers that work together. Thus, these concepts—which may seem easy—are absolutely fundamental to a knowledge of the most sophisticated cutting-edge devices. Pacemakers can really only ever do two things: they sense and they pace. Over and over, as we break down cardiac pacing concepts, they turn out to be fairly simple ideas. We will see this with such potentially confusing topics as fusion and pseudofusion along with automatic versus escape intervals and hysteresis. The key concepts are generally easy.

It is best to start with single-chamber pacing because we can get the basics out of the way before moving on to the much more common dual-chamber pacing modes. Yet single-chamber pacemakers still play an important role in cardiac pacing today. Although rare, AAI pacemakers are appropriate for patients with intact AV conduction (i.e., atrial beats conduct successfully over the AV node to depolarize the ventricles); have a slow, erratic, or otherwise undependable intrinsic atrial rhythm; and do not have atrial tachyarrhythmias, such as (but not limited to) atrial fibrillation. The use of AAI patients in specific patients who meet these criteria may be a wise device choice because it will allow the patient's intrinsic ventricular rate to prevail.

VVI pacemakers are the more common type of single-chamber system, and they are suitable for patients who have a slow underlying rhythm, do not have good or reliable AV conduction (i.e., atrial activity can get delayed or blocked traveling over the AV node down to the ventricles), and have some degree of atrial impairment, including atrial tachyarrhythmias, such as atrial fibrillation. Patients with

The Nuts and Bolts of Implantable Device Therapy Pacemakers, First Edition. Tom Kenny.
© 2015 John Wiley & Sons, Ltd. Published 2015 by John Wiley & Sons, Ltd.

atrial fibrillation and a slow ventricular response are good candidates for VVIR pacing.

In the USA, most pacemakers are dual-chamber systems. The prevailing thought process behind this device selection is simple. A DDD pacemaker can always do less, but a VVI or AAI pacemaker cannot do more. In other words, a patient who may seem a good candidate for an AAI device can be implanted with a DDD device that functions as an AAI system—unless or until the patient ever needs ventricular support. At that point, the device is there and can provide it. Likewise, a good candidate for a VVI pacemaker can obtain that kind of pacing with a DDD device, but if he can benefit from atrial pacing, it is available. Unlike drugs—which are typically prescribed for 30 days and taken daily—pacemakers are implanted and last 5 or 10 years! Most physicians are uncomfortable predicting how their patients' hearts will perform 5 years from today. Cardiac rhythm disorders are often progressive and many other conditions can also affect cardiac rhythm. The bottom line is most doctors prefer to implant the most versatile system they can get even if the patient does not need every single feature today. It is just too difficult to know what will be needed in 5 years. Thus, clinicians should expect to see mostly dual-chamber pacemakers in actual real-world practice, but it is important to know single-chamber basics:

- There are still single-chamber systems being implanted.
- Some dual-chamber pacemakers are for all practical purposes functioning in single-chamber modes, at least some of the time,
- All of these single-chamber concepts will also apply to dual-chamber pacing, that is, clinicians will be able to use all of what is learned in this chapter to just about every pacing situation.

Magnet mode

The so-called *magnet mode* pacing is asynchronous pacing, a type of pacing that clinicians almost never see outside of magnet mode or perhaps in some unusual testing situations. During asynchronous pacing, the pacemaker paces—without any regard to the patient's intrinsic activity. The mode codes for asynchronous pacing are VOO, AOO, and DOO, which shows the pacemaker will pace but there is no sensing and, therefore, no response to sensing.

Historically, asynchronous pacing was actually used for therapeutic purposes. The very earliest pacemakers were all asynchronous systems. That seems hard to imagine today, but going back to the original first-generation devices, asynchronous pacing was far more common than it is today.

Clinicians today see asynchronous pacing mainly in magnet mode. When a magnet is applied above the implanted device, it forces the device into magnet mode or asynchronous pacing. It may never be necessary to revert to magnet mode for a particular pacemaker patient, but there are some good reasons why magnet mode would be used:

- Magnet mode historically was used to assess battery longevity and it can still be used that way today. While clinicians mainly use information from the programmer to get insight into battery longevity, if a programmer is not available, a clinician can *go old school* and simply put a magnet on top of the implanted device. Magnet mode changes as the battery wears down. Referring to the device manual, you can see by the asynchronous pacing rate on an ECG how much battery service life is left.
- Magnet mode may also be useful for troubleshooting scenarios. This is more common with dual-chamber devices.

All manufacturers offer their own magnets, which are typically either donut shaped (round with a hole in the middle) or horseshoe shaped. These are specialized magnets that are exactly the right strength to initiate magnet mode in an implanted device. Magnet mode may not occur if a nonstandard magnet is used.

Magnet mode behavior is not standardized across manufacturers or even within manufacturers. For example, one manufacturer may make several devices with slightly different types of magnet mode. To know what to expect from magnet mode, refer to the device manual (if it is available—many today are online) or contact the Technical Services Hotline of the manufacturer. Most magnet modes are asynchronous pacing at specific rates, for example, 100 ppm VOO at beginning of service life and 80 ppm VOO at elective replacement.

In a single-chamber pacemaker, the pacing interval—which will be discussed in more detail

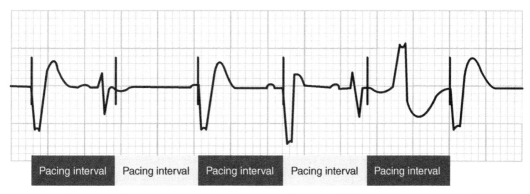

Figure 14.1 This example of asynchronous single-chamber ventricular pacing (VOO) shows pacing spikes marching through at the programmed rate but without any regard to intrinsic activity. The pacemaker is not programmed to sense any intrinsic activity, so it does not respond to sensing.

later—may be defined as the distance between two consecutive pacemaker spikes that reflects the programmed base rate. For instance, if the base rate is set to 60 ppm, the pacing interval will be 1000 ms (60 ppm translates to a 1000 ms interval). When spikes appear on a single-chamber strip at exactly the programmed rate—in other words, pacing intervals—it means that there was no event sensed between spikes that might have reset the timing. This can happen because no intrinsic cardiac event occurred (i.e., there was nothing to sense), or it can happen because the pacemaker is set to an asynchronous single-chamber mode (AOO or VOO) and even if events did occur between spikes, nothing was sensed (see **Figure 14.1**).

What pacemakers do

All any pacemaker can do is sense or pace; those are the only two functions a pacemaker actually performs. The rest of this book will help explain the timing cycles and algorithms that help govern why and when they do these things, but no pacemaker can ever do anything other than sense and pace. In a single-chamber pacemaker, the pacemaker senses and paces in only one chamber of the heart. While this can be the atrium or the ventricle, for the rest of this chapter, we'll talk only about ventricular single-chamber pacing since it is by far more common in real-world clinical practice. Just remember all of these concepts also apply to atrial single-chamber pacing as well.

Sensing is the method by which a pacemaker perceives or *sees* an intrinsic cardiac signal. For instance, if the patient's ventricle is contracting and relaxing at a reasonable rate of 70 bpm and the pacemaker is programmed to 60 ppm, as long as the ventricular rate goes along above the base rate, the pacemaker is going to sense or perceive these ventricular beats and inhibit or withhold the output pulse. The pacemaker essentially goes on standby, monitoring the ventricular rate but not delivering any output pulses. Some patients have pacemakers that are inhibited much of the time; it is not unusual in clinical practice to find patients whose pacing rate is 20 or 30%, meaning the device inhibited its output pulse 70 or 80% of the time.

Many, if not most, pacemaker patients have some underlying rhythm. This brings us to a term that is often misused in the clinic: *pacemaker dependent*. A person is pacemaker dependent if he or she has no underlying rhythm above 40 bpm without a pacemaker. Such a person will be symptomatic or worse without a pacemaker. In the clinic, many patient records are flagged to indicate patients who are *pacemaker dependent*. Sometimes, this label is applied inappropriately to those patients who are paced 100% of the time. In clinical practice, clinicians encounter patients who are literally paced for every single beat, 100% of the time. Such patients may—or may not—be pacemaker dependent. It is hard to know, because pacemaker dependence is not defined by how much of the time the pacemaker paces; rather, it is defined by how fast the patient's intrinsic rhythm is without pacing. In fact, there are patients who are paced 100% of the time who are not truly pacemaker dependent. (To determine pacemaker dependence in a 100% paced patient, slow the programmed base rate in steps and look for the patient's intrinsic rhythm. If the intrinsic rhythm is above 40 bpm, the patient is not pacemaker dependent.)

Sometimes, the pacemaker looks for an intrinsic ventricular contraction but does not *see* one. The device senses no ventricular activity and thus tells the pacemaker to pace, that is, to deliver an output pulse. For example, let's say a patient has a VVI device set to a base rate of 60 ppm and her ventricular rate is less than 60 bpm. The pacemaker will sense a lack of ventricular activity and pace the ventricle at precisely the right time to achieve that 60 ppm rate (which translates to a 1000 ms interval on the rhythm strip).

Whenever a pacemaker paces, the goal is capture. Capture may be defined as a pacing spike leading to the immediate depolarization of the appropriate chamber. For example, delivering a pacemaker spike to the ventricle that results in an immediate depolarization (seen on the ECG as a QRS complex) is capture. Pacing without capture is not of any benefit to the patient. Thus, capture could be considered the cornerstone of pacemaker therapy!

Sensing

The best definition for sensing is an easy one: sensing is the pacemaker's ability to *see* intrinsic activity and, if appropriate, to respond to it. In most single-chamber pacemakers, the response to sensed activity will be inhibition. The pacemaker's sensing function is regulated by the sensitivity setting. Sensitivity is a programmable parameter that the clinician uses to define what signals the pacemaker can *see* and what signals the pacemaker will not *see*. The human body makes a lot of electrical signals or noise, so it is imperative that the pacemaker know what signals to look for. If sensitivity is set so that even very tiny signals are sensed, it is possible that the pacemaker will sense muscle noise and wrongly interpret it as intrinsic cardiac activity. On the other hand, if sensitivity is set so that only very large signals are sensed (and cardiac signals are larger than noise signals), the risk is that some genuine cardiac signals will be overlooked. The best way to get a grasp on sensitivity is to think of it as a wall. Programming sensitivity is defining how tall you are going to build the wall; the height of the wall determines if you can see a person standing behind it or not (see **Figure 14.2**).

Appropriate sensitivity settings can vary by patient; they depend on the patient's intrinsic signals. If a clinician knows that a patient has a ventricular signal of around 6 mV, the *wall* has to be set to something like 5 or 3 mV so that the signal can be seen. If the patient has an intrinsic signal of 6 mV and the sensitivity is set to 7 mV, the patient's intrinsic signal will be obscured and not sensed.

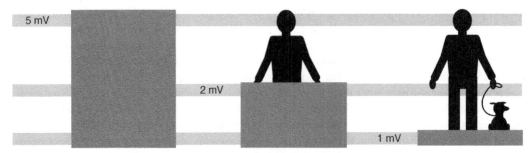

Figure 14.2 This is an intuitive way to understanding sensitivity settings. Imagine a wall of varying height and behind that wall stands a person with a dog. Your ability to see the person and the dog is directly affected by how tall the wall is built. If the wall is very tall, the person is totally obscured; if the wall is very low, the person and the dog are easily seen. If you think of the person as the cardiac signals and the dog as the extracardiac or noise signals, your goal is to build the wall so that you can see the person—but not the dog! Sensitivity is programmed in millivolts; the higher the millivolt setting, the taller the wall and the less sensitive the pacemaker; the lower the millivolt setting, the more sensitive the pacemaker. Using this example, a good sensitivity setting is the one in the middle—you can reliably see the person, but not the dog.

This leads to a bit of terminology that sometimes confuses clinicians, at least at the beginning. To make a pacemaker more sensitive, you *lower the mV setting*. To make a pacemaker less sensitive, you *increase the mV setting*. If you have two pacemakers and two sensitivity settings, the *lower mV setting* is the more sensitive pacemaker. Thus, you make a pacemaker less sensitive by raising the wall and more sensitive by lowering the wall.

When selecting the optimal sensitivity setting, it is important to know the size (in mV) of the patient's intrinsic cardiac signals. The mV setting must be low enough to allow the intrinsic signal to reliably be seen. Signal amplitude can vary and many patients have lower-amplitude signals at least some of the time. So the first goal is to find a low-enough mV setting that will allow the patient's intrinsic signals to be seen every time. This must be balanced with another function of sensitivity: to keep unwanted signals from being sensed. A pacemaker senses based on the mV size of the signal—it really has no way to differentiate an electrical signal that comes from a muscle or from the heart. Thus, the mV setting has to be large enough that it blocks out unwanted signals. Most muscle noise and other extraneous signals within the boy are low-amplitude signals. The best way to balance is to find a mV setting that reliably allows the patient's intrinsic signals to be seen but is still as high as reasonable to block out unwanted signals. Thus, if a patient has an intrinsic ventricular signal of 6 mV, a reasonable mV setting might be 4 mV or even 3 mV—low enough to assure that even lower-amplitude signals were sensed, but still not so low that muscle noise would be sensed.

The goal of sensing is to see all of the signals you want to see and none of the signals you do not want to see.

Intrinsic signal amplitudes are measured at pacemaker implant and can be measured using the programmer after implant. It is not unusual for intrinsic signals to change over time.

Rhythm strips

Most clinicians are familiar with the ECG and even pacing experts rely on ECG rhythm strips to help them care for their patients. However, in the pacing clinic, it is far more common to use intracardiac electrograms (sometimes called IEGMs, EGMs, or electrograms), which are similar but distinctive. A surface ECG relies on electrical signals from the heart that it picks up from the surface of the skin. Nearly all clinicians are familiar with an ECG rhythm strip and can point out the landmarks, even when a pacemaker is involved. An electrogram is a little different. First, it relies on electrical signals that the pacemaker picks up from inside the heart. In a single-chamber ventricular pacemaker, the electrogram comes from signals that the right ventricular lead electrode picks up from the interior of the right ventricle. This creates a somewhat unique perspective that alters the electrogram a bit when compared to an ECG. Pacing clinicians should use EGMs as much as possible, because they offer better insight into pacemaker function. Surface ECGs can seem more familiar, but it is good practice to get used to using EGMs early. And it is good practice to use both the EGM and the ECG together.

Electrograms are presented on the programmer; they come from the pacemaker itself and they can be displayed or printed out from the programmer screen. This allows the programmer to annotate the rhythm strip with markers and other codes that explain what the pacemaker was *thinking* at various points. Annotations are useful because they help clinicians navigate an electrogram quickly, they often provide numerical intervals that save clinicians from a lot of calculation, and they provide a record of how the pacemaker *sees* the patient's rhythm (see **Figure 14.3**). When dealing with an intracardiac electrogram, always compare the electrogram against the ECG (if available, which in this case it is—at the top) and against the annotations and calculated intervals. The tracings and the annotations should agree, and most of the time, they will. But if you ever encounter a situation where the annotations disagree with the tracings, the tracings always win.

The use of annotated EGMs in clinical practice will simplify your work, eliminate a lot of potential mistakes, and provide the most accurate information possible. Annotated EGMs show clinicians what the pacemaker *thinks* and virtually eliminates the need for rate rulers or calculations. One of the best pieces of advice for any clinician thinking of working with pacemakers is to learn to

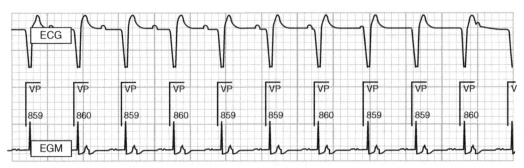

Figure 14.3 The surface ECG on top and the intracardiac electrogram on the bottom do not look much alike, but it is easy to find the landmarks. Notice the wide QRS in the ECG and how it occurs roughly at the same time as the smaller QRS on the EGM. The annotation of VP stands for *ventricular pacing* and indicates that the pacemaker *thinks* it delivered a pacemaker output at that moment. That annotation aligns perfectly with the ventricular depolarizations both above (ECG) and below (EGM). Although the pacemaker spike is not evident on the surface ECG—which sometimes happens—the spike is very prominent in the EGM. Thus, this strip clearly shows ventricular pacing and all three sources of information (ECG, annotations, EGM) agree with each other.

work well with the annotated EGM. The investment in time to learn it upfront will more than pay off in time saved in clinical practice later on.

Inhibition

When a pacemaker senses an intrinsic event, it is tempting to think that it *does nothing* but actually it is doing something very important. When a pacemaker senses an intrinsic event, it may *inhibit* the output pulse. Inhibition refers to withholding the output pulse. While that may look like doing nothing, for the pacemaker, it is actually doing something! It is easier to understand timing cycles if inhibition is regarded as an action. When the pacemaker senses an intrinsic event at a rapid-enough rate, it will actively withhold the pacing output pulse. By contrast, if the pacemaker fails to sense such an event, it will cause the pacemaker to deliver that output pulse. If the pacemaker is programmed to 60 ppm, when the 1000 ms cycle elapses (equivalent to 60 ppm), the pacemaker is going to look within that window of time for intrinsic events. If they occur in that timing window, the pacemaker will inhibit. If no such intrinsic event occurs and the 1000 ms timing cycle elapses, then the pacemaker will pace.

Inhibition is very important in pacing because it brings with it an important benefit, namely, that the patient is not paced unnecessarily. Cardiac pacing is very helpful when it is needed, but only when it is needed. Moreover, the less the pacemaker paces, the less battery energy is used.

Pacemakers today are designed to *fill in the gaps* in a patient's intrinsic rhythm. The pacemaker observes (senses) the patient's native heart rhythm and when needed—and only when needed—fills in a gap with a pacing output. This provides reliable rate support without unnecessary pacing, and it gives the patient's intrinsic rate as much opportunity as possible to take over.

In the early days of pacing, inhibition was an innovation. Pacemakers that inhibited were sometimes called *on-demand* pacemakers or *demand pacemakers* because they paced only on demand. Today, inhibition is used in all pacemakers and the term *demand pacemaker* sounds very old fashioned. But it is important to remember that inhibition is actually a *device feature* that makes good clinical sense. Inhibition is illustrated in **Figure 14.4**.

Pacing

Pacing refers to the delivery of an output pulse with the goal of capture or causing a cardiac depolarization. Any discussion of pacing naturally involves pacing rates, which are usually described in pulses per minute or ppm (some European and other international countries will use *reciprocal minutes* for pacing rates, so that 70 ppm is written 70 min^{-1}). When discussing the patient's intrinsic pacing rate, it is most accurate to talk about beats per minute or

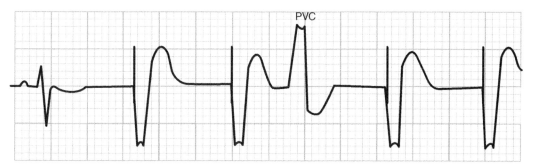

Figure 14.4 VVI pacing showing inhibition when the intrinsic activity occurs at a rate below the programmed base rate (first complex), with ventricular pacing occurring in the next two complexes as the pacemaker *fills in the missing beat* when no ventricular intrinsic events occur. Note that a PVC occurs, which is a type of intrinsic ventricular event. The pacemaker *sees* that and inhibits (withholds the output pulse) until the timing cycle runs out; since no other intrinsic ventricular events occurred, the pacemaker paces.

bpm; when talking about pacing, it is more accurate to use ppm.

The pacing rate may be called many different things, depending on the clinician or the pacemaker manufacturer. Common terms that all means the same thing are pacing rate, programmed rate, base rate, basic rate, programmed base rate, and lower rate limit (LRL). Knowing that these terms all mean the same thing, I prefer to use the term *programmed rate* when talking about single-chamber pacing and reserve some of the other terms for dual-chamber pacing. The most frequently observed programmed rate for single-chamber ventricular pacemakers is 70 ppm. Pediatric pacing rates are higher, sometimes even much higher up to 100 ppm, to correspond with the faster heart rates of young children.

Pacemakers are typically programmed in ppm rates, such as 60 or 70 ppm, but the pacemaker *thinks* in milliseconds and pacing intervals and timing cycles all use ms rather than ppm. Pacing clinicians must learn to use both terms fluently and to *translate* quickly from one to the other. Taking a pacing rate of 60 ppm, this means that the pacemaker will pace 60 pulses in 1 min. It is easy to do the math! If a pacemaker paces 60 pulses in a minute, then it pulses once every second (60 s = 1 min). That means a pacing rate of 60 ppm will correspond to an interval of 1 s, which can be written as 1000 ms (a millisecond is one-thousandth of a second). This illustrates the concept of how to convert ms to ppm and ppm to ms. Nowadays, such conversions are often done automatically by the programmer; in the early days of pacing, most specialists carried around with them a *rate ruler* that was really just a conversion chart that translated ppm to ms and vice versa. There is also a formula, in case you need to do this and have a calculator handy. Whatever value you have (ppm or ms), divide it by 60,000. For instance, if you know the rate is 70 ppm, then 70 divided by 60,000 is 857, so it corresponds to an interval of 857 ms. If you know the interval is 900 ms, then the rate is 67 ppm (900 divided by 60,000 is 66.6). In clinical practice, most pacing specialists get used to common rate conversions and become very adept at translating them in their head.

The pacing interval may be defined as the period of time between a paced event in one chamber and the next paced event in that same chamber without an intervening sensed event. If a pacemaker is programmed to 70 ppm, the pacing interval is going to be 857 ms long. Once a pacing interval starts, there are only two possible outcomes:

- It can time out or expire—that is, the 857 ms will elapse with no sensed event, in which case an output pulse is delivered.
- It can be interrupted—that is, within that 857-ms window, a sensed event will occur, in which case the pacemaker will inhibit the output pulse.

Looking at a paced ECG of a properly functioning pacemaker, there are two main events that occur: sense/inhibit and pace/capture. A sensed event will inhibit the output pulse and reset the timing cycles. If the pacing interval times out, the device will deliver an output pulse (pace) that will cause a cardiac depolarization (capture). No matter how

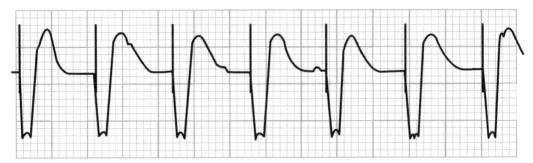

Figure 14.5 Capture in a single-chamber ventricular pacemaker is confirmed with this tracing, because the pacing spike is followed immediately by a ventricular depolarization with the characteristic wide morphology, the notch, and an unusual appearance. In this strip, every pacing output pulse successfully captures the ventricle.

long or complex a single-chamber rhythm strip may appear, clinicians will find only these two types of events. Note that when a pacing interval is interrupted by a sensed event, it resets the interval. For example, if the pacing interval is 857 ms and a sensed event occurs at 801 ms, the timer resets at 801 and begins the next timer for 857 ms.

Capture is the goal of pacing. Capture can be defined as the depolarization of a chamber of the heart resulting in a cardiac contraction *in response to a pacemaker output pulse.* An easy way to confirm capture from a rhythm strip is to identify pacing spikes and see if a cardiac depolarization and contraction occurs immediately after the spike. Paced ECGs usually look different than nonpaced ECGs even beyond the presence of pacing spikes. A paced ventricular beat often has a wider, notched QRS than a nonpaced QRS. P-waves may be inverted with pacing. If a ventricular pacing spike is followed immediately by a QRS that looks *different* from the intrinsic QRS complexes, in particular, if it is wider, is notched, and looks unusual, that gives further evidence of capture.

When the pacemaker is programmed appropriately for the patient, clinicians should see 1:1 capture, which means that every pacing spike causes a cardiac contraction. In other words, 1:1 capture confirms that the pacemaker is successfully pacing the heart every time it tries. One-to-one capture is not an elusive goal; failure to have 1:1 capture should cause the clinician to troubleshoot and solve the problem.

In order to assure reliable 1:1 capture, the clinician must know the patient's capture threshold, the minimum amount of electrical energy required to consistently depolarize the heart. As presented earlier in the book, capture thresholds are stated in two parameters: voltage or pulse amplitude along with milliseconds or pulse width (sometimes called pulse duration). Capture threshold itself is sometimes called the stimulation threshold or the pacing threshold; these terms all mean the same thing (see **Figure 14.5**).

Fusion, pseudofusion, and mass confusion

One of the most confusing aspects of pacing—and not just for beginners—is a phenomenon known as fusion. Because fusion (and its cousin, pseudofusion) is fairly common, the earlier that a clinician can get a grasp of what is going on, the simpler paced ECG analysis is going to be.

Fusion (sometimes called a *sandwich beat*) occurs when the pacemaker delivers an output pulse that contributes to but does not cause an intrinsic beat. In other words, the pacemaker output pulse *collides* with an intrinsic beat. Both occur in the same split second. A fusion beat can have a very unusual (or not-so-unusual) appearance on the ECG. Think of how fusion occurs. An intrinsic beat is starting from around the AV node and the wave of depolarization is starting to radiate downward; at the same moment, the pacemaker output pulse is delivered to the electrode in the ventricular apex and another wave of depolarization travels upward. These two depolarization fronts slam into each other, resulting in the fused beat.

Fusion is a timing problem. But is fusion capture? A fused beat shows both an output pulse and intrinsic activity contributing to depolarization. It is fair to say that fusion contributes to capture. For clinicians, this has important implications! When fusion occurs on a paced ECG, it can be taken as a confirmation of capture. A fused beat is not a classic *captured beat* but a fused beat indicates that the output pulse is capable of depolarizing the heart; in other words, if the heart had not beat on its own at that exact moment, the output pulse would have captured the heart. This is a key concept in understanding pacing: *fusion confirms capture*.

On the other hand, pseudofusion or false fusion occurs when the pacemaker output pulse occurs right on top of an intrinsic beat but does not contribute to that depolarization. Again, this is a matter of timing. In this case, the heart has depolarized on its own, and as the wave of depolarization travels through the heart, it leaves tissue refractory following the depolarization. Refractory tissue is physiologically incapable of depolarizing. So now if the pacemaker output pulse is delivered and hits refractory tissue, nothing happens. The pulse was properly delivered; there was just nothing there to depolarize. On an ECG, pseudofusion looks like an intrinsic beat with a pacemaker spike on top, which is a pretty good picture of what happened! Pseudofusion does not confirm capture, but it does not refute it, either. It just means that the intrinsic event and pacemaker pulse occurred right on top of each other and the heart depolarized on its own. Thus, the difference between fusion (where the output pulse *contributes* to the intrinsic event) is that in pseudofusion, the *output pulse has no effect at all* on the intrinsic event.

Fusion and pseudofusion occur for the same reason: timing. The patient's intrinsic rate is very close to the programmed pacing rate. The pacemaker timing cycle expires and the pacemaker delivers an output pulse in the split second that the heart decides to beat on its own. The most important thing to know about fusion and pseudofusion is that *it is not a capture problem*, it's a timing problem!

When clinicians encounter fusion and pseudofusion, they often try to troubleshoot. Fusion and pseudofusion are not problems with capture and they are not problems with sensing. The answer is actually much simpler: they're timing problems. It's a matter of rates. Fusion and pseudofusion occur when the patient's intrinsic rate and the pacemaker's programmed rate compete with each other. For example, imagine a patient whose intrinsic heart rate is around 70 bpm. Programming his pacemaker to 70 ppm means that the pacemaker and the patient are going to both try to keep the heart at the same speed and sometimes they are going to *bump into each other*.

Fusion and pseudofusion look abnormal, but they are not necessarily harmful to the patient, but they should be corrected. In both fusion and pseudofusion, the patient's heart rate is close to the programmed rate; by lowering the programmed rate a little bit, the patient's heart will have more opportunity to beat on its own, naturally. As a rule of thumb in bradycardia pacing, the more the heart can beat naturally on its own, the better. So allowing a lot of fusion and pseudofusion to go on may deprive the patient of the benefit of having as much intrinsic cardiac activity as possible. Second, fusion and pseudofusion are wasteful of battery energy. This is not a big deal if fusion and pseudofusion occur occasionally (as they often will), but a patient with a mostly fused rate is using battery energy unnecessarily. Another rule of thumb in pacing is conserve battery energy whenever possible as long as it does not compromise patient safety (see **Figure 14.6**).

Timing cycles

Refractory and alert periods

The pacing interval is actually divided into two distinct periods: the refractory period and the alert period. Just like a physiologic refractory period, the pacemaker's refractory period defines a timing cycle when the pacemaker will not respond to intrinsic signals. Even if an intrinsic signal occurs, the pacemaker will not respond to it if it falls in the refractory period. The refractory period itself is divided into two periods: the absolute refractory period and relative refractory period. During the absolute refractory period, the pacemaker is *blind* and incapable of even seeing intrinsic signals. During the relative refractory

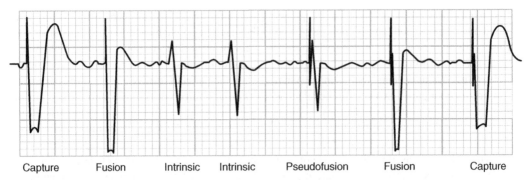

| Capture | Fusion | Intrinsic | Intrinsic | Pseudofusion | Fusion | Capture |

Figure 14.6 Fusion can be distinguished from pseudofusion by the QRS complex. The two capture events show a pacing spike followed by a classic wide, notched paced ventricular depolarization. The two intrinsic events show a typical narrow nonpaced QRS. The fused beats have a QRS complex that is somewhere in between—not as wide and notched as a true captured beat but not as narrow and pointed as an intrinsic beat. Fusion occurs when the pacing output pulse contributes to depolarization but does not cause it. The pseudofusion beat, on the other hand, looks exactly like a nonpaced ventricular complex; the pacemaker output pulse did not contribute at all to depolarization.

period, the pacemaker can perceive or *see* intrinsic events—and it will count them for its data collection—but it will not respond to them. So the pacemaker has no response at all to intrinsic events in the refractory period, although—as we'll learn more later on—it still counts events that occur during the relative refractory period. The relative refractory period is sometimes called the *noise-sampling period* because it allows the pacemaker to perceive (*sample*) stray signals (*noise*) that it assumes are not cardiac in origin.

The refractory period starts with either a paced or sensed event. Put another way, whenever a pacing interval begins, it starts with the refractory period. In a VVI pacemaker, any *ventricular* event starts the pacing interval and starts the refractory period. In a VVI pacemaker, this refractory period is often called the ventricular refractory period (VRP), because it only affects the ventricle. The refractory period always starts with its absolute refractory period, followed seamlessly by the relative refractory period.

The refractory period is programmable and in most single-chamber pacemakers will typically be set to about 250 ms. Note that although the refractory period has an absolute and relative period, these are not independently programmable; the clinician programs the refractory period as a whole and the device subdivides it into absolute and relative segments. The absolute refractory period is the longer portion of the refractory period (see **Figure 14.7**).

The refractory period is a timing cycle that simply starts and stops. The pacemaker does not have to make any *decision* when the cycle times out. When the refractory period times out, the alert period begins. During the alert period, the pacemaker can *see* intrinsic activity and will respond to it. Looking at Figure 14.7, the alert periods are the spaces between the refractory periods. Although the alert period is a critical element in pacemaker timing, it is not a directly programmable parameter. The clinician can only adjust the length of the refractory period (and also the pacing interval by changing the pacing rate). Lengthening the refractory period will shorten the alert period; conversely, by shortening the refractory period, the alert period is lengthened. For example, in a VVI pacemaker set to 70 ppm, the pacing interval is 857 ms. If the relative refractory period is programmed to 250 ms, that means the alert period is going to be 607 ms (857 − 250 = 607). Programming the refractory period to 300 ms will make the alert period be 557 ms (857-300 = 557); shortening the refractory period to 200 ms will change the alert period to 657 ms (857 − 200 = 657).

In a VVI pacemaker, the refractory period of the pacing interval exists to prevent sensing the large T-wave following the QRS complex. If the pacemaker sensed the T-wave, it would inappropriately identify it as an intrinsic ventricular event and withhold the pacemaker output pulse (inhibition),

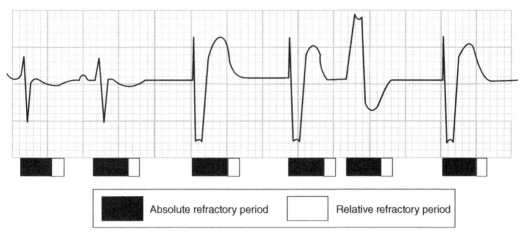

| Absolute refractory period | | Relative refractory period |

Figure 14.7 The refractory period is a programmable parameter that defines the period of time in which the pacemaker will not respond to intrinsic signals. In the absolute refractory period, the device does not *see* intrinsic events at all; in the relative refractory period, it sees intrinsic events and may count them for its data collection, but it will not respond to them. In a VVI pacemaker, any ventricular event (sensed or paced) initiates the refractory period timing cycle.

which would mean the patient would not get the rate support he needed. Looking at the T-waves in Figure 14.7, it is easy to see how the refractory period helps prevent the pacemaker from inappropriately sensing T-waves (a phenomenon known as *T-wave oversensing*).

Automatic and escape intervals

The automatic interval is defined as the interval from one pacing spike to the next consecutive pacing spike with no intervening intrinsic activity. The escape interval is the interval from an intrinsic event to the next paced event with no intervening intrinsic activity. The first difference between an automatic and escape interval is easy: an automatic interval starts with a spike, and an escape interval starts with an intrinsic event. Thus, the automatic interval is the interval from paced event to the next paced event, while the escape interval is the interval from an intrinsic event (which could also be called a *sensed event*) to the next paced event. Thinking of this another way, in a VVI pacemaker, each interval is defined in part by whether it starts with a paced event or a sensed event. The term *automatic* refers to the paced-to-paced interval that is defined automatically by the pacemaker's timing cycle. The *escape* interval is initiated by an escape or intrinsic beat and is terminated by a pacing spike.

An interesting and important fact about pacing is that most of the time, the automatic interval and the escape interval are of the same length.

Rate hysteresis

Hysteresis is a programmable feature that some clinicians may perceive as being complicated. When hysteresis activity appears on a paced ECG, it can sometimes cause confusion. Rate hysteresis is worth mastering, because it is an important feature that helps many patients. The best way to think of hysteresis is as a programmable option that allows the clinician to set the pacemaker to two different programming rates! First, the clinician programs the base rate in the normal way. Using a VVI pacemaker as an example, let's say the base rate is set to 70 ppm, which is a typical setting. With hysteresis programmed on, the clinician can now program a second and slightly lower rate for the hysteresis rate, for example, 60 bpm. The pacemaker now works with both rates—but in slightly different ways. As long as the patient's intrinsic rate is at or above the hysteresis rate, the pacemaker will be inhibited. In this example, the pacemaker will not pace if the patient's intrinsic rate is 65 bpm (even though the base rate is set to 70 ppm). However, if the patient's rate falls below the hysteresis rate, the pacemaker will start to pace at the pacing rate. For instance, if the patient's intrinsic rate is 58 bpm, the pacemaker will pace at 70 ppm.

Thus, the hysteresis rate defines the rate at which the pacemaker will inhibit, while the base rate defines the rate at which the pacemaker will pace. A better way to express this is that the pacing rate defines the automatic interval while the hysteresis rate defines the escape interval. Most of the time, the automatic and escape intervals will be the same, but with hysteresis on, the clinician tells the pacemaker to use two different intervals to define the automatic and escape intervals, respectively. Returning to the example above of a pacing rate of 70 ppm and a hysteresis rate of 60 bpm, that defines the automatic interval as 857 ms (70 ppm translates to 857 ms) and the escape interval as 1000 ms (60 bpm translates to 1000 ms).

Although hysteresis is not often programmed on, many patients can benefit from hysteresis because it allows their own intrinsic rate to take over and control the heart as much as possible. For patients, the most healthful cardiac rhythm is their own natural rhythm as long as it is fast and stable enough to support them. Hysteresis is one of the best (and easiest) pacemaker features to safely encourage intrinsic activity. Another advantage of hysteresis is that it may save battery life by not pacing except when absolutely necessary.

Search hysteresis

Hysteresis may also offer a search function, which can vary somewhat among manufacturers. This function is designed to overcome a potential drawback with hysteresis, namely, that once the pacemaker starts to pace, it will continue to pace at the programmed pacing rate until intrinsic activity interrupts it. Thus, if a pacemaker is programmed to 70 ppm, the patient may be experiencing a run of automatic intervals of 857 ms (857 ms = 70 ppm) that will not stop until intrinsic events occur at or above the rate of 70 ppm. If the patient's intrinsic rate is around 65–68 bpm, this is difficult to achieve and the pacemaker may continue to pace the patient even though the patient has a fairly high intrinsic rate.

The search function allows the pacemaker to periodically extend a so-called hysteresis interval (escape interval) aimed at *searching* for any intrinsic events that might be occurring outside of the faster pacing interval (automatic interval). Another way to think of this is that periodically, the pacemaker will interrupt a run of automatic intervals with an escape interval. The goal is to create a window of time where the patient's own rate has a chance to *take over*. If an intrinsic event falls in the hysteresis interval, then the hysteresis rate prevails. For instance, the pacemaker may be pacing at 70 ppm (857 ms), then a hysteresis interval occurs (1000 ms), and the pacemaker senses an intrinsic event at 882 ms (68 ppm). The pacemaker inhibits the output pulse and the patient's intrinsic rate of 68 ppm is now in control.

In many devices, search hysteresis occurs by clock time, for instance, every 5 min. The search interval can often be programmed so that one, two, or more search cycles occur. If search cycles do not find any intrinsic activity, the device resumes pacing at the programmed base rate until it is time for the next search.

Clinicians have to be cautious with rate hysteresis. Hysteresis can and does cause an inordinate amount of confusion, particularly when a clinician sees a rhythm strip that paces consistently at 70 ppm but then has three beats every 5 min at 50 ppm. This is one of the *frequently asked questions* for any pacemaker manufacturer technical support team. For that reason, hysteresis should only be programmed on when clinicians understand it, expect it, and are familiar with it. In the hospital setting, where many nonpacing experts will see the paced ECG, it may be a good idea to leave hysteresis off unless it is absolutely necessary. Once the patient is home and being treated by a pacing team, hysteresis should be considered if it may benefit the patient. Patients whose intrinsic rate is low or erratic are not good candidates for hysteresis.

Conclusion

Even though single-chamber pacemakers are not all that common in clinical practice, single-chamber pacing concepts are the bedrock of pacing knowledge. Clinicians need to appreciate that pacemakers only do two things: sense (and inhibit) and pace (and capture). The pacing interval in a single-chamber device defines the time between two pacing spikes with no intervening intrinsic events. While clinicians program and talk about rate in pulses per minute or ppm, devices think about rate in milliseconds, so clinicians must become familiar with moving from ppm to ms and back again easily and confidently.

The automatic and escape intervals on a rhythm strip differ by their initiating event: automatic intervals start with a paced event, and escape intervals start with an intrinsic event. Knowing these key concepts—and typical troubleshooting issues like fusion, pseudofusion, and hysteresis intervals—can help clinicians navigate the paced ECG more easily.

The nuts and bolts of single-chamber timing cycles

- When a special magnet is placed on top of the implanted pacemaker, it will cause the pacemaker to revert to *magnet mode*, which is typically asynchronous pacing at a set rate. Magnet mode behavior differs by device. Historically, magnet mode was used to check battery status. Today, it has more limited function but can be used to test device behavior.
- Asynchronous pacing is VOO or AOO (or DOO for dual-chamber modes), which means the device paces but does not sense. It will pace regardless of intrinsic activity.
- On a beat-by-beat basis, pacemakers can only ever do one of two things: they can sense (and inhibit) or pace (and capture).
- Sensing refers to the pacemaker's ability to *see* intrinsic cardiac activity. Actually, all the pacemaker is *seeing* are electrical signals, which it then interprets (based on size of the signal amplitude) as being cardiac or noise (noncardiac). The parameter that helps the device decide what signals are cardiac signals is sensitivity.
- Sensitivity is a programmable feature set in millivolts (mV) that defines the tallest signal amplitude the device can *see*. Programming sensitivity is like building a wall—the taller the wall (the higher the mV setting), the less you can see.
- Programming sensitivity is a balancing act—the setting should be high enough to keep out low-amplitude extracardiac or noise signals but low enough that all true cardiac signals are sensed.
- If you adjust the mV setting higher, you are actually making the device less sensitive. To make the device more sensitive, lower the mV setting.
- When a pacemaker delivers an output pulse, the goal is always capture. Capture can be defined as cardiac depolarization that occurs immediately after and as a result of a pacing spike.
- While most clinicians are comfortable with surface ECGs, it is more common with pacemakers to use electrograms or EGMs, taken from inside the heart. They look different than ECGs but it is important to get comfortable in using them. Most programmers will deliver reports with a surface ECG, an EGM, and annotations. It is important to compare annotations (what the pacemaker is *thinking*) to the tracings. It can also be useful to compare ECG to EGM to get the *big picture*.
- If the annotations and tracings disagree, the tracings always win.
- The pacing rate may also be called the base rate, basic rate, or lower rate limit. Most single-chamber pacemakers are programmed to 70 ppm except when they are implanted in children. Children typically use higher programmed rates, even as high as 100 ppm.
- Clinicians program pacemakers in ppm but devices usually report and *think* in millisecond (ms) intervals. To convert ms to ppm or vice versa, divide by 60,000 or use a rate ruler or other devices. It is important to long-term success in the pacing clinic to get comfortable and confident moving between ppm and ms.
- When a pacing interval starts, there are only two outcomes. It can time out or expire (at

Continued

Continued

which point a pacing output pulse is delivered) or it can be interrupted by an intrinsic event (at which point, it inhibits the output pulse).

- Fusion and pseudofusion can cause a lot of confusion, but they are really straightforward concepts. Fusion occurs when the pacemaker output pulse and an intrinsic event occur at almost exactly the same instant, with the result that the output pulse contributes to the intrinsic event. Fusion confirms capture. Fused beats look like a cross between a genuine paced beat and an intrinsic event.
- Pseudofusion occurs when the pacemaker output pulse falls on top of an intrinsic event in such a way that it has no effect. Pseudofusion looks like an intrinsic event with a spike on top. Pseudofusion does not confirm or refute capture.
- When troubleshooting fusion and pseudofusion, it is important to realize that these are not problems with sensing or capture. They are both timing issues! The patient's intrinsic rate is so close to the programmed base rate that the two are competing and sometimes smash into each other. Troubleshooting fusion and pseudofusion is done the same way: adjust the rate so that it is higher than the patient's intrinsic rate. However, some fusion and pseudofusion may occur occasionally anyway. This type of activity is not unusual and it is not problematic unless it happens frequently.
- Within the pacing cycle, there is a refractory period and an alert period. The refractory period is the period of time in which the pacemaker will not respond to intrinsic activity. In a VVI pacemaker, the refractory period is designed so that the pacemaker will not inappropriately sense a T-wave.
- The refractory is further subdivided into an absolute refractory period (when the device does not even *see* intrinsic events) and a relative refractory period (when the device *sees* intrinsic events and may even count them for its data counts, but will not respond to them).
- In a single-chamber pacemaker, the refractory period is programmable and typically is set to about 250 ms. The absolute and relative portions of the refractory period are usually not independently programmable.
- The pacing interval is composed of the refractory period (say 250 ms) and the alert period. The alert period is not directly programmable but can be adjusted by changing the refractory period setting. For instance, if the pacemaker is programmed to 60 ppm (1000 ms), then a 250 ms refractory period results in a 750 ms alert period (1000 − 250 = 750). Changing the rate or the refractory period will change the alert period.
- The automatic interval is the interval from one pacing spike to the next pacing spike with no intervening intrinsic events. The escape interval is the interval from a sensed event to the next pacing spike with no intervening intrinsic events. The key distinction is what starts the interval: automatic intervals start with a paced event, and escape intervals start with a sensed interval. Most of the time, automatic and escape intervals will be of the same length.
- Hysteresis refers to the ability to program two base rates. The pacing rate defines the automatic interval, while a second *hysteresis rate* defines the escape interval. For example, in a VVI pacemaker set to a base rate of 70 ppm with a hysteresis rate of 50 bpm, the pacemaker will pace at u70 ppm, but if the patient's intrinsic rate is above 50 bpm, it has the ability to inhibit pacing. Hysteresis often involves a search function that periodically imposes an escape interval to *search* for possible intrinsic events within that rate range.
- Hysteresis can be very confusing to clinicians who are not used to pacemakers. On an ECG, it may appear as a run of 70 ppm pacing with two or three intervals every 5 min at 50 bpm (the *search* function).
- Single-chamber pacemakers are not common but single-chamber pacing concepts are crucial for clinicians. First of all, dual-chamber devices sometimes pace in single-chamber fashion if that is appropriate for the patient. Second, all of these concepts apply to dual-chamber pacing.

Test your knowledge

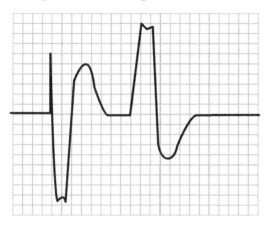

1 In the rhythm strip above, what evidence suggests that the first complex is a paced ventricular event?
   A The pacing spike right before the QRS complex
   B The wider-than-normal QRS complex
   C The notch on the QRS complex that does not appear in an intrinsic beat
   D All of the above

2 What is the second event in this strip?
   A Fusion
   B Pseudofusion
   C Premature ventricular contraction
   D Ventricular capture

3 This second event in the tracing above occurs during the pacemaker's *alert period*. What does the pacemaker do?
   A The pacemaker would pace the ventricle immediately.
   B The pacemaker would sense this event and reset its timing.
   C The pacemaker would not be able to see this event.
   D The pacemaker would be able to see this event, but it just would not respond to it.

4 What type of event starts the automatic interval?
   A Sensed event
   B Paced event

C Atrial event
D Any sensed or paced event

5 If you see fusion on a rhythm strip, what do you know about capture?
   A Fusion proves there is no capture.
   B Fusion confirms capture.
   C Fusion suggests there is capture, but does not prove it.
   D Nothing—fusion tells you nothing about capture.

6 A pacemaker has a sensitivity setting of 5 mV and the doctor wants to make the pacemaker *more sensitive*. Which is an appropriate setting?
   A 4 mV
   B 6 mV
   C First, widen the pulse width, and then program the amplitude to 6 V.
   D Nothing, sensitivity is not programmable.

7 When a magnet is placed over an implanted pacemaker, magnet mode is initiated that typically involves what kind of pacing?
   A Demand pacing
   B Cessation of pacing
   C Asynchronous pacing
   D Pacing according to programmed parameters

8 What is the most accurate definition of a patient who is *pacemaker dependent*?
   A A pacemaker patients who is paced 100% of the time
   B Any patient who has had a pacemaker for more than 5 years
   C A pacemaker patient who becomes symptomatic without pacing
   D A pacemaker patient whose underlying rhythm is ≤40 bpm

9 What pacing rate in ppm is programmed when the patient's pacing interval is 706 ms? (You may use a calculator or any other tools to reach your answer.)
   A 70 ppm
   B 75 ppm

C 80 ppm

D 85 ppm

10 If hysteresis is programmed on, what happens to the escape interval?

A It is longer than the automatic interval.

B It is shorter than the automatic interval.

C It is the same as the automatic interval.

D You cannot ever have an escape interval if hysteresis is on.

CHAPTER 15

Introduction to dual-chamber timing cycles

Learning objectives

- In a few words, state the main goal of dual-chamber pacing.
- Explain how a clinician might program the AV delay in order to maintain AV synchrony.
- Name the four states of dual-chamber pacing.
- State the two drivers of dual-chamber pacing.

Introduction

The first time a clinician encounters dual-chamber pacing in theory and terminology, it can sound like a foreign language. One of the biggest challenges in learning dual-chamber pacing is not so much learning the concepts as it is to persevere in your study long enough—because if you stick with it long enough, you will get it. That is my guarantee. For most people (even very smart people), it is not quick or easy. Most of the concepts of dual-chamber pacing are not intuitive, can seem unnecessarily complicated, and are like nothing you have encountered before. For that reason, take your time, be patient, and do not be afraid to go over these ideas again and again. The best way to approach dual-chamber pacing is to learn to think like a pacemaker! (And most people do not know how to think like a pacemaker without a whole lot of practice.)

In one respect, dual-chamber pacing is like having two single-chamber pacemakers, one in the atrium and one in the ventricle. For that reason, the next two chapters are going to address the atrial and ventricular components of dual-chamber pacing. But before we can get that far, we are going to tackle some of the fundamental ideas on which dual-chamber pacing is built.

In single-chamber pacing, there are two main timing cycles that govern the pacemaker's function. In dual-chamber pacing, there are about 10. These 10 govern the atrial channel and the ventricular channel and how the two channels interact with each other.

Dual-chamber pacing is based on some underlying concepts, atrial and ventricular timing cycles, and ways in which these cycles interact with each other. If you find yourself getting overwhelmed or confused, just backtrack a little and go back over the key concepts. Approaching dual-chamber concepts systematically will help.

The four states of dual-chamber pacing

In dual-chamber pacing, you will only ever encounter four types of complexes. These are sometimes called the *four states* of DDD pacing. They are:
- An atrial sensed event followed by a ventricular sensed event (in other words, no pacing going on at all)
- An atrial sensed event followed by a ventricular paced event (this is an intrinsic atrial beat that does not conduct and depolarize the ventricles so the ventricles have to be paced)

The Nuts and Bolts of Implantable Device Therapy Pacemakers, First Edition. Tom Kenny.
© 2015 John Wiley & Sons, Ltd. Published 2015 by John Wiley & Sons, Ltd.

- An atrial paced event followed by a ventricular sensed event (the pacemaker has to pace the atrium, but the beat conducts over the AV node and depolarizes the ventricles)
- An atrial paced event followed by a ventricular paced event (in this case, nothing is beating on its own—it is all paced).

There are different ways to abbreviate or annotate these various events. For example, AP is sometimes used for atrial paced event; it is sometimes written Ap. Others may abbreviate an atrial sensed event as P or p (for P-wave). The annotations vary from manufacturer to manufacturer and sometimes even from clinician to clinician. Thus, there is no single preferred way to abbreviate these, and you may see them written in different ways.

Each of these four states is associated with specific timing cycles. Mastery of dual-chamber pacing includes a complete understanding of the timing cycles involved in these four states.

It is crucial to remember this key concept: the goal of the dual-chamber pacemaker is to achieve 1:1 AV synchrony. This is not always possible, but to the extent that the dual-chamber pacemaker can *put in the missing beat* to maintain 1:1 AV synchrony, it will try to do that.

In order to maintain 1:1 AV synchrony, the pacemaker may have to do one or both of the following:
- If the atrial rate slows below the programmed base rate, it will have to pace the atrium.
- If the atrial beat does not conduct properly over the AV node to the ventricles, it will have to pace the ventricle.

Thus, the two drivers of pacing in a dual-chamber system are the intrinsic atrial rate and the rate of AV conduction.

General overview of atrial and ventricular pacing in a dual-chamber system

A dual-chamber pacemaker will always pace the atrium whenever the patient's intrinsic atrial rate drops below the programmed rate. For example, if the DDD pacemaker is programmed to pace at 70 ppm and the patient has an intrinsic atrial rate of around 50 bpm, the DDD pacemaker is going to consistently pace the atrium. What this means to

clinicians is that *atrial pacing in a dual-chamber device happens at the base rate.* (There is an exception to this with rate response, but for now, we will assume rate response is turned off.) Pacing clinicians may know the base rate from the programmer or the patient's records, but it is easy to calculate the programmed base rate from the patient's paced ECG. The base rate can be calculated from the distance *between two atrial pacing spikes* (*with no intervening atrial events*). Using an easy example, let's say the distance between two atrial pacing spikes on the tracing was 1000 ms. Since 1000 ms *translates* to 60 ppm, the programmed base rate of that pacemaker is 60 ppm.

Thinking like a pacemaker, there is an entirely different motivation for pacing the ventricle than for pacing the atrium. While the pacemaker will pace the atrium when the atrial rate slows below the programmed rate, pacemakers *will pace the ventricle when AV conduction slows.* The pacemaker determines slow conduction based on a programmable timing cycle called the AV delay (sometimes called the AV interval). The pacemaker does not pace the ventricle based on ventricular timing to other ventricular events; instead, it bases ventricular pacing on the AV delay. This may not be the most intuitive concept, but it is crucial to understand this to grasp dual-chamber pacing.

The AV delay can be defined as the timing cycle between an atrial event (sensed or paced) and the next paced ventricular event. If the ventricles depolarize on their own before the AV delay expires, then the pacemaker will inhibit the ventricular output pulse. On the other hand, if an atrial event occurs and no intrinsic ventricular event occurs, the pacemaker will deliver an output pulse to the ventricle as soon as the AV delay expires. In a way, the AV delay is the electronic version of the natural PR interval. The AV delay is programmable, but it is often set to 200 ms, which is the high end of the intrinsic PR interval.

During the AV delay, the pacemaker will look for ventricular activity. The AV delay can be thought of as an alert period for ventricular events. If the AV delay expires before it senses any ventricular activity, it will cause the pacemaker to *put in the beat that's missing* and pace the ventricle (see **Figure 15.1**).

If you obtain a tracing from a programmer, you have access to annotations. Besides naming the two

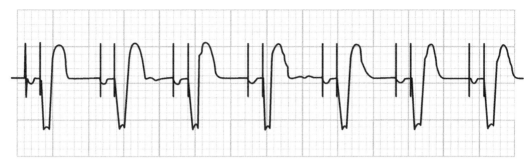

Figure 15.1 This dual-chamber paced strip shows atrial paced events and ventricular paced events (AV pacing). The AV delay is launched after each atrial pacing spike and, in this case, times out before any intrinsic ventricular activity occurs. The result is that when the AV delay expires, the pacemaker delivers a ventricular output pulse.

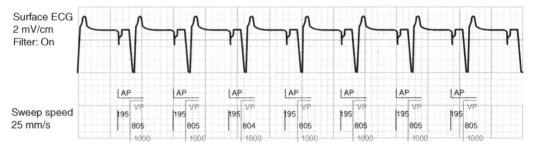

Figure 15.2 In this electrogram, the first number is the AV delay (195 ms) and the second number is the V-to-A interval or, in this case, the time that elapses between the ventricular paced event and the next atrial paced event. The bottom number is the programmed base rate, which is defined as the interval between two atrial pacing spikes with no intervening atrial events. At 1000 ms, the programmed base rate converts to a pacing rate of 60 ppm. The annotations (AP, VP) are color coded on the strip for easy identification. Note that this pacemaker was actually programmed to an AV delay of 200 ms, but there is some *wiggle* in the displayed annotations. This is normal and not a cause for alarm as long as it is a matter of a few milliseconds.

landmarks on the above strip (atrial and ventricular paced events), the annotations will provide interval measurements (see **Figure 15.2**). While clinicians should learn how to calculate intervals using the grids on the paper and also using the caliper method, in real-world clinical practice, most pacing experts rely on the convenience of annotated intervals for their measurements whenever available. Different manufacturers use slightly different annotation systems.

When the pacemaker senses in the atrium and paces in the ventricle, the behavior is also called *atrial tracking* or sometimes just *tracking*. In this case, the patient's intrinsic atrial rate is above the programmed base rate, and thus, the pacemaker inhibits its atrial output pulse. However, for some reason, this atrial beat does not successfully conduct over the AV node and into the ventricles. The AV delay—which starts with the atrial sensed

event—expires, and the pacemaker delivers its ventricular output pulse, which in **Figure 15.3** captures the ventricle.

Atrial tracking behavior can be very advantageous to the patient because it provides 1:1 AV synchrony and allows the patient's natural atrial rate to prevail. However, atrial tracking can be confusing to clinicians. Using the strip in **Figure 15.4** as an example, assume that this is a dual-chamber pacemaker programmed to 60 ppm (1000 ms interval). The pacemaker is pacing at a much faster rate (80 ppm or 750 ms). Why does this occur? Remember to think like a pacemaker! The dual-chamber pacemaker is going to allow the atria to beat on their own as long as they beat faster than the programmed rate. In this example, the patient's atria are beating on their own at around 80 bpm, so the pacemaker is going to inhibit the atrial pacing output. After each atrial beat, the pacemaker

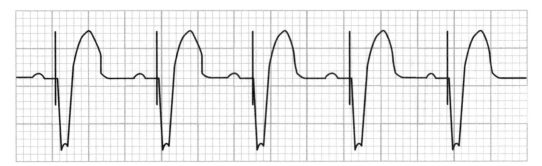

Figure 15.3 The dual-chamber pacemaker tries to maintain 1:1 AV synchrony when the patient has an intrinsic atrial rate above the programmed base rate. In this case, the atrial output pulses are consistently inhibited, because the atria are beating on their own. But in order to make sure each atrial beat has a corresponding ventricular beat, the pacemaker paces the ventricle when the AV delay expires.

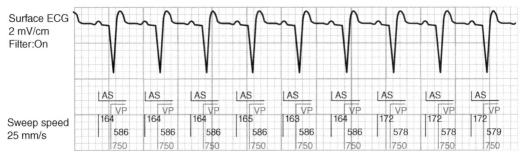

Figure 15.4 This electrogram has a visible but very hard-to-see pacemaker spike. However, a clinician using this annotated strip would know that ventricular pacing is going on because of the annotation (VP means ventricular paced event and signals the delivery of a ventricular output pulse) and because of the immediate ventricular depolarization after the annotation. Atrial sensing is annotated and is easier to see on the strip. The timing cycles are the same: 164 ms is the AV delay, 586 ms is the V-to-A interval (which in this case is a sensed rather than atrial paced event), and 750 ms is the V-to-V interval or paced, which corresponds to a rate of 80 ppm. This is the V-to-V interval because it is color coded for the ventricular channel.

launches an AV delay. It paces the ventricle in response to slow conduction across the AV node, that is, the pacemaker will pace the ventricle to time the ventricular paced event to the preceding atrial event. This maintains 1:1 AV synchrony (which is good), but it also means that the pacemaker is now pacing above the programmed base rate (which can be confusing).

Atrial tracking is a great term for this behavior because the dual-chamber pacemaker will *keep track* of the atrial rate and put in missing beats to maintain 1:1 AV synchrony. Atrial tracking behavior is very commonly observed dual-chamber pacing behavior, but it can still be puzzling, particularly to clinicians who do not see many paced rhythm strips.

While it is not unusual for one dual-chamber pacing state to dominate a patient's rhythm, the

dual-chamber pacemaker can change pacing states in a split second. The pacemaker watches the patient's heart, beat by beat, always ready to fill in the missing beat (see **Figures 15.5** and **15.6**). In that example, the patient's atrial rate suddenly slowed—but the pacemaker preserved 1:1 AV synchrony by pacing the atrium when necessary.

Another common dual-chamber pacing behavior consists of atrial pacing, which conducts reliably to the ventricles (see **Figure 15.8**). Such patients have compromised sinus function but intact AV conduction (that is faster than the programmed AV delay). These rhythm strips can be confusing in that the AV delay may vary across the strip. If the AV delay is measured from a atrial paced event to an intrinsic ventricular event, the AV delay will never be longer than the programmed

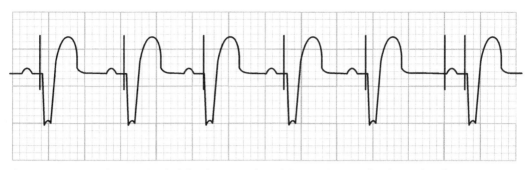

Figure 15.5 In this rhythm strip, the dual-chamber pacemaker exhibits atrial tracking but then—when the intrinsic atrial rate slows below the programmed base rate—paces the atrium. Beat by beat, the pacemaker will try to maintain 1:1 AV synchrony.

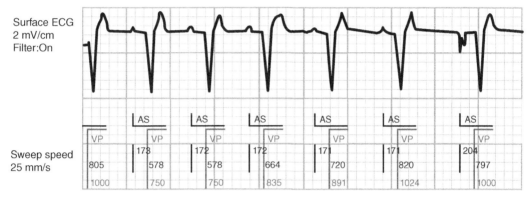

Figure 15.6 In this annotated electrogram for this figure, note that the pacemaker switches smoothly from AS/VP pacing states to AP/VP. Note that the AV delay changes from around 173–204 ms when the pacing state changes. (This represents a little *wiggle* in that the programmed AV delay is 200 ms.)

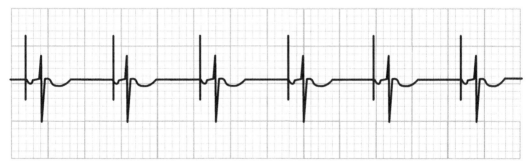

Figure 15.7 The pacemaker paces the atrium because the patient's intrinsic atrial rate is below the programmed base rate. However, each atrial paced event conducts over the AV node and results in a ventricular depolarization, which occurs before the AV delay times out. The result is that the pacemaker inhibits the ventricular output pulse.

value (which is 200 ms in **Figures 15.7** and **15.8**), but it may be shorter! If the patient's AV node can conduct faster than the programmed AV delay, the pacemaker will inhibit the ventricular output. Thus, in Figure 15.8, the AV delay varies from complex to

complex but never exceeds the programmed value of 200 ms.

Another *pacing state* has no pacing at all. If the patient's atrial rate is above the programmed base rate and the atrial beat conducts over the AV

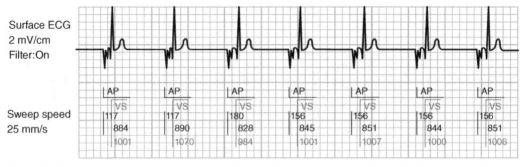

Figure 15.8 The electrogram for this tracing shows the AV delay (first number), then the VA interval (second number), and finally the rate (about 1000 ms). The AV delay varies from complex to complex because it is measured from a *paced event to a sensed event*. (Notice that the AV delay in the first complex is 117 ms, but it is 180 ms in the third complex.) The AV delay will never be longer than the programmed value, but it can be shorter. If the patient can conduct over the AV node faster than the programmed AV interval, the pacemaker inhibits the ventricular output pulse.

node and depolarizes the ventricles faster than the programmed AV delay, the dual-chamber pacemaker remains on standby and inhibits both atrial and ventricular output pulses. If the tracing shows intrinsic activity above the base rate, intact AV conduction, and no pacing—this is fine; in fact, it is the *expected behavior* of the pacemaker. From time to time in clinical practice, clinicians see paced rhythm strips with no pacing at all. Many pacemaker patients do not require 100% or even 50% pacing, so such strips show absolutely appropriate pacemaker behavior. This type of behavior is sometimes called *total inhibition*.

The four states in the real world

It does not take long in clinical practice to see all four states of dual-chamber pacing on a tracing. In fact, you can often find all four in a single tracing from one patient! However, most patients will have one or two states that dominate. A pacing clinician can often look at the most frequently occurring pacing states on an ECG and draw conclusions about the patient's arrhythmia diagnosis. For example, a tracing that shows lots of ventricular sensed events and a mixture of paced and atrial sensed events would indicate the patient had intact AV conduction and intermittent sinus dysfunction. A rhythm strip with consistently ventricular paced events suggests advanced heart block.

If the patient's rhythm strip seems to be at odds with the diagnosis, a couple of things may be going on. First, it could be that the patient's condition and

arrhythmias have changed. A patient may have received a pacemaker 10 years ago for heart block and had intact sinus function but since developed sick sinus syndrome. In this example, it means the clinician can expect to see atrial paced and ventricular paced events today instead of the atrial sensed and ventricular paced events of the past.

The rhythm strip may not align with the diagnosis if the pacemaker is not programmed optimally. For example, sinus node dysfunction with intact AV conduction should result in a strip with mostly atrial paced and ventricular sensed events. If the clinician sees instead a rhythm strip from this patient with a lot of ventricular pacing, this might suggest the device is not programmed appropriately for the patient. For instance, if the AV delay was programmed to a very short value of 150 ms, the pacemaker is going to pace the ventricles because the AV delay times out before the ventricles beat on their own. In such a patient, reprogramming the AV delay to a more typical 200 ms or even slightly longer might give the ventricles enough time to beat spontaneously.

Third, it is not unusual to observe periods of no pacing or minimal pacing, even in patients who are indicated for a pacemaker. Many arrhythmias are intermittent, meaning that they come and go. Sometimes, a run of unpaced activity reflects a spell of normal cardiac activity. However, sometimes, an unpaced strip (atrial sensed and ventricular sensed events) will occur because of an atrial tachyarrhythmia that conducts to the ventricles. For instance, if a dual-chamber pacemaker patient has atrial fibrillation and intact AV conduction, an episode of atrial fibrillation will present on the tracing as atrial sensed and ventricular sensed events. Thus, an unpaced strip may be benign, or it may show a problem. Atrial fibrillation and other high-rate atrial activity will be discussed later in this book. For now, it is important to know that pacemakers cannot pace into atrial fibrillation to *put in a missing beat.*

A fast review: Avoiding common misconceptions

To successfully navigate the world of dual-chamber pacing, clinicians have to dispel some basic misconceptions about how these devices work. Rather than go over these misconceptions, let's focus on some basic true concepts about dual-chamber pacing that you absolutely need to know to understand how these devices work.

There are only four states in DDD pacing, and these states suggest the patient's underlying condition. It is important to master the four states, which are based on two possible events (sensed and paced events) in two chambers (atrial and ventricular). A patient who has sinus node dysfunction will need atrial pacing so pacing states for this type of patient should predominantly show atrial paced and ventricular sensed events and/or atrial paced and ventricular paced events. Likewise, a patient with heart block is going to have a lot of ventricular paced activity. Patients with a healthy sinus node will exhibit a lot of atrial sensed events. If AV conduction is intact, there will be ventricular sensed activity. Sometimes, a patient has intermittent intact AV conduction, in which case there will be a lot of ventricular paced activity with intermittent runs of ventricular sensed activity.

All dual-chamber timing is based on the atrial channel. Because the ventricles are the more important chambers of the heart in terms of cardiac output, it is easy to think that ventricular activity controls pacemaker timing. Not true! Dual-chamber pacemakers use atrial events for all timing. In this way, dual-chamber pacemakers are like the healthy heart that relies on the SA node (located in the right atrium) to time the heart beats. Timing is always atrial—whether you are looking at intrinsic activity in a healthy heart or a dual-chamber paced heart.

To calculate the rate of dual-chamber pacing from a rhythm strip, look for the atrial paced interval. This builds off the previous statement, but it is something that many clinicians miss. If you have only a tracing and want to calculate the paced rate of a dual-chamber device, use the atrial paced interval (the time span between two atrial paced events without an intervening atrial event). It is tempting to want to look at the ventricular events and count from them—but that is not how a pacemaker thinks!

The ventricular rate is timed off the atrial rate. The dual-chamber pacemaker initiates the AV delay following an atrial event (paced or sensed), and when the AV delay times out, the pacemaker will pace the ventricle. Ventricular pacing is timed strictly and solely from the atrial rate. If the DDD patient's atrial rate is entirely paced, then the ventricular rate will occur at the programmed base rate. But if the DDD patient has intrinsic atrial activity at a rate higher than the programmed base rate (leading to atrial sensed events), the ventricular paced rate can be higher than the programmed base rate. The best way to approach this is to think like a pacemaker and only look to the atrial channel for calculating base rate. The ventricular rate then tracks the atrial rate.

There are only two drivers for dual-chamber pacing rate: the patient's intrinsic atrial rate and the patient's intrinsic rate of AV conduction. The dual-chamber pacemaker will pace the atrium if the patient's intrinsic atrial rate drops below the programmed base rate. The dual-chamber pacemaker will pace the ventricle if the AV delay times out and no ventricular activity is sensed. That is all the pacemaker *thinks about* when it comes to rate!

In a dual-chamber pacemaker, you will sometimes see pacing at a rate other than the programmed base rate (even if rate response is turned off). This may seem surprising, but the programmed base rate is not always reflected in the paced rhythm strip. Several things can affect the pacing rate. For the moment, let's set aside rate response and hysteresis, both of which can result in non-base-rate pacing. Instead, let's take the example of a patient with advanced heart block and a dual-chamber pacemaker set to 60 ppm; if she has an intrinsic atrial rate of 62 bpm, the pacemaker will pace the ventricles to keep pace with the atrial rate. The rhythm strip will show ventricular pacing at around 62 ppm.

That's because the patient's intrinsic atrial rate is controlling the atrial channel and ventricular pacing is timed from the atrial channel. Thus, the ventricular paced rate can differ from the programmed base rate. This is not an unusual scenario at all.

Conclusion

To master dual-chamber pacing concepts, you have to learn to *think like a pacemaker*. Pacemakers use a variety of timing cycles to regulate activity. In single-chamber pacing, only a few timing cycles are in play, but there are at least 10 important timing cycles in dual-chamber pacing, and these cycles interact with each other. Thus, it can be important to approach dual-chamber pacing systematically. There are only four states of DDD pacing: atrial paced/ventricular paced events, atrial paced/ventricular sensed events, atrial sensed/ventricular paced events, and atrial sensed/ventricular sensed events. There are only two drivers for dual-chamber timing: the patient's intrinsic atrial rate (which determines if and when the atrium is paced) and the patient's rate of AV conduction (which determines if and when the ventricles are paced). Overall, the dual-chamber pacemaker will consistently attempt to assure 1:1 AV synchrony by filling in the missing beat.

The nuts and bolts of introduction to dual-chamber pacing concepts

- While there are only two main timing cycles for single-chamber pacemakers, dual-chamber pacemakers have at least 10 important timing cycles.
- There are four *states* to dual-chamber pacing involving whether atrial and ventricular events are sensed or paced. These four states are atrial paced/ventricular paced events, atrial paced/ventricular sensed events, atrial sensed/ventricular paced events, and atrial sensed/ventricular sensed events.
- The abbreviations for pacing states or types of events vary by manufacturer and sometimes by hospital or clinic. Thus, an atrial sensed event might be As (atrial sensed event) or P (P-wave).
- A dual-chamber pacemaker always seeks to maintain 1:1 AV synchrony (one atrial event for each and every ventricular event) as much as possible. To do this, it will *fill in the missing beat* when necessary.
- There are two drivers of dual-chamber pacing: the patient's intrinsic atrial rate and the patient's intrinsic AV conduction.
- If the dual-chamber pacemaker patient's intrinsic atrial rate drops below the programmed base rate, the pacemaker will pace the atrium. By the same token, if the patient's intrinsic atrial rate exceeds the programmed base rate, the pacemaker will inhibit the atrial output pulse.

- To calculate the programmed base rate using a paced dual-chamber rhythm strip, measure the atrial paced interval, that is, the time between one atrial paced event and the next atrial paced event (with no intervening atrial events).
- The pacemaker paces the ventricle by timing it to the preceding atrial event. With any atrial event, the pacemaker launches a timing cycle called the AV delay. The AV delay may be thought of a ventricular alert period. If intrinsic ventricular activity occurs during the AV delay, the pacemaker will inhibit the ventricular output pulse. On the other hand, if the AV delay times out and no intrinsic ventricular event occurs, the pacemaker will pace the ventricle.
- Atrial pacing in a dual-chamber device will occur at the programmed base rate. (The exception to this involves rate-responsive pacing, which will be discussed in a future chapter.)
- The AV delay is an important timing cycle; it regulates ventricular pacing. A typical AV delay is programmed to 200 ms. The AV delay may be thought of as the pacemaker's version of the PR interval.
- Different manufacturers use different symbols and codes on the electrogram, but all electrograms offer useful annotations and intervals. These annotations are convenient but should always be checked against the tracings (both intracardiac and surface).

- Atrial tracking refers to the pacemaker's behavior in maintaining 1:1 AV synchrony when the patient's intrinsic atrial rate is higher than the programmed base rate. Up to a point, the pacemaker will pace the ventricle to keep up with the patient's native atrial rate. This can result in faster-than-base-rate ventricular pacing.
- One of the four states of DDD pacing is no pacing at all. This may be benign, in that many pacemaker patients have intermittent arrhythmias and periods when their heart rhythm is relatively normal and requires no pacing. However, this pacing state may also occur when the patient is experiencing an atrial tachyarrhythmia with a ventricular response.
- Clinicians should anticipate what pacing states should predominate in a given patient based on the diagnosis. For example, patients with sick sinus syndrome should have a lot of atrial paced activity. When the actual states of DDD pacing do not align with anticipated events based on the patient's diagnosis, further investigation is warranted. Sometimes, rhythm disorders change or worsen over time. In some cases, the pacemaker may not be programmed optimally for the patient's needs.

Test your knowledge

1 Mrs. Jones has a dual-chamber pacemaker programmed to DDD mode. She has severe sinus node dysfunction with intact and fast AV conduction. What pacing state would you expect to see most frequently?
   A Atrial paced/ventricular paced events
   B Atrial paced/ventricular sensed events
   C Atrial sensed/ventricular paced events
   D Atrial sensed/ventricular sensed events

2 Mr. Smith has a DDD pacemaker and has a good sinus node function with third-degree heart block. What pacing state would you expect to see most frequently?
   A Atrial paced/ventricular paced events
   B Atrial paced/ventricular sensed events
   C Atrial sensed/ventricular paced events
   D Atrial sensed/ventricular sensed events

3 A DDD patient with intact AV conduction experienced several minutes of atrial fibrillation. What pacing state would you expect to see during this spell?
   A Atrial paced/ventricular paced events
   B Atrial paced/ventricular sensed events
   C Atrial sensed/ventricular paced events
   D Atrial sensed/ventricular sensed events

4 How could a DDD pacing strip be used to estimate the programmed pacing rate?

A Measure atrial pacing intervals
B Measure ventricular pacing intervals
C Measure the AV delay
D Measure the VA interval

5 When a patient has a DDD pacemaker and his intrinsic atrial rate falls below the programmed base rate, what does the DDD pacemaker do?
   A Paces the ventricle
   B Paces the atrium
   C Launches the AV delay
   D Inhibits the atrial output pulse

6 When does the AV delay occur?
   A Right after an atrial paced event
   B Right after an atrial sensed event
   C Right after any atrial event (sensed or paced, it does not matter)
   D After a PAC

7 What does *atrial tracking* mean?
   A The pacemaker consistently paces the atrium, regardless of the intrinsic rate.
   B The pacemaker will pace the ventricle to track or keep pace with the intrinsic atrial rate.
   C The pacemaker times atrial events to track or keep pace with the intrinsic ventricular rate.
   D The annotations flag all atrial events and identify them as paced or sensed.

8 What are the two drivers of pacing rate in a dual-chamber device?

  A Intrinsic atrial rate and intrinsic ventricular rate

  B Intrinsic ventricular rate and AV conduction speed

  C Intrinsic atrial rate and AV conduction speed

  D Intrinsic PR interval and intrinsic ventricular rate

9 Which of the following situations might cause a DDD pacemaker to pace at a rate faster than the programmed base rate?

  A Atrial tracking (the patient's intrinsic atrial rate is higher than the base rate).

  B A very short AV delay.

  C Hysteresis.

  D Nothing—the DDD pacemaker will only ever pace at the base rate.

10 A DDD patient's rhythm strip shows no pacing for several minutes. There are multiple explanations for this sort of behavior. Of the rhythms listed below, which would be the most plausible explanation?

  A Normal sinus rhythm at an appropriate rate

  B Sick sinus syndrome

  C Mobitz II

  D None of the above

CHAPTER 16

Dual-chamber timing cycles: the atrial channel

Learning objectives

- Name and briefly define the main atrial channel timing cycles in DDD pacing.
- Define latency and discuss why paced and sensed AV delays might be programmed independently.
- Briefly explain how the DAVID study influenced how clinicians program dual-chamber pacemakers today.
- State what PVARP stands for and its role in dual-chamber timing.
- Name a dual-chamber timing cycle that can help prevent far-field ventricular oversensing.
- Explain how pacemaker-mediated tachycardia gets started and programming tips to prevent it.
- Name the most common trigger for pacemaker-mediated tachycardia.
- Explain the role of magnet application in dealing with pacemaker-mediated tachycardia.
- Define *PVC* the way the pacemaker does.
- Outline how an automatic PMT prevention algorithm works.
- State what the acronym TARP stands for.

Introduction

Dual-chamber pacing is governed by multiple interacting timing cycles, which can be thought of as timing clocks on either the atrial or the ventricular channel. To be sure, the timing cycles in dual-chamber pacing affect both atrial and ventricular activities, but the actual timing cycles are rooted in either the atrial or ventricular side of the device. For beginners or others trying to navigate the complexities of dual-chamber pacing, it helps to think of atrial timing cycles separately from ventricular timing cycles.

Refractory and alert periods

Dual-chamber pacemakers have refractory periods, just like single-chamber pacemakers. To review briefly, a refractory period is a timing cycle during which the pacemaker will not respond to incoming signals. Refractory periods can be subdivided into two components: the absolute refractory period, during which the pacemaker will neither *see* nor respond to incoming signals, and the relative refractory period, during which the pacemaker will *see* (and count) incoming signals, but will not respond to them. In single-chamber or dual-chamber pacemakers, the absolute refractory period is sometimes called a *blanking period*, and the relative refractory period is sometimes called the *noise-sampling period*.

Another commonality between dual-chamber and single-chamber pacemakers is the alert period. In simplest terms, the alert period is the timing cycle during which the pacemaker is looking for intrinsic activity. If intrinsic activity is sensed during the alert period, it may inhibit the output pulse.

Both channels on the dual-chamber pacemaker will have refractory and alert periods. The following

The Nuts and Bolts of Implantable Device Therapy Pacemakers, First Edition. Tom Kenny.
© 2015 John Wiley & Sons, Ltd. Published 2015 by John Wiley & Sons, Ltd.

will go into more detail on some of the unique aspects of the refractory periods on the atrial channel in dual-chamber pacing.

The AV delay

Earlier in this book, the AV delay (sometimes called the AV interval) was presented as the timing cycle that governs the time from an atrial event (sensed or paced) to the next paced ventricular event. This is a correct and serviceable definition, but the AV delay can be a little more complicated than that. There are actually two main types of AV delay depending on whether the atrial event that launches the timing cycle was a sensed or paced atrial event. Thus, we have a paced AV delay and a sensed AV delay, and they have some unique characteristics.

The AV delay was designed to mimic the behavior of the healthy heart, which allows for a brief pause between atrial contraction and ventricular contraction. In the healthy heart, this period allows for *atrial kick*, which contributes to better cardiac output. A good way to think about the AV delay is that it is the electronic version of the normal PR interval. Pacemakers attempt to emulate the behavior of the healthy heart, and the AV delay imitates what the PR interval does in a healthy heart. First, it allows the ventricles a little bit of extra time for extra filling, which assures that they can pump the maximum quantity of blood with each cycle. Second, it allows enough time for the mitral valve to close properly. If the mitral valve does not close entirely or correctly, blood can back up in the heart in a condition known as *mitral valve regurgitation*. This can cause symptoms and it reduces cardiac output. Finally, the AV delay—like the PR interval—allows for optimal hemodynamics.

A properly timed (and programmed) AV delay leads to better hemodynamics and cardiac output. Certain dual-chamber patients have an intrinsic PR interval that is too long. Dual-chamber pacing with a shorter AV delay can actually enhance hemodynamics in these patients and improve cardiac output. In other patients, the AV delay is simply programmed to assure that there is an appropriate pause between atrial and ventricular contractions when the device is pacing.

AV delays are programmable timing cycles, meaning that clinicians can set them to any of a wide range of values. The purpose of programmable parameters in dual-chamber pacing is to allow clinicians the opportunity to fine-tune cardiac pacing to meet the individual needs of patients. While programmability is important, most patients will do well with certain settings. These common settings are often the nominal setting of the device as it is shipped from the factory. It is true that many device settings are left at these nominal values rather than being fine-tuned, but that may be at least partly because the nominal settings happen to work well in the majority of patients.

When programming the AV delay, the clinician can independently program the paced AV delay and the sensed AV delay. AV delays are programmable in milliseconds. The difference is whether the atrial event that launches the AV delay timing cycle is a paced event (paced AV delay) or an intrinsic atrial event (sensed AV delay) (see **Figure 16.1**). Thus, a paced AV delay can be defined as the time between an atrial pacing spike and the next ventricular paced event, while the sensed AV delay is the time between an intrinsic atrial event and the next ventricular paced event. Some device manufacturers and clinicians may call the sensed AV delay the *PV delay*. The paced AV delay is often set to 200 ms, but the sensed AV delay is typically about 25–50 ms shorter. The reason for this timing offset is that when the pacemaker paces the atrium, it launches the AV delay exactly with the pacing spike. When the pacemaker

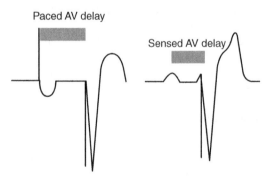

Figure 16.1 The paced and sensed AV delays are independently programmable timing cycles. Note that a typical paced AV delay is programmed to about 200 ms, while a sensed AV delay is about 175 ms. The timing differential owes to the fact that there is a brief time lag (about 25 ms) between the start of the intrinsic atrial event and the time at which the pacemaker senses it and can launch the sensedAV delay.

senses the atrium, on the other hand, there is a very brief lag in time before the event is sensed and the AV delay can be initiated.

This is an important concept. Imagine a dual-chamber device with leads in their typical location—an atrial lead placed in the right atrial appendage and a ventricular lead at the ventricular apex. Now suppose that both sensed and paced AV delays were programmed to 200 ms. For the sensed AV delay, this defines the time from a sensed atrial event to the next paced ventricular event. When an intrinsic atrial event occurs, it will be initiated in the SA node located in the high right atrium. As the pulse travels outward from the SA node, it takes some time for it to reach the right atrial appendage (about 25–50 ms). Thus, the intrinsic atrial event begins before the pacemaker is able to sense it. In this example, where both sensed and paced AV delays are programmed to 200 ms, the *actual sensed AV delay* is going to be about 225 ms (200 ms programmed value + about 25 ms delay). However, the actual programmed AV delay is going to still be 200 ms because the atrial pacing spike is delivered at exactly the same moment that the paced AV delay starts. This timing offset for the sensed AV delay—the timing lag between the point at which the SA node fires and the pacemaker sensed the intrinsic atrial event—is called latency. Latency describes any timing lag in pacing from the point at which a wave of depolarization commences before it is sensed. Latency is most evident in atrial sensing. Because of latency, the sensed AV delay should be programmed to a shorter value than the paced AV delay. Thus, if a clinician programs a sensed AV delay of 175 ms and a paced AV delay of 200 ms, both *actual AV delays* will be about 200 ms. This means that when reviewing a paced ECG, the sensed AV interval is typically going to be shorter than the paced AV interval.

There is no easy way to measure atrial latency for the purposes of programming the pacemaker, but for most patients, the value is going to be about 25–50 ms. In routine practice, most physicians will program the sensed AV delay to 25, 30, or 50 ms shorter than the paced AV delay with values that derive from their practice and experience rather than a specific test.

Once an AV delay (paced or sensed) is launched, only two things can happen. If the AV delay times out and no intrinsic ventricular activity is sensed, the dual-chamber pacemaker will deliver a ventricular output pulse. The other thing that can happen is that intrinsic ventricular activity will be sensed during the AV interval, which will cause the pacemaker to inhibit the ventricular output pulse.

Optimizing AV delay

In 2002, a landmark clinical trial known as the DAVID study found that right ventricular pacing in heart failure patients made their heart failure worse, increasing both morbidity and mortality [1]. This study is very well known among pacing experts because the results were counterintuitive and surprised even the experts. DAVID was so influential that in the past decade, even pacing experts seem to have come to the conclusion that pacing the right ventricle should be avoided to the greatest extent possible. Clinicians will often demand that pacemakers be programmed in such a way as to *minimize right ventricular pacing*.

The DAVID study is actually misunderstood by many pacing experts. The patients in the DAVID study all had some degree of left ventricular dysfunction upon entry into the study; in other words, they were heart failure patients. None of these patients had a standard indication for pacing, that is, they did not actually need pacing. Furthermore, patients in the DAVID study were paced at around 100% of the time. The thought process behind this was that constant pacing might benefit failure patients. What the DAVID investigators found was that constant, unnecessary right ventricular pacing in heart failure patients made their heart failure worse.

It is not hard to understand why. The typical dual-chamber pacemaker patient has a right ventricular lead placed in the right ventricular apex or the right ventricular outflow tract (RVOT). When the pacing pulse is delivered, it is delivered to the apex or the RVOT. The pulse creates a wave of depolarization, but it is not going from the AV node outward and downward to both the right and left ventricles (which is natural), but rather from the apex or RVOT upward and from the right ventricle to the left ventricle. This creates something known as mechanical dyssynchrony, which means that the right and left ventricles contract out of synch with each other. Right ventricular pacing causes at least a degree of mechanical dyssynchrony because the right ventricle is going to contract slightly ahead of the left ventricle. In patients who already have a compromised left ventricle (and likely some mechanical dyssynchrony to begin with), this just makes it worse. The take-away message from the DAVID study is that for patients with heart failure, right ventricular pacing poses real problems and can worsen their cardiac dysfunction.

But does the average patient indicated for dual-chamber pacing have heart failure and some degree of mechanical dyssynchrony? Today, such patients should be prescribed a cardiac resynchronization therapy (CRT) device, which paces the right and left ventricles together. A patient with impaired left ventricular function should not get a conventional dual-chamber pacemaker that will subject him to right ventricular pacing. To be fair, dual-chamber pacemaker patients who had normal left ventricular function at implant may develop left ventricular dysfunction over time. Clinicians must be mindful that patients with dual-chamber pacemakers may indeed have heart failure and then right ventricular pacing has to be taken into account. But this is not the typical dual-chamber pacemaker patient!

Many clinicians will argue that the best approach to dual-chamber pacing in general is to *minimize right ventricular pacing*, but it is my opinion that it is clinically better and more efficient to *optimize the AV delay*. Aggressively minimizing right ventricular pacing may deprive patients of necessary ventricular pacing support. For some patients, there will be a balancing act where the clinician must weigh the value of ventricular pacing against its potential risks of causing or worsening mechanical dyssynchrony.

Optimizing the AV delay can be a balancing act. As an example, assume that a patient has a heart block, a normal left ventricular function, and an intrinsic PR interval of about 385 ms. A heart block and a prolonged PR interval are conventional pacing indications. The clinician can program the AV delay to 400 ms, which will *minimize right ventricular pacing*, but such a long AV delay means the patient will have suboptimal hemodynamics and likely a reduced cardiac output. The patient will also be deprived of ventricular pacing support and may have symptoms from such a slow ventricular rate. What happens if we instead *optimize the AV delay*? By programming a more normal AV delay of around 200 ms, the patient will have enhanced

hemodynamics and better cardiac output but will experience right ventricular pacing at an activity-appropriate rate. This will likely improve the patient's symptoms and well-being. Some clinicians might argue that it is risky to pace this patient in the right ventricle, but remember that in our example the patient has normal left ventricular function and does not have mechanical dyssynchrony. It would be better clinically for this patient to experience right ventricular pacing when needed.

The matter can get a little trickier if that same patient had an intrinsic PR interval of 250 or 275 ms. Here, clinical judgment has to determine how long an *optimal* AV delay can be in a specific patient. The clinician needs to consider the patient's overall health, left ventricular function, and how active the patient is. The point is that the DAVID study evaluated unnecessary constant right ventricular pacing in patients who already had heart failure and did not have a pacing indication—and that population by definition is not the typical dual-chamber pacemaker patient!

That being said, there is wisdom in limiting right ventricular pacing to the amount the patient actually needs. Unnecessary atrial and ventricular pacing should be avoided. But rather than focusing on reducing right ventricular pacing by all means possible, we should concentrate on optimizing the AV delay and getting the patient's hemodynamics and cardiac output to the best values they can be. This will result in getting the patient only the amount of right ventricular pacing he or she actually needs.

Postventricular atrial refractory period

The postventricular atrial refractory period, known as PVARP (pronounced pee-varp), is an atrial timing cycle that is initiated by any type of ventricular event (sensed or paced). During the PVARP, the atrial channel becomes refractory and will not respond to incoming signals for a specific period of time, usually programmed to around 250–275 ms. In mastering dual-chamber pacing concepts, it is important to think of the PVARP as an *atrial timing cycle*—even though it is initiated by a ventricular event and has the word *ventricular* in its name.

The main objective of the PVARP is to prevent the atrial channel from sensing and responding to signals from the ventricle. In dual-chamber pacing, both atrial sensing and ventricular sensing are going on, and it is important that events are sensed by the appropriate channel. A ventricular event—such as an intrinsic ventricular contraction or a ventricular paced event—could easily generate a signal large enough to be picked up by the atrial channel, which would then inappropriately interpret it as an atrial event. Thus, when ventricular events occur (paced or sensed), the PVARP is launched to *blind* the atrial channel and prevent it from *seeing* ventricular activity that it could potentially misinterpret. PVARP also prevents the atrial channel from sensing far-field ventricular contractions, retrograde P-waves, and other stray signals (see **Figure 16.2**).

Just as refractory periods in single-chamber pacemakers could be divided into an absolute and a relative refractory period, the PVARP also has an absolute and a relative period. The absolute portion of the PVARP is the time during which no signals are *seen* by the atrial channel, which is called the post-ventricular atrial blanking (PVAB) period. During this time, the atrial channel cannot sense anything at all. This is followed by the relative portion of the PVARP, which is typically just called the PVARP; during this time, the atrial channel can *see* and sense incoming signals (and count them for the device's diagnostic data collection), but it will not respond to them. Not only is the PVARP value programmable (which is the whole timing cycle, PVAB + PVARP), but in many devices, the clinician can independently program the PVAB setting. A typical PVAB value is around 100 ms. Thus, with a PVARP set to 250 ms and a PVAB programmed to 100 ms, the absolute atrial refractory period (PVAB) will be 100 ms and the relative refractory period will be 150 ms (100 + 150 = 250 ms) (see **Figure 16.3**).

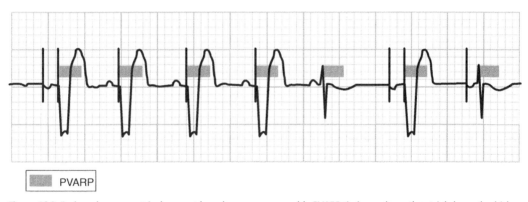

PVARP

Figure 16.2 Each and every ventricular event launches a programmable PVARP timing cycle on the atrial channel, which makes the atrial channel refractory so it will not respond to incoming signals.

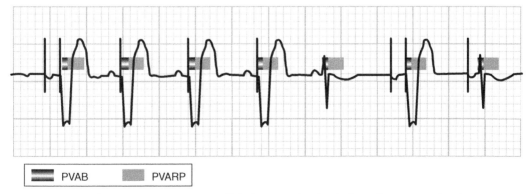

PVAB   PVARP

Figure 16.3 PVAB refers to the programmable atrial blanking period or the absolute refractory period on the atrial channel. The total PVARP value is programmable as well.

By far the main benefit of PVARP is its role in minimizing or even eliminating a phenomenon known as pacemaker-mediated tachycardia (PMT), sometimes called endless loop tachycardia, discussed in detail in the following text. The main goal behind the PVAB portion of the PVARP is to prevent the atrial channel from seeing and inappropriately interpreting ventricular signals as atrial activity (this is called far-field R-wave oversensing and is a common cause of inappropriate mode switching).

PVARP: preventing PMT

The main purpose of PVARP is to minimize or prevent PMT. PMT will be discussed in much greater detail in the next section. As the name suggests, PMT is a type of tachycardia this is sustained in part by the pacemaker. Once PMT gets started, the pacemaker will actually keep it going. The goal of the PVARP is to prevent the atrial channel from responding to these triggering events and thus averts a potential episode of PMT.

PVAB: preventing far-field R-wave oversensing

Far-field R-wave oversensing, sometimes called far-R oversensing, occurs when the dual-chamber pacemaker's atrial channel senses ventricular activity and inappropriately interprets it as atrial activity. This can result in inappropriate inhibition of the atrial output pulse, leading to loss of AV synchrony and no atrial contribution to ventricular filling. PVAB is the timing cycle designed to minimize or prevent far-field R-wave oversensing.

To understand the importance of preventing far-R oversensing, we have to jump ahead a bit to discuss mode switching. Mode switching is an automatic algorithm in dual-chamber pacemakers that—in simple terms—is activated by atrial tachycardia or atrial fibrillation. When the pacemaker detects atrial tachycardia or atrial fibrillation, it will automatically *switch modes* or turn off atrial tracking for the duration of the high-rate atrial activity. When the patient's intrinsic atrial rate comes back down to the normal range, the pacemaker *switches modes* again and resumes atrial tracking. This is an accurate but overly simple description of mode switching, which is generally a very useful algorithm for

dual-chamber pacemaker patients. However, when far-R oversensing is going on, the pacemaker is sensing every atrial event plus it is also sensing every ventricular event and labeling it an atrial event. This phenomenon is called *double counting*. This is going to cause the pacemaker to *see* atrial tachycardia that is not there—and mode switch, resulting in no more atrial tracking. Since this is oversensing, there was no clinical need to stop atrial tracking. In fact, it deprives the patient of AV synchrony! So for that reason, the PVAB is an important timing cycle to reduce the risk of far-field R-wave oversensing (which at the very least messes up timing cycles and, worse, can even cause an inappropriate mode switch and unnecessary loss of AV synchrony).

PMT

The PVARP timing cycle prevents PMT by preventing the tracking of so-called retrograde P-waves. Normal or antegrade P-waves go from top to bottom of the heart, that is, from the atria to the ventricles. Retrograde P-waves, by contrast, are not true P-waves at all, but rather ventricular events that go backward through the heart, from the ventricles to the atria, where they are inappropriately *seen* by the atrial sensing of the dual-chamber pacemaker as atrial events (see **Figure 16.4**). When PMT occurs, it creates an endless loop; each ventricular event is counted by the atrial channel and tracked by the ventricle, driving the pacemaker to pace the ventricle faster.

PMT requires certain specific conditions to happen; some patients are not susceptible to it. In order to experience PMT, a patient must have:
- A dual-chamber pacemaker (PMT never occurs with single-chamber pacemakers)
- Physiologic retrograde conduction (not all patients have this)
- Retrograde conduction time longer than the programmed PVARP
- A triggering event that interrupts AV synchrony
First, PMT requires a dual-chamber pacemaker because PMT involves tracking retrograde P-waves. Only dual-chamber pacemakers offer atrial tracking. When the dual-chamber pacemaker starts to track these retrograde P-waves, it drives the ventricular pacing rate up.

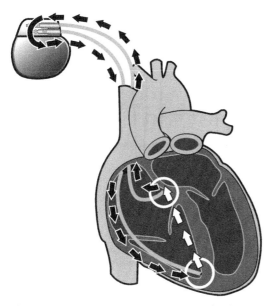

Figure 16.4 Normal conduction is indicated by the dark line. Retrograde or VA conduction is shown by the lighter line. These retrograde signals conduct backward into the atria where they are sensed and counted by the pacemaker (double counting), which then paces the ventricle fast enough to track them. The pacemaker then contributes to ventricular tachycardia by pacing the ventricle to *keep up* with a misinterpreted atrial rate. In addition, there may be intrinsic cardiac activity contributing to the PMT as well.

Second, the patient must have retrograde or VA conduction (also called retrograde VA conduction or RVAC). Only about 60% of patients have retrograde conduction in the first place, and many who do have retrograde conduction have it only intermittently. Retrograde conduction is often transient, that is, it exists for a time but goes away on its own. There is some evidence to suggest that retrograde conduction may relate to catecholamine levels in the blood, specifically to epinephrine levels. This means that even patients with known retrograde conduction may only have it under certain conditions. For this reason, pacemaker clinics rarely test patients in advance to see if they have retrograde conduction—there would be too many false-negatives. Thus, the wisest and most practical clinical approach is to assume that every dual-chamber pacemaker patient is at risk for retrograde conduction and program the device accordingly.

There is a myth in clinical practice that patients with complete heart block are immune to PMT

because they do not have intact AV conduction. Actually, it is possible to have the so-called unidirectional heart block, which means that conduction is blocked one way but not the other. This is extremely rare, but there are individuals who have complete AV block (no A to V conduction) but intact VA conduction. For that reason, clinicians should take appropriate steps to program all dual-chamber pacemaker patients (even those with heart block) with appropriately long PVARPs to protect them from PMT.

PMT can only occur when retrograde conduction is longer than the PVARP, that is, when retrograde conduction is taking place outside of the atrial refractory period. For most patients, retrograde conduction time is around 235 ms, but this can vary among patients. If a patient has retrograde conduction of 235 ms, a PVARP value of 250 ms will protect him, but a PVARP of 225 ms will not.

Finally, PMT requires some kind of triggering event that breaks AV synchrony. Typical triggers are PVCs, loss of atrial capture, atrial undersensing, and magnet removal. In a healthy heart, the atria contract and then are physiologically refractory; the ventricles contract and then are physiologically refractory. Even in a paced heart, as long as AV synchrony is maintained, the *physiologic refractory periods* of the cardiac tissue are going to act as a natural defense to retrograde conduction. For example, the ventricles contract, and even if the patient had retrograde conduction, the refractoriness of the ventricular tissue is going to prevent retrograde conduction. Thus, as long as AV synchrony is intact, the patient will not experience retrograde conduction and thus cannot develop a PMT. When AV synchrony is broken, for instance, by a PVC, then retrograde conduction may be possible because the tissue is no longer physiologically refractory. Think of a series of cardiac contractions: A, V, A, V, A, V, and then a PVC. This PVC is a ventricular event that occurs against the background of the now-responsive (nonrefractory) cardiac tissue—allowing for retrograde conduction. While PVCs can cause PMT, today, the most common trigger for PMT is loss of atrial capture (see **Figure 16.5**).

Because PMT is only possible in a subset of dual-chamber pacemaker patients and, even then, requires these four specific conditions to align precisely, it is not very common, but clinicians do

Loss of atrial capture   Retrograde conduction possible

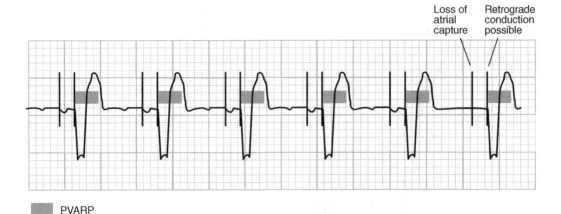

PVARP

Figure 16.5 For a dual-chamber pacemaker patient with retrograde conduction, loss of atrial capture can trigger a PMT. In this strip, the loss of atrial capture breaks AV synchrony. This means that atrial tissue will be physiologically refractory. When the ventricular spike causes ventricular depolarization, retrograde conduction is now possible because the atrial tissue is not refractory and the PVARP has timed out.

encounter it and need to be equipped to trouble-shoot. The good news about PMT is that there is a way to program the dual-chamber pacemaker to prevent it. When the PVARP interval exceeds the patient's retrograde conduction time, PMT simply cannot happen.

The retrograde conduction time is the interval it takes a ventricular event to conduct backward and get sensed by the atrium; there are ways to measure this that will be discussed later. For now, know that a typical retrograde conduction time is around 235 ms. If the PVARP is longer than 235 ms (and a 25 ms margin is not a bad idea, either), then the retrograde P-wave will fall into the PVARP. That means that the pacemaker may *see* the retrograde P-wave, but it will not respond to it; that is to say, it will not try to track it. Thus, PVARP cannot prevent retrograde conduction, but it can effectively stop the dual-chamber pacemaker from responding to sensed retrograde P-waves if they fall into the PVARP.

Of course, PMT can still occur if the patient's retrograde conduction time exceeds the PVARP value. In that case, the retrograde events will fall outside the PVARP timing cycle and be sensed by the atrial channel and inappropriately considered atrial events—causing the pacemaker to try to track them. While most patients with retrograde conduction will have extremely consistent retrograde conduction times around 235 ms, there can

be significant variation among patients. There may be times when it will be necessary to measure retrograde conduction times to assure appropriate programming of the PVARP.

Retrograde P-waves can sometimes be seen on a surface ECG. They have the opposite deflection of true sinus P-waves (because they are moving in the opposite direction with respect to the positive pole of Lead II). RVAC times can be measured intraoperatively or using the programmer in a follow-up visit. This test may be automated by the programmer, but it can also be done *old school* as follows:

- Temporarily program the pacemaker to a rate above the patient's intrinsic rate to force constant pacing.
- Once 100% pacing is established, temporarily program the mode to VVI. (This breaks AV synchrony, setting up the scenario for retrograde conduction.)
- Monitor the patient's atrial rhythm on a simultaneous surface ECG and an atrial electrogram, looking for atrial sensed events that are actually derived from ventricular events. The annotations on the electrogram are very useful for this. Compare ventricular events on the surface ECG with the atrial electrogram, which reports what the pacemaker sees.
- When ventricular events and atrial counting can be linked, measure the VA conduction interval.

This is usually around 235 ms. Program the PVARP to the patient's actual VA conduction time plus a safety margin of around 50 ms.
* Upon conclusion of the test, revert the device to previously programmed rate and mode.

Identifying PMT

When PMT occurs, it typically occurs at the maximum tracking rate or MTR. This is a great clue in identifying PMT: PMT presents on the ECG as a run of ventricular pacing at the MTR. (Note that PMT can never be faster than the MTR, but in patients with long retrograde conduction, it may be slightly below the MTR. This is very rare but possible.) A great definition of PMT is tracking, usually at the MTR or upper rate limit, secondary to retrograde conduction (see **Figure 16.6**).

Another clear indication of PMT is an abrupt transition from relatively normal base-rate pacing to atrial sensing/ventricular pacing at the MTR. If this occurs in one single beat, it is almost definitely PMT. More evidence of PMT involves the presence of a triggering event that breaks AV synchrony, such as loss of atrial capture or a PVC.

Symptoms are not always a reliable indicator of PMT. In fact, symptoms may not even occur; it depends on the patient's overall health and pump function. A relatively healthy, physically fit young person may tolerate PMT well and be completely asymptomatic, but a geriatric patient with ischemic heart disease may have moderate or even severe symptoms.

Stopping PMT

There will be times when clinicians will be called upon to stop an ongoing episode of PMT. In this case, let's assume the patient has atrial tracking (atrial sensing/ventricular pacing) at the programmed MTR of 120 ppm. Since PMT is essentially *tracking* secondary to retrograde conduction, the best way to break an episode of PMT is to *stop tracking*. There are several ways to do this (e.g., programming the pacemaker to a nontracking mode, such as VVI) but the fastest and easiest approach is to apply a magnet over the implanted device. Magnet application initiates magnet mode, which, by definition, involves asynchronous pacing. Asynchronous pacing is pacing without sensing, and without sensing, there is no atrial tracking; this will break the endless loop of PMT in a single beat!

While magnet application is a fast, foolproof way to break PMT, one of the initiating triggers of PMT is magnet removal! A clinician who applies a magnet, stops the PMT, and then simply removes the magnet may end up seeing the PMT come right back. For that reason, during magnet application, the clinician needs to take steps to prevent PMT. Once those steps are in place, then the magnet can be removed.

Preventing PMT

The first and most obvious strategy in preventing PMT is to program a sufficiently long PVARP value. This is usually around 250 or 275 ms, but when a clinician is troubleshooting PMTs, retrograde conduction times should be measured to be sure that the PVARP value is sufficiently long. Once the retrograde conduction time is known, program the PVARP to a value that exceeds the patient's retrograde conduction time. A safety margin of 25 ms or more can be helpful as well.

But while a long PVARP value will prevent PMT, the PVARP length cannot be extended indefinitely. As with most dual-chamber pacemaker parameters,

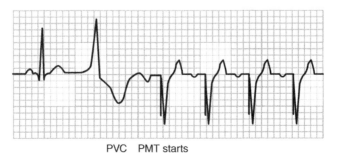

PVC   PMT starts

Figure 16.6 A typical example of PMT initiated by a PVC. Note that the PMT starts abruptly and tracks the atrial rate. The inverted P-waves contrast with the positive P-wave in the first complex; these are retrograde P-waves.

the clinician has to balance this length with the other settings. For instance, you cannot program the pacemaker to pace at 60 ppm and have a PVARP setting of 800 ms! And as pacing clinicians know, every time you adjust a parameter to solve one problem, you open the door to causing new (but different) problems. PVARP programmability is a very good first step, but it may not be the cure-all for PMT in some patients.

Another good strategy that some clinicians overlook is identifying the PMT trigger and eliminating the cause. For example, if the patient's trigger for PMT is loss of atrial capture, taking steps to assure reliable atrial capture will further prevent PMT. Ironically, PMT often occurs in the pacemaker clinic during atrial capture tests. Atrial capture testing is performed by lowering the atrial output stepwise until *capture is lost*. In other words, atrial capture testing by definition sets up a PMT trigger! If the patient has retrograde conduction, it is quite possible that an ordinary atrial capture test will initiate PMT. Knowing that an atrial capture test might be useful to help prevent PMT but that conducting such a test can cause PMT means that the clinician must proceed cautiously and be prepared to use a magnet to break the PMT if it occurs. Many device clinicians who conduct atrial capture testing are surprised when PMT occurs, but it is actually not an unexpected phenomenon if the patient has retrograde conduction. Just be prepared to identify the PMT, use the magnet to stop it, and then program the device as needed.

Dual-chamber pacemakers today offer a variety of specialized PMT options and even PVC options aimed at preventing or terminating PMTs. These special algorithms exist in all dual-chamber pacemakers but may use unique terminology and have slight variations.

Automatic PMT prevention algorithms

Many years ago, the most frequent trigger of PMT was by far the PVC. PVCs occur naturally in most patients, they cannot be prevented, and they absolutely will break AV synchrony. PVCs are less problematic for pacemaker patients today than they were a couple of decades ago because of automatic PMT prevention algorithms built into today's dual-

chamber pacemakers. These automatic algorithms may or may not be active in the pacemaker as it comes out of the box, but it is generally good clinical practice to be sure they are programmed on from the outset for all patients. PMT algorithms can be a little complicated to discuss because each manufacturer's algorithm works slightly differently and uses different terminology. That being said, there are some basic concepts in PMT prevention that all of these PMT prevention features share.

All PMT prevention algorithms are based on the pacemaker's ability to detect PVCs. A clinician with an ECG can identify a PVC because of three main distinguishing characteristics: the PVC occurs early in the cycle, it is not preceded by an atrial event, and it has a wide, bizarre morphology. Pacemakers identify a PVC using a somewhat different approach. When the pacemaker *sees* two ventricular events without an intervening atrial event (sensed or paced), it calls the second ventricular event a PVC. This is the *pacemaker definition* of a PVC. The pacemaker does not consider morphology at all.

PMT prevention algorithms are designed to automatically extend the PVARP value for one cycle whenever a PVC is detected. For example, the pacemaker paces the ventricle and launches the PVARP. Before the PVARP times out, the pacemaker senses a ventricular event, which it labels a PVC. This causes an automatic prolongation of the PVARP for that one cycle. This is not a permanent pacing parameter change; PVARP reverts in the next cycle to its programmed value.

There are nuances to this algorithm that vary by manufacturer along with terminology, but the general principle is that upon identification of a PVC (as the pacemaker defines it), the PVARP is automatically extended. A good way to think of this is + PVARP on PVC. The duration of this extension varies by company and device, and it is not programmable. It is preset as part of the algorithm. For instance—and this is certainly not the case with every algorithm—a sensed PVC will cause the PVARP to automatically extend to 400 ms for one cycle. This cannot prevent a retrograde P-wave, but it can cause the retrograde P-wave to fall in the extralong PVARP, meaning the pacemaker will not try to track it.

These PMT prevention algorithms are highly effective and have eliminated a lot of PVC-triggered

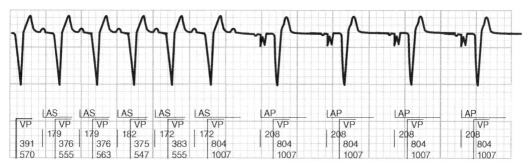

Figure 16.7 Pacemaker-mediated tachycardia occurs at the programmed MTR and is detected by the device when a certain number of beats are detected. At that point, the automatic PMT termination algorithm extends the PVARP, causing the retrograde P-wave to fall into the PVARP and not be tracked. This restores normal dual-chamber pacing. Note the horizontal lines associated with the electrogram annotations. The horizontal lines represent atrial and ventricular refractory periods. The extended PVARP occurs in about the middle of the strip, restoring normal pacing in a single beat.

episodes of PMT. Note that when the PVARP is automatically extended in response to a PVC, the atrial alert period is shortened by the amount of the extension.

While all devices allow for automatic prolongation of the PVARP in response to a PVC, some manufacturers offer other options to manage PMT. These options vary by manufacturer and can be fairly complex. While these specialty variations on PMT algorithms can be very helpful in managing certain individual patients, they are in widespread use because the majority of patients do not need them. The +PVARP on PVC algorithm included in all dual-chamber pacemakers works well for most patients. If a clinician ever has to troubleshoot PMT in a particularly challenging patient, these specialty algorithms come in very handy.

The main limitation of +PVARP on PVC is that it works only on PVC. It will not prolong the PVARP in response to a loss of atrial capture, which is a common trigger for PMT.

Automatic PMT termination algorithms

Most dual-chamber pacemakers also have automatic algorithms designed to stop a PMT that is already in progress. These algorithms basically work by searching for PMT, which the pacemaker defines as atrial tracking at the programmed upper rate limit (MTR) for a certain number of beats. The number of beats may or may not be programmable

and can vary by manufacturer. In general, the algorithm is going to seek 8–16 beats at MTR before it *decides* that the episode is PMT. Once PMT is detected, the pacemaker will automatically extend the PVARP (again, the amount of prolongation can vary among manufacturers). This prolonged PVARP should cause the retrograde P-wave to fall into the PVARP and not be tracked (see **Figure 16.7**).

The PMT termination algorithm can be very helpful, but it must be remembered that it does not work to prevent PMT, only to stop one once it starts. For example, in a patient with regular loss of atrial capture, the PMT termination algorithm would break a PMT, but the next loss of atrial capture would trigger a new PMT. The +PVARP on PVC does not extend the PVARP in response to loss of atrial capture. At present, there are no algorithms that automatically prevent PVARP when atrial capture is lost. For that reason, it is important to assure reliable atrial capture to prevent PMT.

Total atrial refractory period

The total atrial refractory period, usually just called TARP, is the interval on the atrial channel during which the pacemaker will not respond to incoming signals. TARP can be calculated by adding the AV delay interval plus the PVARP. TARP is not directly programmable for the pacemaker, but the clinician can determine its length by the programmed values of AV delay and PVARP. As an example, if the pacemaker is programmed to an AV delay of 200 ms and a

PVARP of 250 ms, then the TARP is 450 ms (200+250=450). For the time being, the most important take-away about TARP is that it is the point at which a pacemaker will exhibit 2:1 block. To calculate when pacemaker 2:1 block will occur, convert the TARP to rate. In our example, 2:1 block would occur at 133 bpm (450 ms converts to 133 bpm).

This phenomenon and its implications will be discussed more in the chapter on upper rate behaviors.

Atrial alert period
Both atrial and ventricular channels can only ever be refractory or alert. On the atrial channel, when the refractory period (TARP) is over, the alert period begins. When the alert period ends, the refractory period (TARP) begins. The purpose of the alert period is to allow the pacemaker to seek out and be *alert* to intrinsic activity so that it might respond. For example, the atrial alert period is the time when the pacemaker is looking for intrinsic atrial signals that, if detected, will cause the pacemaker to inhibit the atrial output pulse. The alert period also defines when the pacemaker will pace.

If no intrinsic events in the atrium are sensed during the atrial alert period, when the alert period expires, the pacemaker will deliver a pacing output to the atrium.

Conclusion

Mastering the atrial timing cycles of dual-chamber pacing is no easy task, because the dual-chamber pacemaker relies on the atrium to drive its timing. Understanding the AV delay, the PVARP, and the alert period is crucial to being able to successfully program and follow implantable dual-chamber systems. While PMT may not seem like an *atrial timing cycle*, it is atrial tracking at the upper rate limit secondary to dual-chamber pacing and deserves serious study. While PMT is not very common outside the clinic, clinicians will encounter it during atrial threshold testing in clinic. Automatic PMT detection and termination algorithms have made it easier and more automatic to deal with PMT, but a basic understanding of how and why PMTs occur will help clinicians deal with this phenomenon quickly and effectively.

The nuts and bolts of dual-chamber timing cycles: the atrial channel

- The AV delay or AV interval is the dual-chamber pacemaker timing cycle that is launched with an atrial event (sensed or paced). During the AV delay, the pacemaker looks for intrinsic ventricular activity; if an intrinsic ventricular beat is sensed, the pacemaker inhibits the ventricular output. On the other hand, if the AV delay expires and no intrinsic ventricular activity was sensed, then the ventricular output pulse will be delivered.
- Dual-chamber pacemakers pace the ventricle in response to the atrial channel; the key timing cycle for this is the AV delay.
- The AV delay is the electronic version of the PR interval and promotes good hemodynamics by allowing sufficient time for ventricular filling and *atrial kick*.
- The AV delay is programmable and a sensed AV delay (following a sensed atrial event) and a paced AV delay (following a paced atrial event) can be independently programmed. Typical

values for paced and sensed AV delays are 200 and 175 ms, respectively.
- The paced AV delay is usually shorter than the sensed AV delay because of atrial latency. When an intrinsic atrial event occurs, it takes a brief span of time (about 25–50 ms) from SA node firing to the point at which the pacemaker can sense the wave of depolarization. Remember that the atrial lead is typically in the atrial appendage and the SA node is located in the high right atrium. When the high right atrium fires, there is a brief lag time before the electrode on the lead in the atrial appendage can sense the signal.
- Since the landmark DAVID clinical trial in 2002, many clinicians are adamant about minimizing right ventricular (RV) pacing. Rather than taking this extreme view, clinicians ought to focus on optimizing the AV delay. After all, some patients absolutely require RV pacing. Optimizing the AV delay

means allowing an AV interval sufficiently long to give the ventricles opportunity to beat on their own, without compromising hemodynamics (by making the AV delay too long) or denying the patient pacing support that he or she might need.

- The reason that many clinicians are wary about excessive RV pacing is that in patients with heart failure, unnecessary RV pacing can make their heart failure worse. The mechanism behind this is mechanical dyssynchrony. When the pacemaker paces the right ventricle, it causes the right and left ventricles to contract out of synch with each other. This does not appear to be a problem for some patients, but in patients with some degree of mechanical dyssynchrony or left ventricular dysfunction to begin with, it can make that condition worse.
- Although it is beyond the scope of this book, patients who need pacing and have heart failure, mechanical dyssynchrony, or compromised left ventricular function can still get the therapy they need. It involves pacing both the right and left ventricles simultaneously. Cardiac resynchronization therapy (CRT) devices are available and can deliver appropriate pacing support for such patients.
- Optimizing the AV delay is a balancing act because an excessively long AV interval can compromise hemodynamics. On the other hand, a very short AV delay may cause ventricular pacing that is not absolutely necessary. AV delay optimization has to be done on an individual patient-by-patient basis and requires expert clinical judgment.
- The postventricular atrial refractory period (PVARP) is an atrial timing cycle that is launched by any type of ventricular event (sensed or paced). It is important to think of PVARP as an atrial clock, not a ventricular clock.
- PVARP is programmable and typical values range from 250 to 275 ms.
- In simplest terms, the purpose of PVARP is to prevent the atrial channel from responding to signals from the ventricle.
- Like any refractory period, PVARP can be divided into an absolute and refractory period.

The tricky part is nomenclature. The absolute portion of the PVARP is called the postventricular atrial blanking period (PVAB). The relative portion of the PVARP is called PVARP. And the whole timing cycle (PVAB+PVARP) is called the PVARP. This may sound confusing at first, but it becomes more familiar with time.

- The purpose of the PVAB is to prevent the atrial channel from sensing a ventricular event and then inappropriately *thinking* it is atrial activity—the PVAB simultaneously with the ventricular event. Remember that ventricular signals are very large and could easily be picked up by the atrial channel if it were not for the blanking period. This type of inappropriate sensing is sometimes called *far-field R-wave oversensing* or just *far-R oversensing*.
- Far-R oversensing can result in double counting of atrial signals; that means the pacemaker will *think* the atrial is beating on its own far more rapidly than it actually is. A dual-chamber pacemaker will then try to track this rapid atrial rate, resulting in high ventricular rate pacing. It is possible for far-R oversensing to lead to inappropriate ventricular pacing up to the maximum tracking rate (MTR).
- PVAB is often independently programmable and is typically set to 100 ms.
- For most devices, the clinician can program the PVARP (the total absolute and refractory segments) and PVAB, which indirectly allows for programming of the relative portion of PVARP. For example, if the clinician programs a PVARP value to 250 ms and then sets PVAB to 100 ms, the relative portion of the PVARP is 150 ms (100+150=250).
- The objective of the PVARP timing cycle is to prevent pacemaker-mediated tachycardia (PMT) or endless loop tachycardia. PMT is atrial tracking secondary to retrograde conduction.
- PMT does not occur in all patients; in fact, it may not be possible in many patients. To experience a PMT, a patient must have a dual-chamber pacemaker, retrograde conduction, and a triggering event that breaks AV synchrony.

Continued

Continued

- The three most common triggers for PMT are loss of atrial capture (this can occur during an atrial capture test in the clinic), PVC, and magnet removal.
- Retrograde conduction refers to *backward* conduction along the heart's electrical pathways, in other words, conduction that goes from the ventricles toward the atria. Antegrade or normal conduction goes forward from the atria to ventricles. About 60% of patients have some degree of retrograde conduction, which is typically intermittent and transient (it comes and goes). Although extremely rare, it is possible for a patient to have complete heart block (lack of antegrade conduction) and retrograde conduction!
- A PMT occurs because the pacemaker is trying to track *retrograde P-waves.* Retrograde P-waves may show up on an ECG as P-waves with the opposite deflection from genuine sinus P-waves. They occur because conduction from the ventricles goes back up to the atrium. This causes the pacemaker to sense the retrograde P-wave (which it counts as a normal P-wave) and try to track it. This causes the pacemaker to pace the ventricle at high rates, up to the MTR.
- There are two easy ways to identify a PMT from a tracing. First, PMT starts abruptly, from one beat to the next. Second, PMT often (not always but very often) occurs at the MTR.
- In years past, PVCs were the most common trigger for PMTs. Today, all devices have built-in algorithms to identify and protect the patient from PVCs. The pacemaker defines a PVC as two ventricular events without an intervening atrial event. When a PVC is detected (as the pacemaker defines it), it automatically prolongs the PVARP so that the dual-chamber pacemaker will not respond to it and try to track retrograde P-waves.
- Today, the most common trigger of PMTs is loss of atrial capture, which is more likely to occur in clinic than outside. Atrial capture tests require, by definition, lowering the atrial pacing output to the point that capture is lost. For some patients, this routine and important test will provoke PMT.
- PMT can be interrupted when it is occurring by magnet application. Magnet application causes magnet mode or asynchronous pacing. To get PMT to stop, a clinician only needs to stop tracking. This can be done by asynchronous pacing (fastest and easiest way is magnet application) or by reprogramming the mode to a nontracking mode, such as VVI.
- To prevent PMT, a sufficiently long PVARP value has to be programmed. It may be necessary to measure the patient's retrograde conduction interval to find the right value. Prolonging the PVARP will cause future retrograde P-waves (which cannot be prevented in some patients) to fall into the PVARP and thus not be tracked.
- If PMT is broken by magnet application, care must be taken when removing the magnet as magnet removal can trigger PMT! While the magnet is in place, extend the PVARP. Then when the magnet is removed, the new PVARP value is in place.
- To test for retrograde pacing, force 100% pacing, program the pacemaker temporarily to VVI pacing, and then monitor the rhythm on a surface ECG and simultaneous atrial channel electrogram. Look for atrial sensed events on the electrogram that are clearly derived from ventricular events on the ECG. Use electrogram annotations to see what the pacemaker is labeling an atrial sensed event. Once you can link ventricular events to atrial double counting, measure the VA conduction interval. It is usually going to be very regular and in the vicinity of 235 ms in duration. When the test is over, be sure to restore previously programmed values.
- While it is not particularly difficult to measure retrograde conduction in terms of technique and technology, it can be difficult to observe retrograde conduction at your convenience. Retrograde conduction is transient, meaning that it comes and goes, and it is unpredictable.
- Dual-chamber pacemakers today have automatic PMT prevention algorithms that automatically extend the PVARP upon detection of a PVC. While manufacturers have

different nuances in the algorithm, including the duration of the PVARP extension, they can all be thought of as + PVARP on PVC.

• Dual-chamber pacemakers also offer automatic algorithms that terminate an ongoing PMT. The device detects PMT by searching for atrial tracking at the MTR or programmed upper rate limit for a certain number of beats. (The number of beats may or may not be programmable and varies with manufacturers; it is in the neighborhood of about a dozen beats.) When the dual-chamber pacemaker identifies a PMT, it will automatically extend the PVARP, causing the retrograde P-wave to fall into the PVARP and not be tracked. This will break the PMT.

• The biggest drawback to PMT termination algorithms is that they only work for PMTs triggered by a PVC. There is no PMT termination algorithm for a PMT triggered by loss of atrial capture. This is in part because the pacemaker does not readily identify loss of atrial capture; the pacemaker *thinks* that every output pulse results in capture.

• TARP stands for the total atrial refractory period, and it is made up of the AV delay plus the PVARP. In many cases, TARP itself is not directly programmable, but the clinician can set it indirectly by programming AV delay and PVARP. For instance, if the AV delay is 200 ms and the PVARP is 275 ms, then TARP is 475 ms (200 + 275 = 475).

• TARP, converted to rate, is the point at which 2:1 block will occur. For instance, if TARP is 475 ms, then 2:1 block will occur 126 ppm (475 ms translates to a rate of 126 ppm). This will be covered in greater detail later.

• The atrial channel is always either in TARP (AV delay + PVARP) or alert. If the pacemaker is programmed to 60 ppm (1000 ms) and the patient has a 200 ms AV delay and a 250 ms PVARP (450 ms), then the atrial alert period is 650 ms (1000 − 450 = 650).

• During the atrial alert period, the atrial channel is looking for intrinsic atrial activity. If such activity is sensed, it will inhibit the atrial output pulse.

Test your knowledge

1 The clinician programs the paced AV delay in Mr. Smith's pacemaker to 200 ms. What would be a recommended value for programming the sensed AV delay?
   A 225 ms.
   B 175 ms.
   C 400 ms.
   D There is no such thing as a sensed AV delay.

2 Why is it important to optimize the AV delay when programming a pacemaker?
   A To enhance hemodynamics
   B To allow sufficient time for ventricular filling and atrial kick
   C To prevent unnecessary ventricular pacing
   D All of the above

3 TARP is the total atrial refractory period. What does it consist of?
   A AV delay + PVARP
   B PVAB + PVARP

   C AV delay + atrial alert period
   D AV delay + retrograde conduction time

4 What is the most important take-away from the DAVID clinical trial?
   A Never pace the right ventricle.
   B Never pace the left atrium.
   C People with heart failure benefit from constant pacing.
   D Right ventricular pacing can worsen heart failure.

5 To have PMT, a patient must have a dual-chamber pacemaker, a retrograde conduction, and a triggering event that breaks AV synchrony. Which of the following is NOT a PMT trigger?
   A Loss of atrial capture
   B PVC
   C Magnet application
   D Magnet removal

6 The postventricular atrial blanking (PVAB) period is designed for what function?
  A To terminate PMT once it starts
  B To prevent far-field R-wave oversensing
  C To prevent PMT
  D To allow for the ventricular filling

7 A typical setting for which parameter is 100 ms?
  A PVAB
  B PVARP
  C AV delay
  D TARP

8 Which of the following is true about retrograde conduction?
  A It is very rare and occurs in only about 10% of patients
  B It is highly irregular.
  C It is transient.
  D It appears to be related to sodium levels in the body.

9 In general terms, how do PMT prevention algorithms work?

  A They prevent retrograde conduction.
  B They extend PVARP for one cycle when a PVC is detected.
  C They shorten PVARP for one cycle when a PVC is detected.
  D They mode switch.

10 Mrs. Miller's pacemaker is programmed to an AV delay of 200 ms and a PVARP of 250 ms and a base rate of 60 ppm. How long is the alert period of this pacemaker?
  A 800 ms.
  B 750 ms.
  C 550 ms.
  D There is not enough information provided to figure this out.

Reference

1 Wilkoff, B.L., Cook, J.R., Epstein, A.E., et al. (Dec 25, 2002) Dual-chamber pacing or ventricular backup pacing in patients with an implantable defibrillator: the dual chamber and VVI Implantable Defibrillator (DAVID) trial. *JAMA: The Journal of the American Medical Association*, **288** (**24**), 3115–3123.

CHAPTER 17

Dual-chamber timing cycles: the ventricular channel

Learning objectives

- Define crosstalk in general and explain the role of the ventricular blanking period in preventing a specific type of crosstalk.
- Describe the *crosstalk detection window* and how it prevents crosstalk inhibition.
- State the formula that can be used to calculate the VA interval if you know the programmed base rate and the paced AV delay setting.
- Explain briefly what the dual-chamber pacemaker does during the ventricular alert period.
- Name the dual-chamber timing cycles that are initiated by each of these events: paced atrial event, sensed atrial event, paced ventricular event, and paced atrial event.
- Define the maximum tracking rate and state a commonly programmed value for this parameter.

Introduction

The ventricular timing cycles in a dual-chamber pacemaker are actually fewer in number and a little less complex than the atrial timing cycles. To recap, atrial timing cycles include the AV delay (sensed AV delay and paced AV delay), the PVARP (broken down into PVAB and PVARP), and the atrial alert period. Timing cycles on the ventricular side are relatively straightforward by comparison. The real complexity of dual-chamber pacing comes as the clinician recognizes that the pacemaker has simultaneous atrial and ventricular timing cycles. This is

a little bit like playing the piano—the right hand and the left hand do not do the same thing! However, with practice, clinicians can learn to think like a pacemaker.

Ventricular blanking period

The ventricular blanking period (VBP) is one of those dual-chamber timing cycles, like PVARP, that are initiated by an event on one channel but affect activity on the other channel. In the case of the VBP, an atrial output pulse initiates the timing cycle that causes an absolute refractory period (blanking period) to go into effect on the ventricular channel. With every paced atrial event, there is a brief VBP. This VBP is a total blind spot during which the ventricular channel will simply not see and not respond to any intrinsic events.

It is a bit more complicated than it sounds. Thinking back to the atrial timing cycles, a paced AV delay is launched with every atrial output pulse. The purpose of the paced AV delay (or any AV delay) is to search for intrinsic ventricular activity. Yet at the same moment the pacemaker initiates the paced AV delay to look for intrinsic ventricular events, it will also start a very short VBP or blanking period where such events would not be detected! (This only applies to the paced AV delay, not the sensed AV delay.)

The purpose of the VBP is to prevent a phenomenon called *crosstalk*. The best all-purpose definition of crosstalk for dual-chamber pacemakers is sensing of something in one chamber of

The Nuts and Bolts of Implantable Device Therapy Pacemakers, First Edition. Tom Kenny.
© 2015 John Wiley & Sons, Ltd. Published 2015 by John Wiley & Sons, Ltd.

the heart (atrial or ventricular) by the opposite channel. One example of crosstalk is far-field R-wave oversensing (when the atrial channel inappropriately senses ventricular activity and interprets it as intrinsic atrial events). In this case, it is possible for an *atrial* pacing spike to be sufficiently larger than the *ventricular* channel might *see* it. Remember that devices sense only electrical energy from signals and then have to assume where they originate. If the dual-chamber pacemaker's ventricular channel senses an atrial output pulse, it is going to *see* it as a sensed ventricular event. This can lead to what might be a big problem—ventricular oversensing. Oversensing always leads to underpacing, which means that the patient may not get the ventricular pacing support he or she needs. The danger associated with any form of crosstalk is the so-called crosstalk inhibition. Thus, if the atrial output pulse is sensed by the ventricular channel, the ventricular channel will inappropriately label it an intrinsic ventricular event and withhold the ventricular output pulse; this is an example of crosstalk inhibition.

To understand why crosstalk inhibition can occur, imagine a heart with a right atrial and a right ventricular lead. The right ventricular lead is set to a sensitivity setting of 3.5 mV. Think of this as a receiver; the ventricular lead electrodes are waiting for incoming electrical signals. The pacemaker does not identify signals by morphology; it simply looks at signal magnitude or size. Any signal that is 3.5 mV or larger will be interpreted by the ventricular channel as being a ventricular event. Now imagine that the atrial lead is pacing the right atrium with an output pulse of 3.5 V. The relationship of 3.5–3.5 mV is a thousandfold difference! The atrial output pulse is one thousand times bigger than what the ventricular channels identify as a ventricular event. Naturally, if such a huge signal occurs, it will be like a tsunami, and the ventricular channel will definitely see it and recognize it inappropriately as an intrinsic ventricular event. Crosstalk can occur virtually at any time, but some things make it even more likely:

- A very sensitive ventricular lead
- A very high atrial output pulse
- Atrial and ventricular lead placement in close proximity to each other

Remember that the VBP is launched only together with the paced AV delay; there is no VBP with a sensed AV delay. There is a simple reason for this. An atrial output pulse is measured in volts; even a low output pulse is going to be around 1 V and that is huge compared to the ventricular sensitivity setting, which is going to be around 3.5 or 4 mV. However, an intrinsic atrial event is associated with a vastly smaller signal. A typical atrial sensed event is going to have a signal size of around 2 or 3 mV. Plus, remember the signal originates in the atrium and dissipates as it spreads outward; the electrical energy that reaches the ventricular electrodes will be much too small to be sensed.

The atrial output pulse may be large compared to the ventricular sensitivity threshold, but it is very brief. By imposing a very short blanking period—the VBP—the pacemaker prevents the atrial output from being seen. A typical VBP is about 15–20 ms long.

On an ECG, crosstalk inhibition will show up as paced atrial activity followed by no paced ventricular activity (see **Figure 17.1**). If ventricular events occur at all, they will be intrinsic and will most likely be slow. On an electrogram, the programmer will annotate atrial paced events followed by ventricular sensed events, although the sensed events will not be there on the tracing.

It would be unusual to see a tracing like Figure 17.1 in clinical practice today because there are things that can help prevent crosstalk inhibition. An important safety feature, ventricular safety pacing, is described in the following text. Moreover, the VBP value is programmable and can be extended. While a blanking period of 20 ms works well for many patients, there are times when it should be programmed to a longer value. In some advanced devices today, the clinician can set up the VBP so that it adjusts itself automatically based on atrial output (higher outputs, longer VBPs) and ventricular sensitivity (higher sensitivity, longer VBPs).

Thus, the VBP is the initial portion of the ventricular alert timing cycle on the ventricular channel *following a paced atrial event* (see **Figure 17.2**). There is no VBP following a sensed atrial event.

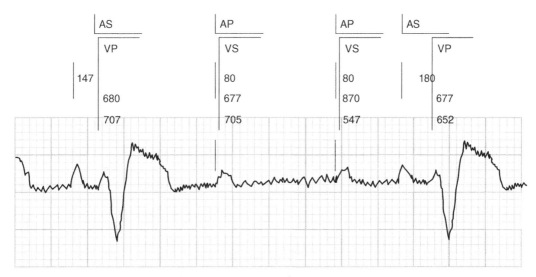

Figure 17.1 Crosstalk occurs in the second and third complexes of this tracing. Atrial pacing outputs inhibit the ventricle inappropriately. Note that the programmer annotates ventricular sensed events that do not show up on the tracing. According to the annotations, the *ventricular sensed events* (actually oversensing) occur just 80 ms after the atrial output pulse. This is much too fast to represent any kind of sensing of a normal impulse over the AV node. However, the 80 ms timing was longer than the VBP of about 20 ms, so the atrial spike fell outside the VBP and thus was inappropriately sensed by the ventricular channel.

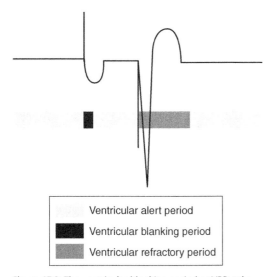

Ventricular alert period
Ventricular blanking period
Ventricular refractory period

Figure 17.2 The ventricular blanking period or VBP only occurs after an atrial output pulse and is the short initial period immediately preceding the ventricular alert period.

Ventricular safety pacing

The best way to understand ventricular safety pacing is to think of the paced AV interval as composed of three distinct timing cycles: the VBP, a crosstalk sensing window (also called a crosstalk detection window), and the ventricular alert period (see **Figure 17.3**). The VBP is programmable and together the VBP plus the crosstalk sensing window will equal 65 ms. As the VBP changes, the device automatically adjusts the crosstalk sensing window to keep the total at 65 ms.

The crosstalk sensing window is an interesting timing cycle. If any intrinsic ventricular event is sensed during the crosstalk sensing window, the pacemaker commits to delivering a ventricular output pulse in 100–120 ms (varies by manufacturer and device) as timed from the atrial pacing output pulse. Anything sensed on the ventricular channel during this interval commits the pacemaker to deliver a ventricular output pulse when the window expires. This commitment to ventricular pacing is sometimes called *safety pacing*. The concept behind the crosstalk sensing or detection window is that if a signal occurs in this time period, the pacemaker decides to *play it safe* and pace the ventricle. This feature is available from various manufacturers and works slightly differently for each; however, the underlying principle of a special sensing window and safety pacing is the same (see **Table 17.1**).

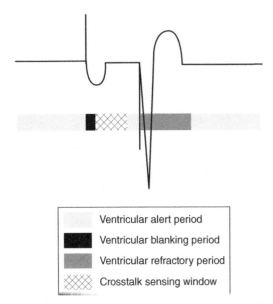

Ventricular alert period

Ventricular blanking period

Ventricular refractory period

Crosstalk sensing window

Figure 17.3 Ventricular safety pacing divides the paced AV interval into three distinct timing cycles: the VBP (typically 15–20 ms), the crosstalk sensing window (typically 45–50 ms), and then the alert period. The VBP + crosstalk sensing window always equals 65 ms. As the VBP changes, the crosstalk sensing window adjusts automatically to keep the total duration 65 ms. Signals that occur during the VBP are not seen; signals that are sensed during the alert period will cause ventricular inhibition. However, signals sensed during the crosstalk sensing window cause the pacemaker to commit to ventricular pacing.

Table 17.1 Responses to incoming signals on the ventricular channel during the paced AV interval, based on the three components of the paced AV delay (VBP, crosstalk sensing window, and alert period)

Timing cycle	Approximate duration	What happens when an incoming signal occurs
VBP	15–20 ms, programmable	It is ignored (the ventricular channel is blind)
Crosstalk sensing window	45–50 ms so that the total with VBP is 65 ms	The pacemaker commits to delivering a ventricular output pulse at 100–120 ms after the atrial output pulse
Alert period	About 135 ms, varies with programmed paced AV delay	The ventricular output pulse is inhibited

Thus, the crosstalk sensing window effectively prevents crosstalk inhibition. It does not prevent crosstalk—crosstalk may still occur. It simply does not allow the dual-chamber pacemaker to inappropriately inhibit ventricular pacing if and when such crosstalk occurs.

One might wonder what would happen if a ventricular event is sensed during the crosstalk sensing window. The most likely scenario for this to happen would be a PVC that falls in the crosstalk detection window. The pacemaker will sense this and then commit to pacing the ventricle. This is actually not a problem, although when there is a true ventricular event, then safety pacing will result in pseudofusion. Pseudofusion, as you may remember, is not clinically detrimental and occurs when a pacing spike and an intrinsic event occur simultaneously and the spike does not contribute to the depolarization.

On the other hand, if the ventricular channel senses the atrial output pulse late and it falls in the crosstalk detection window, the ventricular output pulse will be delivered and will most likely capture the ventricle because it will meet with responsive (not refractory) ventricular tissue.

Thus, the crosstalk sensing window with safety pacing allows the pacemaker to avoid crosstalk inhibition, even in those cases where crosstalk occurs outside the VBP. This is almost a *belt-and-suspenders* approach to preventing crosstalk inhibition. The VBP will prevent most crosstalk inhibition, but if a signal falls outside the VBP, then the crosstalk detection window and safety pacing will prevent crosstalk inhibition. Because of these features, rhythm strips of crosstalk inhibition are more likely to be found in textbooks than in clinics.

It is important to remember that the crosstalk sensing window only occurs following a paced atrial event; there is no VBP and no crosstalk sensing window following intrinsic atrial activity. After an intrinsic atrial event, the entire sensed AV interval is an alert period. There will never be ventricular safety pacing after a sensed atrial event.

Ventricular refractory period
The ventricular refractory period, sometimes called the V-ref, has what should now start to be an expected definition. In fact, the V-ref in a dual-chamber device is the same as the V-ref in a single chamber device.

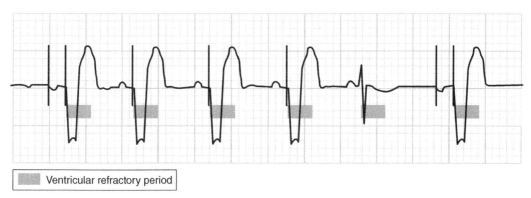

Ventricular refractory period

Figure 17.4 The ventricular refractory period is initiated by either a sensed or paced ventricular event. It has a programmable duration and is typically set to about 250–275 ms.

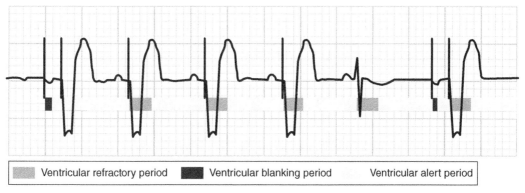

Ventricular refractory period   Ventricular blanking period   Ventricular alert period

Figure 17.5 The ventricular refractory period is initiated by a sensed or paced ventricular event; when it expires, the ventricular alert period begins. During the ventricular alert period, the ventricular channel actively seeks intrinsic ventricular activity. If an atrial paced event occurs, the ventricular alert period is briefly interrupted by the ventricular blanking period.

The V-ref is the timing cycle on the ventricular channel initiated by a sensed or paced ventricular event during which the pacemaker will not respond to incoming signals (see **Figure 17.4**). Like other refractory periods, the V-ref has an absolute segment (during which incoming signals are not even seen) and a relative refractory period (during which incoming signals may be seen but there is no response to them). While there is an absolute and relative component of the V-ref, these are less crucial to understanding timing cycles. The V-ref is programmable and typically is set to 250–275 ms.

Ventricular alert period

During the ventricular alert period, the pacemaker is actively searching for intrinsic ventricular activity that, if detected, will inhibit the ventricular output pulse. The ventricular alert period occurs immediately after the V-ref following any ventricular event (paced or sensed). This means that the ventricular alert period occurs after the V-ref all the way through a sensed atrial event (see **Figure 17.5**). If an atrial paced event occurs, the ventricular alert period is briefly interrupted by the VBP, but then resumes when it times out.

The VA interval

The VA interval, sometimes called the V-to-A interval, is a calculated timing cycle on the ventricular channel defined by the time period from a sensed or paced ventricular event to the next atrial paced event. An important dual-chamber formula involves the VA interval; it states that the programmed base rate equals the AV delay (in this case, we'll just use the paced AV delay) plus the VA interval (see **Figure 17.6**). When the VA interval expires—provided that no intrinsic atrial activity has been sensed—the dual-chamber pacemaker will pace the atrium.

For instance, let's take a dual-chamber programmed to a base rate of 60 ppm with a paced AV delay set to 200 ms. The 60 ppm base rate is translated to 1000 ms. This means the base rate (1000 ms) will equal the AV delay (200 ms) and the VA interval. So even if a clinician does not know the VA interval, it can be easily calculated from the base rate and the paced AV delay. In this case, the VA interval has to be 800 ms (1000 = 200 + 800). While the base rates of the pacemaker and the AV delay are programmable

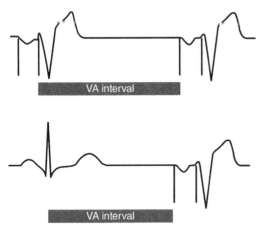

Figure 17.6 The VA interval commences with any ventricular event (sensed or paced) and ends with an atrial output pulse. The VA interval is a calculated timing cycle and is not directly programmable. However, it can be changed by adjusting the base rate and/or the AV delay.

parameters and can be changed, the VA interval is a *calculated rate*. It cannot be directly programmed, although it can be indirectly programmed by changing the AV delay value and/or the base rate.

Dual-chamber timing cycles start to get tricky when we overlay the various simultaneous timing cycles on top of each other. In a dual-chamber pacemaker, there are always simultaneous atrial and ventricular timing cycles happening. For now, let's consider what other timing cycles occur together with the VA interval. First, since a paced or sensed ventricular event always launches the VA interval, the beginning of any VA interval is going to include the ventricular refractory period. When the ventricular refractory period times out, it initiates the ventricular alert period. So the VA interval also includes a ventricular alert period. Switching over to the atrial channel, the ventricular event launches PVARP, a refractory period. When PVARP times out, it initiates the atrial alert period.

Thus, the VA interval encompasses both an atrial and a ventricular alert period. This is going to be very important as we go on, but for now, it is important to see that this VA interval involves several timing cycles going on in the two chambers. For a simplified overview, see **Table 17.2**. Note that this applies only to certain timing cycles. (There is actually more going on than is shown below!)

Knowing these timing cycles and being able to describe what happens on atrial and ventricular channels simultaneously as specific events occur allow you to *think like a pacemaker*. This is the crucial first step in mastering dual-chamber pacing!

Just to make things confusing, the VA interval is sometimes called the atrial escape interval or AEI.

Table 17.2 A few timing cycles on the atrial and ventricular channels during the VA interval

Cardiac event	VA interval	Atrial channel	Ventricular channel
Sensed or paced ventricular event	Starts VA interval	Starts PVARP (PVAB + PVARP), which times out	Starts V-ref, which times out
		When PVARP times out, atrial alert period begins	When V-ref times out, ventricular alert period begins
Paced atrial event	Ends VA interval	Starts atrial refractory period	Starts ventricular blanking period
Sensed atrial event	Interrupts VA interval	Inhibits atrial output pulse and begins sensed AV delay	Begins ventricular alert period

It is important to recognize that many timing cycles overlap and the pacemaker is always doing something on the atrial and ventricular channels.

Table 17.3 This is a highly simplified overview of the main timing cycles associated with the only four events possible in dual-chamber pacing (atrial and ventricular paced and sensed events)

Event	Atrial channel	Ventricular channel
Sensed atrial event	Begins the sensed AV delay	Ventricular alert period
Sensed ventricular event	Begins PVAB that then goes into PVARP	Begins V-ref that then goes into ventricular alert Begins the VA interval
Paced atrial event	Begins the paced AV delay Ends the VA interval	Begins the VBP that goes into the crosstalk detection window and then ventricular alert
Paced ventricular event	Begins PVAB that then goes into PVARP	Begins the V-ref that then goes into the ventricular alert Begins the VA interval

This name comes from the fact that when the AEI (or VA interval) expires, an atrial output pulse is delivered (atrial escape). For now, we will stick with calling it the VA interval (which is more intuitive), but it will be encountered in the field and in other textbooks as the AEI.

Going back to Figure 17.6 for a moment, what would happen if a PVC occurred about in the middle of the VA interval? First, we know it would be sensed because it would fall in the ventricular alert period when the pacemaker is looking for intrinsic ventricular activity. Because the pacemaker considers it a sensed ventricular event, it will restart the VA interval (the VA interval begins anew every time there is a paced or sensed ventricular event). This will launch PVARP on the atrial channel simultaneously with V-ref on the ventricular channel. In other words, a sensed ventricular event during the ventricular alert period of the VA interval will inhibit both channels and restart the VA interval.

Maximum tracking rate

This is the last timing cycle in the dual-chamber pacemaker to be presented here, and for many patients, it is one of the most important. The maximum tracking rate (sometimes called max track or MTR) is also known as the upper rate limit (URL) or the upper tracking limit (UTL). The best definition of MTR is that it defines the fastest rate at which the ventricles can be paced in response to intrinsic atrial activity. A dual-chamber pacemaker will never pace the ventricle faster than the MTR, no matter how fast the intrinsic atrial rate becomes. For instance, if the MTR is set to 120 ppm, the

ventricular pacing rate will never exceed that. The MTR is programmable and is typically set to 120 or 130 ppm, but when programming this value, the physician should consider the patient's age, overall condition, activity level, and underlying cardiac status. The timing clock for the MTR starts with a sensed or paced ventricular event.

Putting it all together

The complexities of dual-chamber pacing occur because the two channels have simultaneous timing cycles based on whether or not the channel sensed an intrinsic event or not. While this can seem daunting at the outset, it can really help to review the main type of events and the timing cycles associated from them. There are only two channels: atrial and ventricular. There are only two things the pacemaker can actually do: paced and sense (inhibit). That leaves us with only four possible dual-chamber pacing states: atrial paced/ventricular paced, atrial paced/ventricular sensed, atrial sensed/ventricular paced, and atrial sensed/ventricular sensed (see **Table 17.3**).

Conclusion

There are fewer ventricular timing cycles than atrial timing cycles. Clinicians need only be mindful of the ventricular refractory period and the ventricular alert period. The VA interval or AEI is a calculated rather than programmable timing cycle that will become increasingly important in future sections. The VA interval can be calculated by converting the programmed base rate to an interval and then subtracting the AV delay interval. Ventricular timing cycles are important in the prevention of crosstalk. Technically, crosstalk occurs any time one channel inappropriately senses activity that occurs on the other channel. In the past, this often occurred when an atrial output pulse (which could be 3.5 V in magnitude) was inappropriately sensed by the ventricular pacing electrode (which might have a sensitivity setting of 3.5 mV or a thousand times smaller). Crosstalk led to oversensing that, in turn, causes underpacing in a phenomenon called *crosstalk*

inhibition. To prevent crosstalk inhibition, the dual-chamber pacemaker today offers a VBP following an atrial output pulse plus a crosstalk detection window. If an event is sensed in the crosstalk detection window, the pacemaker commits to delivering a ventricular output pulse as *safety pacing*. This output pulse is delivered about 100–120 ms after the atrial spike. Knowing these timing cycles can help the clinician to understand all of the multiple things a pacemaker *thinks* about during pacing.

The nuts and bolts of dual-chamber timing cycles: the ventricular channel

- The timing cycles on the ventricular channel are fewer in number and less complex than atrial timing cycles, but the complexity of dual-chamber pacing resides in the fact that atrial and ventricular timing cycles may occur simultaneously and events in one channel can initiate timing cycles on the other channel.
- The ventricular refractory period consists of a short ventricular blanking period (VBP) followed by a relative refractory period.
- The purpose of the VBP—during which the ventricular channel is blind to all events—is to prevent the ventricular lead from picking up the atrial pacing spike and inappropriately interpreting it as a ventricular event.
- Whenever one channel inappropriately picks up signals from the other channel, it is called crosstalk. Probably the most well-known (and most troublesome) form of crosstalk occurs when the ventricular channel picks up an atrial pacing spike and inappropriately labels it an intrinsic ventricular event. This is a form of ventricular oversensing.
- Oversensing always leads to underpacing. (By contrast, undersensing leads to overpacing.) Oversensing caused by double counting due to crosstalk is called crosstalk inhibition.
- The typical VBP is about 15–20 ms long and it is initiated with an atrial pacing spike.
- The *paced* AV delay interval is divided into three distinct phases: the VBP, the crosstalk detection window (also called the crosstalk sensing window), and a ventricular alert period. During the VBP, the pacemaker will

not sense or respond to anything. During the alert period, the ventricular channel is looking for intrinsic ventricular signals that would inhibit the ventricular output pulse. During the crosstalk detection window, the pacemaker can see signals, and if it detects what seems to be an intrinsic ventricular event, it commits to pacing. A ventricular output pulse will be delivered in about 100–120 ms.
- The crosstalk detection window occurs immediately after the VBP. The total time of the VBP plus the crosstalk detection window is 65 ms. In some devices, the VBP may be programmable, but all devices limit the VBP and crosstalk detection window to a total time span of 65 ms.
- Any event sensed during the crosstalk detection window that the pacemaker considers ventricular activity will force the pacemaker to pace the ventricle *for safety's sake*. The ventricular output pulse will be delivered 100–120 ms (depends on device), timed from the start of the VBP.
- If the event sensed during the crosstalk detection window turns out to be crosstalk, the pacemaker spike will provide the safety of ventricular pacing and prevent crosstalk inhibition. On the other hand, if the event turns out to be a true intrinsic ventricular event, then the ventricular spike will fall on the intrinsic event. This will lead to pseudofusion. Pseudofusion is not harmful to the patient.
- The *sensed* AV delay interval consists of a ventricular alert period. There are no blanking or crosstalk detection intervals.

- The ventricular refractory period (sometimes called the V-ref) is initiated by a sensed or paced ventricular event and is typically programmed to 250–275 ms.
- When the V-ref expires, then the pacemaker launches the ventricular alert period. During the ventricular alert period, the pacemaker seeks intrinsic ventricular events.
- The VA interval, sometimes called the V-to-A interval, is the timing cycle that begins with any ventricular event (sensed or paced) and ends with a paced atrial event. In a patient with consistent atrial sensing, there will be no VA intervals.
- The VA interval can be calculated. Convert the programmed base rate into milliseconds (e.g., 60 ppm = 1000 ms) and then subtract the paced AV delay (e.g., 200 ms). In such a case, the VA interval = 800 ms (1000 minus 200).

- The VA interval is not directly programmable, but it can be affected by changes in the base rate and the AV delay settings.
- Dual-chamber pacing involves simultaneous events and clocks on both the atrial and ventricular channels. For instance, a sensed atrial event will initiate the sensed AV delay on the atrial channel and the ventricular alert period on the ventricular channel. A paced atrial event launches the paced AV delay interval (atrial channel) and the VBP followed by the crosstalk sensing window (ventricular channel).
- Sensed and paced ventricular events launch the PVAB on the atrial channel (which then transitions into the PVARP) and simultaneously the ventricular refractory period on the ventricular channel. When the ventricular refractory period expires, the ventricular alert period begins.

Test your knowledge

1 What event will initiate a VBP on the ventricular channel?
   A An atrial paced event
   B An atrial sensed event
   C A ventricular paced event
   D A ventricular sensed event

2 Which statement best describes the main purpose of the VBP?
   A To prevent crosstalk
   B To stop the ventricular channel from picking up the atrial pacing spike
   C To avoid ventricular oversensing, double counting, and inappropriate inhibition
   D All of the above

3 Which of the following is an example of *crosstalk* in a dual-chamber pacemaker?
   A Pacemaker-mediated tachycardia
   B Ventricular undersensing
   C Far-field R-wave oversensing
   D Mechanical dyssynchrony

4 You are handed an electrogram strip with a run of crosstalk. The pacing states are annotated. What will you predominantly see?

   A Atrial paced event/ventricular sensed event
   B Atrial paced event/ventricular paced event
   C Atrial sensed event/ventricular sensed event
   D Atrial sensed event/ventricular paced event

5 On that same electrogram, what will you see predominantly on the tracing?
   A Atrial tracking with rapid ventricular response
   B Rapid atrial pacing with ventricular response
   C Atrial paced events with no ventricular events
   D Ventricular paced events with no atrial events

6 How many milliseconds is the VBP plus the crosstalk sensing window together?
   A 15–20 ms
   B 40–100 ms
   C 65 ms
   D 100–120 ms, depends on the manufacturer

7 What happens when the ventricular channel senses what it thinks is a ventricular event during the VBP?
   A It commits to pacing the ventricle in 100–120 ms.
   B It launches the AV delay.

C It immediately delivers a ventricular output pulse.

D Nothing—the VBP cannot even see a ventricular event.

8 What happens when the ventricular channel senses what it thinks is a ventricular event during the crosstalk detection window?

A It commits to pacing the ventricle in 100–120 ms.

B It launches the AV delay.

C It immediately delivers a ventricular output pulse.

D Nothing—the crosstalk detection window cannot even see a ventricular event.

9 What is a typical setting for the ventricular refractory period in a dual-chamber pacemaker patient?

A 40 ms.

B 250 ms.

C 800 ms.

D It is not programmable but is based on the VA interval.

10 A dual-chamber pacemaker is programmed to 70 ppm (which converts to 857 ms). In this patient, both paced and sensed AV delay intervals are programmed to 200 ms. What is the VA interval?

A 657 ms.

B 1057 ms.

C 800 ms.

D There is not enough information provided to figure this out.

CHAPTER 18

Paced ECG and EGM analysis

Learning objectives

- List the key steps to take when analyzing a paced ECG or EGM systematically.
- Explain how to analyze atrial capture in a dual-chamber rhythm strip when the patient has consistent intrinsic atrial activity.
- Briefly state why functional noncapture can actually be appropriately captured.
- Provide the rationale for evaluating a dual-chamber device in DDD mode rather than evaluating VVI and AAI modes.
- Define *failure to output* and how this may show up on a rhythm strip.
- Explain the main differences in analyzing single-chamber versus dual-chamber rhythm strips in terms of the systematic approach.

Introduction

Pacing experts must be confident in their ability to analyze and interpret paced ECGs and electrograms (EGMs). After all, pacing clinicians deal with these tracings all day long, and sometimes, they provide diagnostic clues that cannot be found anywhere else. The paced ECG can be a little daunting at first—it has all of the complexity of a normal ECG but with the interaction of a very powerful *third party*, namely, the pacemaker. An EGM can look deceptively familiar, but even with its annotations and cycle lengths, it can still be tricky to interpret properly. ECG and EGM analysis is a cornerstone of the pacing clinic, so it pays to devote serious time and effort in mastering this art.

There are a couple of things that will make it easier.

First, the paced ECG or EGM has to be analyzed systematically. Without a system, a clinician will just note random things that jump out and may miss the whole point. With a system, you have a step-by-step guide of what to look for first, what to look for next, and so on and finally how to put it all together. When people struggle with paced ECG analysis, it is almost always because they do not attack the rhythm strip systematically. Fast and accurate ECG and EGM analysis requires a system. In this chapter, we are going to concentrate on building that system so that it becomes second nature. The time you invest in learning this system will pay off big dividends in future years of paced ECG and EGM analysis.

Second, the call it paced ECG and EGM *interpretation* for a reason. Pacing clinicians sometimes confront rhythm strips that require a bit of speculation. For instance, you may have access only to a very short run of an arrhythmia and you need to base conclusions on a few complexes—although you would like to see more. Rhythm strips in actual clinical practice are not as nice and clean as they are in this textbook, so sometimes you may have to deal with an imperfect tracing. And finally, sometimes, things on a rhythm strip are subject to multiple interpretations. This latter case is rarer in clinical practice but becomes almost a sporting event at pacing conventions when experts try to best their peers. So as you move forward in paced ECG and EGM interpretation, remember that there is a little bit of art mixed in with the science.

The Nuts and Bolts of Implantable Device Therapy Pacemakers, First Edition. Tom Kenny.
© 2015 John Wiley & Sons, Ltd. Published 2015 by John Wiley & Sons, Ltd.

Gathering information

Let's start with a very typical scenario: a pacemaker patient comes to the device clinic and the clinician is going to check out the paced ECG and EGM. Before getting started, the clinician should try to get this background information, which should be readily available:

- The type of pacemaker the patient has (single chamber or dual chamber)
- The currently programmed mode and other programmed settings
- Patient history, particularly as to how it relates to the device's programmed settings
- Other patient information that may relate to pacing, such as whether or not the patient has intermittent atrial tachyarrhythmias
- The age of the pacemaker (new implant or chronic system?)

Next, establish the best lead on the surface ECG for the tracing, that is, the lead that is going to get the best P-waves and QRS complexes on the tracing. Routinely use the marker channels and annotations on the tracing; not only are they useful information, but they tell you what the pacemaker *thinks*. When doing an in-clinic analysis, turn on the intracardiac EGM and compare it against the surface ECG. While the EGM and ECG will not always match exactly, they should both be telling the same story.

These steps help to lay the foundation for an in-clinic paced ECG and EGM analysis. With a little practice, an experienced clinician can run through these points fairly quickly—and they can be enormously helpful as the strips are analyzed.

You can't beat the system

The system is surprisingly simple, but if you use it consistently, you will see how powerful this little checklist can actually be. Note that if you're analyzing a dual-chamber pacemaker, you will have to do certain steps for both atrial and ventricular channels:

- Gather information (described in previous section; the crucial information is the mode).
- Measure the intervals in milliseconds.
- Convert the rate (milliseconds) to ppm.
- Check capture.
- Check sensing.
- Check the patient's underlying rhythm.
- Document, document, and document.

This system is a little bit arbitrary in that different clinics or physicians may opt to use a slightly different sequence. For example, I prefer to check capture before sensing because, to my mind, capture is hemodynamically the more important element to check. However, I am certain that some clinicians would say it is better to check sensing before capture. In the end, it does not matter as much as the fact that you develop a systematic approach so that nothing is overlooked and you don't rush to a conclusion without gathering all of the evidence carefully. You can also state this checklist in a more abbreviated way that may be easier to memorize:

- Mode
- Rate
- Capture
- Sensing
- Underlying rhythm
- Document findings

In real-world clinical practice, most clinicians obtain rhythm strips from actual pacemaker patients, affording the luxury of knowing a bit about the device, the patient, and the programmed settings. Rhythm strips sometimes are analyzed *blind* with minimal to no background information. Device clinicians must become familiar with the look and annotations of the various device manufacturers; they differ somewhat (see **Figure 18.1**). For dual-chamber devices, be sure to obtain the atrial and ventricular EGMs. When viewing multiple rhythm strips, make sure that the activity aligns appropriately, that is, a ventricular event on the surface ECG should be evident at or very close to the same time on the ventricular EGM (see **Figures 18.2** and **18.3**).

Questions for analysis

When analyzing a paced rhythm strip or an EGM, the clinician should go through a systematic list of questions. This list assumes that the clinician is reviewing a dual-chamber pacemaker. The order of these questions is not as important as that all of them are addressed:

- Do you see atrial pacing spikes?
  - If so, are they followed immediately by an atrial depolarization? (If they are, that shows appropriate atrial capture.)
  - If they are not, that *suggests* loss of atrial capture. Note that loss of capture can be intermittent.

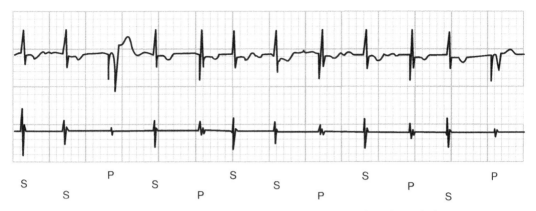

Figure 18.1 The patient has a Guidant VVI pacemaker. The annotations below use the code S and P for sensed and paced events; since it is a single-chamber pacemaker, these only refer to ventricular events. Note that while the surface ECG above and the EGM below have distinctly different looks, they are both *telling the same story*.

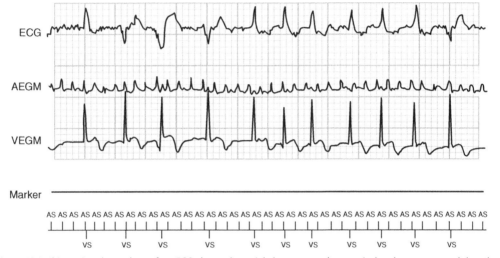

Figure 18.2 This tracing shows the surface ECG above, the atrial electrogram, the ventricular electrogram, and then the markers. In this case, AS stands for atrial sensed event and VS for ventricular sensed event. Although this tracing comes from a dual-chamber pacemaker patient, there is no pacing in this particular portion of the tracing. The rapid atrial activity and irregular ventricular response indicate this patient is experiencing atrial fibrillation. The marker channel explains how the pacemaker categorizes these events.

As we will see later, atrial events are not always evident on the tracing.
  ○ Another way to confirm atrial capture is to see if the atrial pacing spike resulted in a normal-looking QRS complex. If a normal QRS occurs at an appropriate interval after the atrial spike, this suggests that the spike depolarizes the atria and conducted down over the AV node and depolarized the ventricles. One of these things (atrial depolarization or normal-looking QRS) is sufficient to confirm atrial capture.
• Do you see ventricular pacing spikes?

  ○ If so, are they followed immediately by a ventricular depolarization? (If they are, that shows appropriate ventricular capture.)
  ○ If they are not, that suggests loss of ventricular capture. Note that loss of capture can be intermittent.
• Do you see intrinsic P-waves?
  ○ If so, do they inhibit atrial pacing? (If they do, that shows appropriate atrial sensing.)
  ○ If they do not inhibit atrial pacing, that suggests atrial undersensing.
• Do you see intrinsic R-waves?

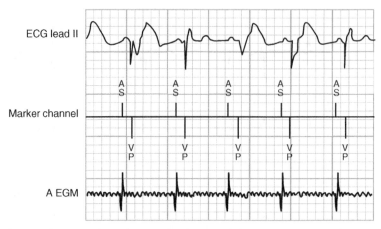

Figure 18.3 This dual-chamber pacemaker is shown with only an atrial electrogram and the marker channel in the middle. The patient appears to have intrinsic atrial activity that does not conduct over the AV node, necessitating ventricular pacing. The prominent and sharp waveforms on the atrial electrogram are atrial events; notice how they align with the markers (AS) and the surface ECG; to the atrial lead, the intrinsic atrial event *looks bigger* than the background ventricular activity.

- If so, do they inhibit ventricular pacing? (If they do, that shows appropriate ventricular sensing.)
- If they do not inhibit ventricular pacing, that suggests ventricular undersensing.
- Can you measure the base rate?
  - The paced atrial interval (the interval from one paced atrial event to the next paced atrial event) will be equivalent to the base rate. This requires that you have two consecutive paced atrial events.
  - Note that pacing is not always at the base rate—it may be higher (for instance, if atrial tracking is going on) or lower (if hysteresis is active). If you see pacing at a rate other than the base rate, you should be able to figure out why it is not pacing at the base rate.
- Do you see a paced AV interval?
  - If possible, measure the interval from an atrial paced event to the next ventricular paced event with no intervening events.
  - This value should match the programmed paced AV delay.
- Do you see a VA interval? (That is the interval from any ventricular event, paced or sensed, to the next paced atrial event with no intervening events.)
  - If possible, measure the VA interval.
  - Note that the VA interval plus the AV interval should equal the interval associated with the

base rate. For instance, if the base rate is 60 ppm, that translates to a base rate interval of 1000 ms. If the AV interval is 200 ms, then the VA interval should be 800 ms.
- Can you evaluate the patient's underlying rhythm?
  - Is it consistent with the patient's diagnosis? For instance, you should not expect to be seeing a lot of intrinsic atrial activity in a patient with sick sinus syndrome.
  - Does the patient appear to have a reliable escape rate?
- What is the final interpretation?
  - Do not jump the gun—wait until you have all of the information before putting it together.
  - You want to be able to determine if the pacemaker is operating normally or if there is some type of inappropriate pacemaker behavior.

Navigating the paced ECG: Things to look out for

The goal of a systematic approach to paced ECG analysis is to make sure the clinician considers all of the information that a tracing contains before reaching any conclusions. It is very easy for certain events to stand out and lead a clinician to a false conclusion. The following are some common pitfalls and ways to navigate clear of them when analyzing a paced ECG.

Functional noncapture

Obviously, capture is a crucial element in paced ECG analysis, and noncapture is a serious problem that requires immediate attention. When a pacing spike is not followed immediately by a depolarization above, it *suggests* but *does not prove* loss of capture. When a pacing spike without a subsequent depolarization appears on a tracing, the clinician has to ask whether capture was possible. If the heart is refractory when the spike is delivered, the event is called *functional noncapture*, which means the failure to capture owed to cardiac function rather than a device problem (see **Figure 18.4**).

Figure 18.4 actually shows what can be called an *appropriate atrial capture*. This may seem strange considering the circled event, but atrial capture occurred each and every time that it could. The real problem in this strip is that the intrinsic atrial event that preceded the circled spike was not appropriately sensed. Thus, this strip shows both atrial undersensing and appropriate atrial capture.

The key take-away from the potential pitfall of paced ECG interpretation is that functional noncapture almost always indicates a sensing problem, specifically undersensing. Expressed another way, sensing problems can lead to functional noncapture.

Not enough information

Sometimes, a rhythm strip does not provide adequate information for a full assessment of capture and sensing. For example, a clinician working with a dual-chamber pacemaker patient who has consistent AS/VP pacing will not see any examples of atrial pacing on the rhythm strip and will not be able to evaluate atrial capture. Moreover, with a rhythm strip of nothing but ventricular pacing, it will be impossible to evaluate ventricular sensing. For in-clinic rhythm strip evaluations, there are ways to temporarily reprogram the pacemaker to force certain types of events, such as atrial pacing, to occur long enough for evaluation. Using the programmer, the clinician can set up temporary pacing parameters that are in force for the duration of the test. Temporary programming offers the important advantage of reverting back to previously programmed parameters with the touch of a button (see **Table 18.1**).

For example, in a rhythm strip from a dual-chamber pacemaker where certain parameter settings are known (base rate 60 ppm, paced AV delay 160 ms, sensed AV delay 140 ms), a wealth of information can be gleaned even if there is no pacing going on and the strip looks like normal sinus rhythm. The clinician knows the AV delay intervals; using calipers, he or she can determine if the intrinsic ventricular events fell into the AV delay. (Set the calipers to 140 ms and place one end of the calipers on the start of the intrinsic P-wave; this shows the sensed AV delay interval.) If the ventricular event fell inside the sensed AV delay, and the pacemaker did not pace the ventricle, then ventricular sensing was appropriate. Using the information, the clinician can calculate the VA interval by converting 60 ppm to 1000 ms and subtracting the

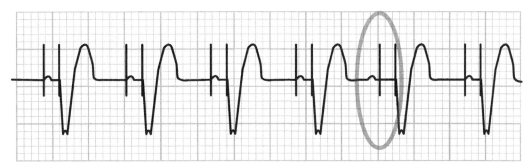

Figure 18.4 A good habit for paced ECG analysis is to pencil in the events right on the strip. The first three atrial events are paced atrial events. The fourth atrial event is a sensed atrial event. The fifth complex shows an atrial sensed event followed by an atrial pacing spike and no depolarization (circled). While this suggests loss of capture, it is important to dig deeper. Notice that the atrial spike was preceded by an intrinsic atrial event. Would it have been possible for an atrial output pulse to capture the atrium right after it had just contracted? No, because the atrial tissue at this point is physiologically refractory. No atrial pacing spike, no matter how large, could cause an atrial depolarization. Thus, this atrial pacing spike does not show *loss of capture* but rather *functional noncapture*.

Table 18.1 It is important to evaluate atrial and ventricular capture and sensing in a dual-chamber pacemaker

Desired test	Atrial	Ventricular
Capture	If you have consistent atrial sensing, increase the base rate to force atrial pacing and evaluate capture	If you have consistent ventricular sensing, shorten the paced and/or sensed AV delay to force ventricular pacing and evaluate capture
Sensing	If you have consistent atrial pacing, decrease the base rate to allow intrinsic atrial activity to emerge and evaluate sensing	If you have consistent ventricular pacing, lengthen the paced and/or sensed AV delay to allow intrinsic ventricular activity to emerge and evaluate sensing

If you do not get the information you need to test for capture and sensing, these temporary programming steps are often helpful.

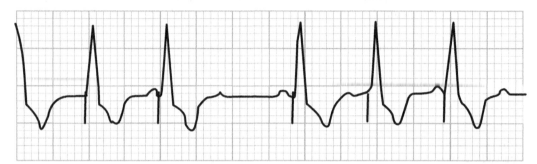

Figure 18.5 This is a tracing from a VVI pacemaker. Note that all ventricular pacing spikes result in a ventricular depolarization; capture is appropriate. However, there is a gap between the second and third ventricular events. This could be ventricular oversensing—in fact, it probably is. But check the marker channel to make sure it is not a failure to output, a rare but potentially serious device problem.

paced AV delay to reach 840. During the VA interval, the pacemaker is searching for the next atrial event. By setting calipers to 840 ms and putting one point of the caliper on the ventricular event (the V in the VA interval), the clinician should determine if an intrinsic atrial event fell in this VA interval; if it did and if that intrinsic P-wave inhibited atrial pacing, then atrial sensing is normal. While not every rhythm strip will allow the clinician to assess everything, it is remarkable how much can be analyzed with even a few pieces of information. However, there are limits. Such a rhythm strip would not allow the clinician to reach any conclusions about appropriate capture.

Failure to output

Figure 18.5 depicts a rhythm strip from a VVI pacemaker. It is very tempting to glance at this type of strip and assume that the flatline gap between the second and third complexes relates to a sensing problem, specifically that the pacemaker has oversensed something that is really not there. When a pacemaker oversenses, it inhibits an output pulse that the patient actually needs. Think of it this way: oversensing leads to underpacing! However, there is the possibility that this kind of event can be caused by the pacemaker's failure to output. This is rare, but it is such a serious problem that it warrants double checking. The best way to determine if a gap in a rhythm strip is oversensing or failure to output is to turn on the marker channel. The markers will tell you how the pacemaker *saw* things. If the marker channel reveals a ventricular sensed event, that is a clear case of ventricular oversensing. The pacemaker thought a ventricular event occurred (although none did) and inappropriately inhibited ventricular pacing. However, if the marker channel shows a ventricular paced event, it indicates a failure to output. Failure to output means that the pacemaker is generating an output pulse, but for some reason, it is not getting down the lead and to the heart properly.

Clean atrial capture

Atrial capture is suggested when an atrial pacing spike results in an atrial depolarization. This is very easy to see in textbooks and very rare to see in actual clinical practice. However, there is a way to confirm atrial capture in some situations even if the rhythm strip is equivocal. In **Figure 18.6**, atrial capture clearly occurs in the third, fourth, and fifth complexes by virtue of the fact that the ventricles depolarize. In the first two complexes, the patient has an intrinsic atrial beat that conducts over the AV node and depolarizes the ventricle. The same thing happens after the pacing spikes—the ventricles depolarize at the proper time and have the same normal, narrow morphology as they did following an intrinsic atrial event. This is a roundabout way of confirming appropriate capture, even if the atrial spike and depolarization are not clear. Thus, there are two ways to confirm atrial capture: clear, clean P-waves after an atrial pacing spike and consistent intrinsic ventricular conduction.

Obviously, there are some drawbacks to both of these atrial capture confirmation methods. The first, getting a clean P-wave after an atrial pacing spike, is not all that common in clinical practice. I would estimate that about half of all in-clinic rhythm strips will not show clean spikes and atrial capture. This is something clinicians should look for but will not always find.

The second method—finding consistent intrinsic ventricular conduction after atrial pacing—can only occur in patients with intact AV conduction.

Thus, it only works if the patient does not have AV block.

Dual-chamber strategies

Some clinicians will evaluate dual-chamber pacemakers by temporarily programming the device to VVI pacing (to check the ventricular channel) and then AAI pacing (to check the atrial channel). This is a very common approach and one that should be avoided. By temporarily programming a dual-chamber pacemaker to VVI and then AAI pacing, the device is forced to act as a single-chamber ventricular and then a single-chamber atrial system. This might seem a logical way to evaluate ventricular capture and sensing, on the one hand, and then atrial capture and sensing, on the other hand. However, there are serious drawbacks to this method. A dual-chamber pacemaker is not an AAI + VVI device combination. DDD mode is far more complex than just simultaneous AAI and VVI pacing. If a clinician follows the patient by *breaking down* the DDD device into an AAI and a VVI device:
- Pacemaker-mediated tachycardia will not occur, even if the patient has it or is susceptible to it.
- Crosstalk inhibition will not occur.
- The patient may be put at risk, for example, a patient with heart block should not be subjected to AAI pacing.

A DDD pacemaker should be evaluated as a DDD device. Evaluating it as a VVI and an AAI system does not provide real insight as to how it functions and can cause the clinician to miss potential device

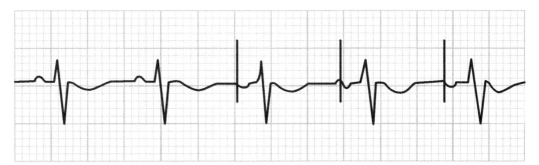

Figure 18.6 An AAI pacemaker rhythm strip reveals appropriate atrial sensing (first two complexes) and appropriate atrial capture (third and fifth complexes). The fourth complex (second atrial spike) shows atrial fusion, where an atrial output pulse *collides* with an intrinsic atrial event. In real-world clinical practice, seeing clear evidence of an atrial spike leading to atrial depolarization can be difficult if not impossible to see. Atrial capture is confirmed by the fact that the atrial beat conducts to depolarize the ventricles.

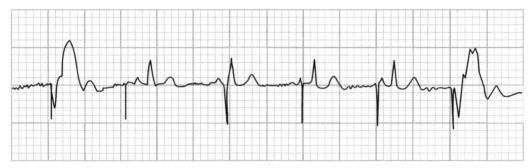

Figure 18.7 This strip comes from a VVI pacemaker and show ventricular pacing spikes. The first and last events on this strip show appropriate ventricular capture. Measure the pacing rate by measuring the V-to-V interval. The V-to-V intervals between complexes three and four, four and five, and five and six show the programmed base rate. The interval between the second and third pacing spike is much longer, because the pacemaker sensed the intrinsic ventricular event and inhibited the ventricular output pulse and reset timing. That shows appropriate ventricular sensing. However, the third, fourth, and fifth ventricular pacing spikes failed to capture the ventricle and were followed by an intrinsic ventricular event (note how the paced and sensed ventricular events have different morphologies). The question is why did the pacemaker fail to sense these intrinsic ventricular events? Before suspecting ventricular undersensing, the clinician should ask, "Should the pacemaker sense these ventricular events?" The answer is no because they fall into the ventricular refractory period. Thus, ventricular sensing in this strip is appropriate.

problems. It may also be uncomfortable or even harmful to the patient.

Pacemaker refractory periods

Whenever clinicians fail to see capture on an ECG under evaluation, the next question has to be: Should there have been capture? Sometimes, apparent noncapture is misleading and turns out to be functional noncapture (which is a sensing problem). The same thing can occur with sensing. Whenever clinicians suspect a sensing problem on an ECG under evaluation, the next question should be: Should this event have been sensed (see **Figure 18.7**)? In this example, ventricular sensing is appropriate. Every ventricular pacing output pulse launches the ventricular refractory period. Thus, the spike initiated a refractory period that effectively stopped the pacemaker from seeing the intrinsic ventricular event. These events could not have been sensed because of the pacemaker's imposed refractory period. In Figure 18.7, the main thing to report is intermittent ventricular loss of capture rather than a sensing problem.

Strategies to force capture

As discussed previously, sometimes, a rhythm strip does not contain all of the pieces of information required for a thorough assessment. A patient may present at the clinic with a nonpaced rhythm strip, but the physician at the clinic still has to evaluate capture. As mentioned earlier, there are ways to force capture.

In the first example, a patient has a dual-chamber pacemaker and the clinician needs to evaluate appropriate atrial capture. As discussed earlier, this can be done fairly easily, namely, by increasing the base rate. Let's run through such a situation in a step-by-step way:

- Once it is determined that the base rate has to be increased to force atrial pacing in order to evaluate atrial capture, look at the rhythm strip and measure the patient's intrinsic rate. This will give a good idea of how fast the base rate needs to be set to overdrive the sinus node and force pacing.
- As a rule of thumb, increase the base rate by about 15 ppm in the first step. Do not set an extremely high rate, which can be uncomfortable for the patient and could even cause problems. For instance, if the patient has a pacemaker set to 60 ppm and his intrinsic rate is around 63 bpm, setting the base rate to 75 (60 + 15) is a good starting place. This should force pacing.
- Do not permanently reprogram the base rate. Instead, use the temporary parameters or temporary settings feature. All manufacturers offer an easy way for the clinician to program many parameter values on a temporary basis. Using temporary

values offers two main advantages: first, it allows you to restore the original values with the press of one button, and second, you don't have to remember the previously programmed parameter settings. They are stored in memory. When this test is complete, restore the base rate back to the original setting.

Once atrial pacing occurs, the clinician can determine if atrial capture is appropriate or inappropriate. To assess ventricular capture, the clinician has to force ventricular pacing, which can be done by shortening the sensed AV delay (or the paced AV delay if atrial pacing is occurring):

• Once the clinician has decided to assess ventricular capture, the sensed AV delay has to be shortened. It can be helpful to measure the patient's intrinsic PR interval and to compare it to the sensed AV delay. As an example, let's assume the sensed AV delay is programmed to 150 ms and the patient's intrinsic PR interval is about 130 ms. Taking the sensed AV delay down to a value of around 100 ms will almost surely force ventricular pacing. Again, take care that you decrease the AV delay sufficiently to force pacing but not to an extremely low value.

• Use the temporary settings for this change.

• Once ventricular pacing occurs, the clinician can assess appropriate capture and, when the evaluation is concluded, return the pacemaker to its previously programmed AV delay setting.

In the event that a change in the base rate or a shortening of the AV delay does not produce atrial or ventricular pacing, respectively, it may be necessary to make another change (increase the base rate slightly or decrease the AV delay slightly). Do not make big changes.

The system in steps

Every patient is unique and clinicians evaluating paced rhythm strips may hit certain variations, but here are the steps in the system, one by one:

1 Look at all of the available data that you have; the most important information includes the device mode, programmed base rate, and programmed AV delay intervals. It also helps to know if the pacemaker is new or old and why the patient is indicated for pacing.

2 Start out with the base rate. If you know it, *translate* it into milliseconds. If you do not know it, see

if you can find an atrial interval (atrial paced event to next atrial paced event with no intervening atrial events) to calculate it.

a Be aware that pacemakers may not always pace at the base rate! For instance, if the pacemaker is rate responsive, it may be pacing at the sensor-driven rate. If there is a lot of higher-rate atrial activity, a dual-chamber device may be tracking the atrium. If hysteresis is turned on, the pacemaker may be pacing at the hysteresis rate.

b If the pacemaker is not pacing at the base rate, determine why.

c If the patient is not being paced at all, it means his or her rhythm is faster than the programmed base rate. Confirm that this is true. For instance, a patient with an intrinsic rhythm of 50 bpm and a pacemaker set to 70 ppm should be pacing.

3 Identify the events on the strip, using annotations, EGMs, and/or the tracing—use all of the tools in your toolbox. Note that you should see agreement across the various strips. The ECG should tell the same story as the annotations and as the EGMs, although they will not always look alike.

4 Evaluate appropriate capture. You have enough to evaluate capture if you see pacing spikes. In a dual-chamber strip, evaluate atrial and ventricular capture separately. Capture is appropriate if you see pacing spikes followed by depolarizations.

a Be on the lookout for potential pitfalls: fusion and pseudofusion.

b Watch out for functional noncapture.

c If you don't have pacing in one or both chambers, force pacing to evaluate capture.

i To force pacing in the atrium, increase the base rate.

ii To force pacing in the ventricle, shorten the AV delay.

d Evaluating atrial capture can be tricky, because clear P-waves are not always present on paced rhythm strips. Two things confirm normal atrial capture: an atrial depolarization (if you have the luxury of a strip with clear P-waves) and a normal QRS indicating the atrial spike traveled over the AV node and depolarized the ventricles. When deciding if atrial capture is appropriate, one or the other is sufficient—you don't need both!

e Verify on annotations (if available) that what you are seeing is the same thing the pacemaker is seeing.

5 Evaluate appropriate sensing by determining if an intrinsic event falls into a timing cycle where it should be sensed and if that leads to output inhibition. Start with ventricular sensing and the sensed and paced AV delay values (if known). If you know the AV delay, set the calipers to the interval and put one end of the calipers on the paced or sensed AV event and determine if the intrinsic ventricular event fell into the AV delay and, if so, if it inhibited a ventricular output. That would be appropriate sensing.

a If you do not know the programmed AV delay settings, you may have to estimate them at around 150 ms.

b If you do not have intrinsic ventricular events, lengthen the AV delay until they emerge.

c Confirm with annotations (if available).

6 Evaluate appropriate sensing by calculating the VA delay (base rate interval minus the paced AV delay). Measure that interval on the calipers and put one end of the calipers on a ventricular event and see where the other leg of the calipers falls. If an intrinsic atrial event occurs in that VA interval and its appearance inhibits an atrial output, then atrial sensing is appropriate.

a If you have consistent atrial pacing, you may be able to force intrinsic atrial activity by lowering the base rate in small steps (about 15 ppm per step) using temporary settings.

b Verify that the annotations (if available) agree with what you are seeing.

7 If possible, evaluate the patient's underlying rhythm. This is not always possible in pacemaker-dependent patients. If you know the patient's history and diagnosis, you should determine if the underlying rhythm is consistent with that information.

Table 18.2 summarizes these steps for single-chamber and dual-chamber systems.

Eyeballing versus the system

Many clinicians like to *eyeball* a rhythm strip, because they have the notion that what appears on a tracing is going to be clear, obvious, and jump out at them. I cannot stress enough that taking a *scan* or *glance-and-go* approach to analyzing paced rhythm strips does not work. Paced rhythm strips contain a wealth of information,

Table 18.2 The aforementioned description of the steps of the systematic approach to paced ECG analysis is very useful for study, but in the hectic world of the busy device clinic, this is a summary of the key points you need to bear in mind

Single chamber	Dual chamber
Mode	Mode
Rate	Rate, AV delay, VA interval
Capture	Capture (A and V)
Sensing	Sensing (A and V)
Underlying rhythm	Underlying rhythm

The biggest difference between single chamber and dual chamber (besides the fact that dual-chamber pacemakers require assessments of both atrial and ventricular capture and sensing) is that dual-chamber pacemakers require the clinician to know rate, AV delay, and VA interval, while single-chamber pacemakers only require the clinician to know the rate.

but the information is in the details. Some weird-looking rhythm strips turn out to be perfectly appropriate—and some very appropriate-looking strips turn out to be quite problematic and abnormal (**Figures 18.8** and **18.9**).

The following strips are examples of why you cannot eyeball a rhythm strip and get real information. In these next strips, look at the strip first off and get an impression. That's what most people who *eyeball* tracings do. But then go through the captions and see what is really hidden. It's surprising!

Rhythm strips

Pacemaker clinicians deal with various models of devices from five different manufacturers. All of the current device manufacturers have been in business for decades, which means that there are many device models, old and new, that will be evaluated in a clinic. Over time, clinicians will gain experience with old and new EGMs and rhythm strips and will become familiar with the various annotation codes used by different companies. Many of these terms, although unique to a manufacturer, are intuitively understandable. Manufacturers offer manuals and software guides to help clinicians learn to navigate their proprietary EGMs and programmer screens.

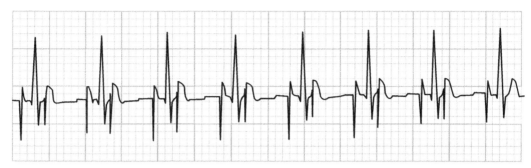

Figure 18.8 This is an ECG from a dual-chamber pacemaker patient. She is paced at 60 ppm and her paced AV delay has been temporarily set to 350 ms (sensed AV delay is 250 ms) to force intrinsic ventricular activity to emerge. Atrial pacing is appropriate (there are atrial pacing spikes and normal-looking QRS complexes, so even without a clear P-wave, atrial capture is confirmed). This is followed by an intrinsic ventricular event and then what appears to be a pacemaker spike in the T-wave. Using calipers, the distance between the atrial spike and the ventricular spike is 350 ms. Can ventricular capture be confirmed? The answer is no, because the ventricular pacing spike falls after an intrinsic ventricular event when the heart is physiologically refractory. This is functional noncapture. There are intrinsic ventricular events on the strips: is ventricular sensing appropriate? Clearly, it is not because these intrinsic ventricular events are overlooked. This strip shows appropriate atrial capture and ventricular undersensing.

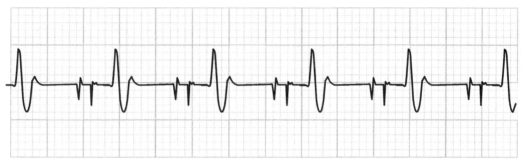

Figure 18.9 This tracing comes from a dual-chamber pacemaker patient with a programmed base rate of 50 ppm and a paced AV delay of 200 ms. Glance at the strip and you're tempted to see pacemaker spikes that get no results and some intrinsic activity. The intrinsic ventricular events are wide and bizarre, indicating that these are escape beats. At first glance, it looks like nothing is working right with this pacemaker. But hang on! The pacing interval is 1200 ms, so the VA interval is 1000 ms (1200 minus 200). Start with capture. There is no clear case for atrial capture (atrial spikes occur but there are no P-waves evident and no ensuing normal-looking QRS complexes). Likewise, there is no ventricular capture; the ventricular pacing spikes do not result in an immediate ventricular depolarization. The escape beats are ventricular intrinsic events that show the patient's underlying rhythm. The paced atrial event is 200 ms, which defines the length from atrial spike to ventricular spike. The VA interval is 1000 ms and starts with a sensed or paced ventricular event and ends with the next atrial pacing spike. However, if you measure this strip from the ventricular spike, 1000 ms falls before the next atrial spike! Since a VA interval can start with a paced or sensed ventricular event, the escape beats might start the VA interval. Indeed, if you time the 1000 ms starting with the intrinsic ventricular event, it ends with the atrial pacing spike. This means that the paced ventricular event may have launched the initial VA interval, but when the intrinsic escape beat occurred, it reset the VA interval. This shows appropriate ventricular sensing! This strip actually came from a patient who had recently started taking an antiarrhythmic agent that changed her pacing thresholds.

Conclusion

Device clinics deal with paced rhythm strips all day long, and device clinicians need to become confident and familiar with analyzing these tracings. The great pitfall in evaluating paced rhythm strips is that considerable information can be contained in even very short tracings and clinicians can be tempted to think that with a glance they have mined all of the information from it. A systematic approach is absolutely essential to gaining confidence in accurate paced rhythm strip interpretation. In a nutshell, clinicians should evaluate mode, rate, capture, sensing, and the patient's underlying rhythm. Some pitfalls in rhythm strip interpretation include things like functional noncapture or unclear P-waves, which can make it challenging to assess appropriate atrial capture. By learning and employing a systematic approach, clinicians are more likely to get the whole story from a rhythm strip and can confidently analyze tracings knowing that nothing will be inadvertently overlooked.

The nuts and bolts of paced ECG and EGM analysis

- Paced rhythm strips must be approached and analyzed systematically, and the basic system can be summed up: mode, rate, capture, sensing, and underlying rhythm. Eyeballing rhythm strips can result in mistaken assessments.
- Clinicians should gather as much information as possible before analyzing a rhythm strip in terms of knowing the patient's history (is the device old or new? Why was the patient indicated for pacing in the first place?), the device (manufacturer, model, mode), and some key programmed settings (base rate, paced and sensed AV delays).
- If the clinician is evaluating a tracing that includes a surface ECG, annotations, and one or two electrograms, these strips should all align with each other. They may not look alike, but they should all be telling the same story. The annotations are the best source of information in terms of what the pacemaker is *thinking* and how it *sees* and categorizes events. However, the surface ECGs and EGMs are the best source of information for what the heart is actually doing.
- When analyzing a device, it is important to know if it is a single-chamber or a dual-chamber device. For single-chamber devices, the clinician must assess mode, rate, capture, sensing, and underlying rhythm. With dual-chamber systems, it is a little more complicated. The clinician must know the programmed base rate, sensed and paced AV delays, and (using that information for calculation) the VA interval. When assessing capture and sensing in a dual-chamber device, capture and sensing must be evaluated for both the atrial and ventricular channels.
- Avoid the temptation of programming a dual-chamber device temporarily to AAI and then VVI mode. This shortcut can miss important problems (such as pacemaker-mediated tachycardia). If the device functions as a DDD system, it should be evaluated as a DDD system.
- Annotations and markers are available from programmers from all device manufacturers, but the codes can vary somewhat.
- Atrial pacing can be tricky to confirm on paced tracings, in that a clear-cut atrial depolarization may not be present. If a spike is followed by an immediate atrial depolarization (that is easy to see), that confirms atrial capture. In the event that is not evident on the strip, atrial capture can be confirmed if the atrial spike leads to a normal-looking QRS complex at an appropriate interval. This means the atrial spike depolarized the atria and the wave of depolarization traveled outward over the AV node and into the ventricles, leading to a normal-looking QRS complex.
- A wide, bizarre-looking QRS complex indicates an escape beat and not a conducted beat.
- Appropriately sensed intrinsic events should inhibit the pacemaker output pulse. If they are not sensed, that is *undersensing* and it leads to overpacing. By contrast, if events are sensed that are not there, that is called *oversensing* and it leads to underpacing.
- The VA interval is the time interval from a ventricular event (sensed or paced, it does not matter) to the next *paced* atrial event. The VA interval is not programmable and can be calculated by deducting the paced AV delay from the base rate interval. For instance, if the base rate is set to 60 ppm (1000 ms) and the paced AV delay is set to 200 ms, then the VA interval is 800 ms (1000 minus 200).
- Sometimes, a pacing spike will appear on a rhythm strip with no depolarization following

it. This may be loss of capture, but look carefully. If the spike falls in the heart's physiologic refractory period, this is called functional noncapture. The spike did not capture, but it was impossible for capture to occur because of where the beat fell. Functional noncapture is actually a sensing problem.
- Loss of capture and loss of sensing can be intermittent problems, that is, they can be problems that come and go. This makes them more difficult to find.
- Clinicians may not always have or be able to get all of the information they need to make a comprehensive rhythm strip evaluation. For instance, clinicians may be asked to analyze a strip from a patient about whom little is known. In some cases, it may not be possible to assess sensing because intrinsic activity either will not appear or might be too dangerous to get. For instance, some patients have little to no underlying rhythm.
- To assess capture, the clinician must have pacing. If no pacing is occurring, pacing can be forced. In a single-chamber device or for the atrial channel of a dual-chamber device, force pacing by increasing the base rate. As a rule of thumb, increase the base rate to about 15 ppm and observe. If necessary, increase more but go in small steps. To force ventricular pacing in a dual-chamber pacemaker, decrease the AV delay (sensed and/or paced, depending on the patient's rhythm).

- To assess sensing, the clinician must see intrinsic activity. This is not always possible in all patients. It can be attempted in single-chamber devices or for the atrial channel of a dual-chamber device by decreasing the base rate. This should be done in the same increments, about 15 ppm lower to start and then in small steps. Do not decrease the base rate below a tolerable rate for the patient, even if no intrinsic activity occurs. To see intrinsic ventricular activity in a dual-chamber pacemaker, increase the AV delay.
- When making changes to the pacemaker for testing purposes, use temporary settings or temporary pacing features. This allows you to restore the prior settings with one touch.
- A failure to output occurs when the pacemaker *thinks* that it paced (and the pacing annotations will show a paced event) but the output somehow does not travel from the pulse generator to the heart. While rare, this is indicative of a serious problem.
- When evaluating sensing, the clinician must consider not only whether or not an event was sensed but whether or not sensing should have occurred. For example, the pacemaker should not be expected to sense an event that falls in a pacemaker refractory period.
- Avoid the temptation to glance at a strip and render a judgment. Many strips—especially unusual-looking ones—can contain a lot of buried information that is not evident at first glance.

Test your knowledge

1 A clinician needs to analyze appropriate atrial sensing in a dual-chamber pacemaker. The problem is that the device paces the atrium consistently. What can be done?
   A Increase the base rate about 15 ppm.
   B Decrease the base rate about 15 ppm.
   C Extend the AV delay.
   D Program the device to AAI.

2 The same clinician has to analyze ventricular sensing in a dual-chamber pacemaker and the device paces the ventricle constantly. What is the best method to allow intrinsic ventricular activity to emerge?

   A Increase the base rate about 15 ppm.
   B Decrease the base rate about 15 ppm.
   C Extend the AV delay.
   D Program the device to AAI.

3 What does ventricular functional noncapture look like on a dual-chamber rhythm strip?
   A A ventricular spike followed by a ventricular depolarization
   B A ventricular spike with no following ventricular depolarization at a time when capture was not possible

C Any ventricular spike with no following
   ventricular depolarization

D A pacing spike on top of an intrinsic
   ventricular event

4 The doctor tells you that Mr. Jones has a
   dual-chamber pacemaker with atrial oversensing. What would you expect to see on the
   tracings?

   A Lots of atrial pacing even though there was
      intrinsic atrial activity

   B No atrial activity at all

   C Atrial pacing spikes that did not capture the
      atrium or conduct to the ventricles

   D Little to no atrial pacing with some intrinsic
      atrial activity

5 You are trying to confirm atrial capture on a
   rhythm strip but there are no clear atrial events.
   What else can you look for?

   A A wide, bizarre QRS complex will confirm
      atrial capture.

   B A ventricular pacing spike appearing after
      the paced AV delay expires confirms atrial
      capture.

   C A normal-looking QRS complex after the
      atrial pacing spike confirms atrial capture.

   D The annotations may confirm atrial capture.

6 Mr. Marx has a DDD pacemaker programmed
   to a base rate of 55 with sensed and paced AV
   delays both set to 180 ms. What is his VA
   interval?

   A 910 ms.

   B 1270 ms.

   C 1000 ms.

   D The VA interval is programmable; it depends
      on what it was programmed to.

7 A ventricular pacing spike on a dual-chamber
   rhythm strip falls right after an intrinsic

ventricular event. How should this be
interpreted?

   A Loss of ventricular capture.

   B Ventricular oversensing.

   C Ventricular undersensing.

   D It is the normal and expected behavior of
      the device since the spike fell in the
      physiologic refractory period.

8 Mrs. Anderson is a chronic DDD patient who
   has always done well at her checkups. Today,
   the rhythm strips show intermittent loss of
   both atrial and ventricular capture. What
   should the clinician suspect is behind the
   problem?

   A Lead fracture.

   B Insulation failure.

   C Loose connection at the pulse generator
      header.

   D Mrs. Anderson may have changed her
      medications.

9 What might explain a DDD rhythm strip
   showing pacing at a rate other than the
   programmed base rate?

   A Hysteresis

   B Rate response

   C Atrial tracking

   D Any of the above

10 What happens when a VA interval starts but is
    interrupted by a PVC in the middle?

    A Nothing; the VA interval will not see a PVC
       that occurs at any point in the VA interval.

    B The PVC will reset the VA interval (start it
       over).

    C The PVC will initiate the AV delay and
       cause atrial pacing in about 150 ms.

    D It depends on what PVC algorithm is
       programmed.

CHAPTER 19

Upper-rate behavior

Learning objectives

- Briefly explain the importance of understanding upper-rate behavior in dual-chamber pacing and name the two types of upper-rate responses.
- Name the two timing cycles which function essentially as *speed limits* for pacing rate and which channels they each apply to.
- Point out the advantages and potential disadvantages of atrial tracking in a dual-chamber pacemaker.
- Explain how to optimize upper-rate behavior in dual-chamber pacemakers.
- Name at least two points to consider whenever programming a maximum tracking rate.
- State some of the risks associated with upper-rate behavior in pacing.
- Give the formula for calculating the Wenckebach interval and 2:1 block and explain why they occur.
- Define TARP and explain how it is calculated.
- Name the most frequent causes of both appropriate and inappropriate mode switching.

Introduction

In previous chapters, the role of the maximum tracking rate or MTR was presented. As a review, the MTR is the maximum rate at which the ventricle can be paced in response to intrinsic atrial activity. Pacemakers attempt to preserve 1:1 AV synchrony as much as possible, which means that if a pacemaker is programmed to 60 ppm but the patient's intrinsic atrial rate is 70 bpm, the pacemaker will *decide* that it is better for the patient to try to match each of those faster intrinsic atrial events, one-to-one, to ventricular paced events, even if it means pacing above the programmed base rate. Atrial tracking is an excellent feature for preserving 1:1 synchrony. The MTR sets the *speed limit* for this function. Typically programmed to around 130 bpm, the MTR will not allow the pacemaker to pace the ventricle faster than 130 bpm.

This begs the question: what happens if the patient's intrinsic atrial rate exceeds the MTR? That's where upper-rate behaviors come in. Upper-rate behaviors are the device's methods for dealing with intrinsic atrial rates above the MTR.

Speed limits

Dual-chamber pacemakers can have two built-in *speed limits* that limit how fast the pacemaker can pace. While 1:1 AV synchrony is important to preserve hemodynamics and assure optimal cardiac output, pacing at excessively fast rate can be uncomfortable for the patient, cause symptoms, and even compromise hemodynamics and cardiac output. The two main speed limits are the MTR, mentioned previously, and the maximum sensor rate or MSR.

The MTR governs how fast the ventricle can be paced in response to intrinsic atrial activity, in other words, how fast the ventricle can go to track the atrium. It is an absolute speed limit, in that the pacemaker will simply not pace the ventricles faster than the programmed MTR. Thus, if a pacemaker is programmed to a base rate of 60 ppm with a 130 ppm MTR, ventricular pacing will never exceed 130 ppm even if the patient's intrinsic atrial rate is 160 or 180 bpm or higher. The key to understanding the MTR is that it is the speed limit for the

The Nuts and Bolts of Implantable Device Therapy Pacemakers, First Edition. Tom Kenny.
© 2015 John Wiley & Sons, Ltd. Published 2015 by John Wiley & Sons, Ltd.

ventricular channel. It puts the brakes on ventricular pacing only.

The MSR is only available in rate-responsive pacemakers, but that includes most pacemakers today. The full functionality of rate response will be discussed in detail in a later chapter, but for now, it is important to recognize that the MSR is the other speed limit for pacing rate. Rate-responsive pacing is based on some kind of sensor that indicates the patient's activity level; the more active the patient, the faster the rate-responsive pacemaker will pace. Rate-responsive pacing allows patients to run or climb stairs or exercise—even climb mountains—because it adjusts the rate to activity level, that is, to metabolic demand. However, no matter how much activity the sensor detects, the MSR sets the absolute speed limit for how fast the pacemaker will pace in response to sensor input. A typical MSR setting is 120 ppm (it is often programmed to the same value as the MTR, but independent programming is possible). Sensor-indicated rates (rate-responsive pacing) can be defined as atrial pacing above the programmed base rate in response to sensor input, in order to better meet the patient's activity level and metabolic demand.

What is important to realize about MSR is that in a dual-chamber pacemaker, the MSR puts the brakes on the atrial channel.

This makes sense in that the MTR governs tracking, which is *ventricular pacing* in response to intrinsic activity, while the MSR governs rate response, which is driven by *atrial pacing*.

Atrial tracking and the MTR

Atrial tracking can be a highly beneficial feature because it preserves 1:1 AV synchrony even with fluctuations in the patient's intrinsic atrial rate. Throughout a normal day, reasonably active patients will experience spells of sinus acceleration. Sinus acceleration might occur with postural changes (sitting to standing), with low levels of activity (getting in and out of the car), with greater activity (climbing stairs, exercise), with surprise or emotion, or even without an obvious cause. The average heart rate for an adult during a slow moderate walk is around 90–100 bpm. Sympathetic stimulation and certain comorbid conditions, such as heart failure, can also cause sinus acceleration.

Atrial tracking is a highly important feature because it preserves 1:1 AV synchrony throughout these *ups and downs* of the day.

The drawback of atrial tracking occurs when the patient's intrinsic atrial rate gets very high. Tracking an intrinsic atrial rate of 90 or 100 bpm can be helpful to the patient, but tracking an intrinsic atrial tachyarrhythmia can be uncomfortable and even dangerous for the patient.

Dual-chamber pacing with atrial tracking is particularly beneficial to patients with complete heart block. Complete heart block means that the patient has functioning atria and ventricles, but they work independently of each other. They are dissociated. Typically, the ECG shows sporadic atrial activity and occasional ventricular escape beats. There is no pattern; the rhythm strip can seem almost random. A dual-chamber pacemaker is an ideal device for this patient:

- It senses the patient's intrinsic atrial activity and *tracks it* by pacing the ventricle to time up to the intrinsic atrial activity.
- It gives the patient 1:1 AV synchrony.
- If need be, it can pace the atrium as well to make sure the patient's rate is always appropriate.

On a rhythm strip, atrial tracking will appear as sensed atrial events followed by paced ventricular events at a rate at or above the programmed base rate but not higher than the MTR. For instance, in a pacemaker programmed to 70 ppm with an MTR of 150 bpm, atrial tracking behavior (ventricular pacing) can occur at 70–150 ppm, but never more than 150 ppm.

The optimal MTR has to be customized for individual patients; clinicians need to consider their age, activity level, and left ventricular function. Perhaps the most crucial (and most overlooked) consideration is that setting a patient-specific MTR will determine the rate of any pacemaker-mediated tachycardias (PMTs). PMTs occur at the upper-rate limit. That means that the MTR value is the same rate at which PMTs will occur, if they occur. For example, programming an MTR to 140 ppm means that should a PMT occur, it is going to be 140 ppm. Thus, clinicians need to realize that programming a high MTR could potentially subject the patient to higher-rate PMTs. Of course, not all patients are susceptible to PMTs, and even among those who could get them, they will not necessarily occur. But

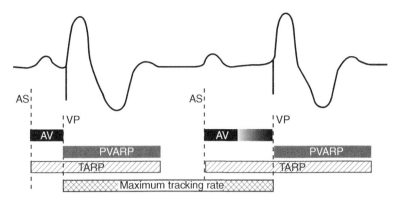

Figure 19.1 The MTR is an absolute speed limit. In this case, the second atrial event launches the AV delay. When that AV delay expires, the pacemaker should have paced—but that would have fallen inside the MTR timing cycle. Since the MTR is an absolute speed limit, it automatically extends the AV delay so that ventricular pacing will not exceed the MTR. The prolongation of the PR interval defines Wenckebach behavior and is an example of the so-called pacemaker Wenckebach.

the potential exists and should be taken into account when trying to establish the right MTR value for a given patient.

Another key consideration for finding the best MTR for a particular patient involves how well the patient would tolerate a sudden drop in pacing rate after a sinus tachycardia. For example, imagine an MTR is programmed to 160 ppm. At the point at which the intrinsic atrial rate exceeds 160 bpm, the MTR—being an absolute speed limit—will no longer allow tracking. This causes an abrupt drop in the rate. Upon hitting the MTR, the brakes come on and the patient's rate may go from MTR to base rate in one beat (about 1 s). The higher the MTR, the more pronounced the drop! Consider how a patient would handle that! Most patients can tolerate a drop from 100 to 70 ppm better than a drop from 150 to 70 ppm. That is one reason many clinicians will program an MTR value to 100 or 120 ppm.

A handy formula that can be used when calculating MTR is the target heart rate zone, which is also used for setting heart rate limits for exercise. The formula is simple: 220 minus 80% of the patient's age. Thus, if the patient is 60 years old, the target heart rate is 172 (220 minus 60×0.8 or 220 minus 48). However, this number applies to physically fit, active patients. If your 60-year-old patient is sedentary and frail and has left ventricular dysfunction, hypertension, and limited mobility, this target rate is much too high, but it gives you an estimate of what it should be in a fit person.

The MTR timing cycle starts with any ventricular event (sensed or paced) and runs to the next ventricular paced event. The MTR will override other timing cycles, if necessary, to preserve its speed limit (see **Figure 19.1**).

Upper-rate behavior

Upper-rate behavior is a broad general term that describes how dual-chamber pacemakers deal with high intrinsic atrial rates. *By far, the best upper-rate behavior is atrial tracking that preserves 1:1 AV synchrony, also called 1:1 tracking.* That is the optimal device behavior for patient comfort and well-being, for optimal cardiac output, and for good hemodynamics. The problem is that 1:1 tracking is not always possible.

The two main types of upper-rate behaviors are pacemaker Wenckebach (sometimes called pseudo-Wenckebach) and 2:1 block. Pacemaker Wenckebach is named for the Wenckebach type of heart block and is actually a way that the pacemaker mimics the normal behavior of the healthy heart when beating at very high rates. While the term *fixed-ratio block* is actually more accurate, most clinicians refer to the other type of upper-rate behavior as 2:1 block. As the name suggests, 2:1 block means that the pacemaker will *track* only every other intrinsic atrial event (two intrinsic atrial events to one ventricular event); in other words, 1:1 AV synchrony is gone and the pacemaker will pace at a rate that is half that of the intrinsic atrial rate.

Total atrial refractory period

The key to understanding upper-rate behaviors involves some math based on a timing cycle that is not even directly programmable. The total atrial refractory period (TARP) is defined as the AV delay + the postventricular atrial refractory period (PVARP). Think of TARP as the entire span of time during which the atrial channel is refractory or unresponsive to incoming signals. You can calculate TARP easily for any device if you know the programmed PVARP setting and the sensed AV delay (if there are separate sensed and paced AV delays, use the sensed AV delay value since we are dealing with tracking sensed atrial events). TARP is not directly programmable, but clinicians can indirectly program it by changing the PVARP and/or the sensed AV delay interval.

TARP is the point at which the pacemaker will exhibit 2:1 block.

For example, a dual-chamber pacemaker is programmed that has a sensed AV delay of 150 ms and a PVARP of 250 ms. The TARP value is 400 ms (sensed AV delay + PVARP or 150 ms + 250 ms). Convert 400 ms to rate (150 ppm) and that is the point at which 2:1 block occurs.

Another important—and easy calculation—is the ventricular pacing rate. If the point at which 2:1 block occurs is 150 ppm, the ventricular pacing rate

at that point is going to be 75 ppm (half of the 2:1 block rate).

The clinical implications of 2:1 block must be seriously considered. Using the earlier example (TARP 400 ms or 150 ppm), the clinician has to recognize that if the patient's intrinsic atrial rate exceeds 150 bpm, the pacemaker is going to track only every other intrinsic atrial event. This will result in a loss of 1:1 AV synchrony and a ventricular pacing rate of about 75 ppm. What's more, 2:1 block occurs abruptly, so the patient will have been paced at or around 150 ppm and then the rate will—in a single beat—drop to 75 ppm.

Pacemaker Wenckebach

Pacemaker Wenckebach or pseudo-Wenckebach behavior gets its name because it resembles physiologic Wenckebach behavior. Physiologic Wenckebach rhythms show a progressive prolongation of the PR interval. The PR interval widens and widens to the point that an atrial event *falls into the PR interval* and is missed (see **Figure 19.2** for an example of 4:3 Wenckebach (four atrial beats for every three ventricular beats)). In order not to violate the MTR (remember, the MTR is an absolute speed limit), the pacemaker has to extend the AV delay, creating the pacemaker version of Wenckebach behavior. Pacemaker Wenckebach can only occur when the intrinsic atrial rate exceeds the MTR.

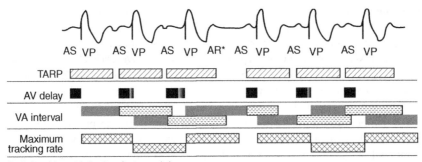

*intrinsic atrial event during the refractory period.

Figure 19.2 As the intrinsic atrial rate speeds up, the MTR imposes limits that prolong the AV delay until eventually one atrial event *falls into the PVARP* and is not married to a corresponding ventricular event. This is an example of pacemaker Wenckebach or pseudo-Wenckebach with a 4:3 pattern (four atrial events to every three ventricular events). This is a normal and expected behavior of a dual-chamber pacemaker in response to an intrinsic atrial rate that is bumping over the MTR *speed limit*. Note that the fourth atrial sensed event falls in the TARP (PVARP) and the pacemaker does not respond to it.

Pseudo-Wenckebach behavior has some noticeable characteristics:
- It shows a progressive widening of the AV delay until an atrial event falls into the PVARP and is missed.
- Beats occur in a clear, discernible, and repeated pattern (so-called group beating) such as the 4:3 pattern in Figure 19.2.
- Although the rhythm is paced, it looks like physiologic Wenckebach.
- The ventricular pacing rate will not exceed the programmed MTR.

The earlier example is fairly common in clinical practice and shows 4:3 Wenckebach behavior. This means every fourth atrial event is not tracked, but the patient is getting 1:1 AV synchrony every three out of four beats (75% of the time). As the patient's intrinsic atrial rate increases, the Wenckebach pattern will change from 4:3 to 3:2 and finally to 2:1, which is no longer Wenckebach at all but rather 2:1 block.

The atrial continuum

Pacemaker Wenckebach is caused by an intrinsic atrial rate above the MTR. As the patient's intrinsic atrial rate increases:
- 1:1 AV synchrony will be preserved up to the MTR.
- Above the MTR but below the 2:1 block rate, pacemaker Wenckebach occurs.
- Above the 2:1 block rate, 2:1 block occurs.

For example, imagine a dual-chamber pacemaker with a TARP of 400 ms and an MTR of 120. TARP can be directly converted by dividing by 60,000 into the 2:1 block rate; in this case, 400 ms is equivalent to 150 ppm. Thus, with a TARP of 400 ms, it can be determined that 2:1 block will occur at 150 ppm. For this particular pacemaker:
- 1:1 AV synchrony will be preserved as long as the intrinsic atrial rate is below 120 bpm.
- If the intrinsic atrial rate exceeds 120 bpm but is less than 150 bpm, pacemaker Wenckebach occurs.
- If the intrinsic atrial rate exceeds 150 bpm, then 2:1 block occurs (and the ventricular pacing rate drops to 75 ppm).

This sequence is often described as the atrial continuum, in that as the intrinsic atrial rate changes, the pacemaker's upper-rate behaviors change. Using the earlier example, the atrial rate continuum is illustrated in **Figure 19.3**. For a hypothetical patient with complete heart block, the clinician can roughly predict the type of pacing states and rates that will occur as the patient's intrinsic atrial rate changes.

Two-to-one block

Let's start with an example: imagine a patient with an MTR of 120 ppm and a TARP of 50 ms (equivalent to 120 ppm). In this case, both MTR and 2:1 block rate are the same: 120 ppm. As long as the patient's intrinsic atrial rate stayed below 120 ppm, there was 1:1 tracking. Imagine that this patient was exercising. Typically, most patients feel pretty well with 1:1 tracking and they can be active without being symptomatic. But as soon as the patient's intrinsic rate exceeded 120 (the MTR and the TARP), the patient experienced 2:1 block. From one beat to the next, the patient's ventricular pacing rate dropped by half (from 120 to 60 ppm) and the patient lost 1:1 AV synchrony. For most patients, this is a very rough transition and can even provoke symptoms. Most device clinicians can understand why the pacemaker is doing what it is doing

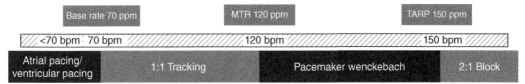

Figure 19.3 The atrial rate continuum in a hypothetical patient with complete heart block. When the patient's intrinsic atrial rate is at or below the programmed base rate of 70 ppm, atrial paced event/ventricular paced event pacing at the base rate occurs. If the intrinsic atrial rate increases above the programmed based rate but below the MTR, that is, >70 but <120 ppm, then 1:1 atrial tracking will occur with pacing states of atrial sensed events and ventricular paced events. If the atrial rate exceeds the MTR of 120 ppm, pacemaker Wenckebach occurs up to the TARP rate, in this case 150 ppm (400 ms). When the intrinsic atrial rate exceeds TARP, in this case, when it is >150 ppm, the 2:1 block occurs. The transitions along the continuum can be abrupt.

in this example, but physiologically, this can be very uncomfortable for the patient.

Two-to-one block is not very physiological. It is uncomfortable for the patient and may limit their activities and lifestyle. However, at very high intrinsic atrial rates, 2:1 block is unavoidable. It is a necessary evil when the patient's intrinsic atrial rate gets very high—which can happen. But the main goal of the device clinician in upper-rate behavior programming is to delay 2:1 for as long as is reasonably possible.

Upper-rate programming strategies must recognize that the best pacemaker behavior is 1:1 atrial tracking. Patients feel better and have the best cardiac output and hemodynamics when 1:1 AV synchrony is preserved. At the other end of the spectrum is 2:1 block; think of that as the worst pacemaker behavior in that it makes patients uncomfortable and symptomatic; it does not support optimal cardiac output or hemodynamics. The pacing expert is often faced with a situation where the patient's intrinsic atrial rate is too high to allow for the best solution (1:1 atrial tracking); you simply cannot track at very high atrial rates because it involves rapid ventricular pacing. But there are techniques to use to delay 2:1 block. So what falls between our *best-case scenario* (1:1 atrial tracking) and our *worst-case scenario* (2:1 block)? Pacemaker Wenckebach!

To be sure, pacemaker Wenckebach is not the *best choice* or the optimal pacing technique. But for patients with rapid intrinsic atrial rates, it represents the best available compromise between the best-case and worst-case scenarios. Comparing 4:3 pseudo-Wenckebach behavior, where every fourth atrial event is dropped to 2:1 block, where every other atrial event is dropped, it is clear that pacemaker Wenckebach is a better choice than 2:1 block even if it is not the best choice. (The best choice is not available for patients with intrinsic atrial rates above the

MTR.) Think of Wenckebach pacing as a *buffer* to help patients as then transition from intrinsic atrial rates above MTR but before they go into 2:1 block. Another way to think of this is to use the version of the atrial rate continuum shown in **Figure 19.4**. If you know the base rate, MTR, and TARP, you can use Figure 19.4 to determine the atrial rate points when Wenckebach behavior and 2:1 block will occur.

The Wenckebach window

Using the atrial rate continuum drawings shown in Figures 19.3 and 19.4, it is apparent that between the best-case scenarios (1:1 atrial tracking) and the worst-case scenarios (2:1 block), there is a Wenckebach zone, which represents a reasonable compromise for the patient. Think of this time period as the Wenckebach Window. When programming the pacemaker, the clinician should try to program as large a Wenckebach Window as reasonable for the patient.

If the MTR and the TARP are the same value (as used in an example earlier, where the MTR was 120 ppm and the TARP 500 ms), the Wenckebach Window is closed. The pacemaker will literally transition from 1:1 tracking up to 120 ms and then go into 2:1 block. In other situations, the Wenckebach Window may be barely cracked. So how do we open up the Wenckebach Window for patients? The Wenckebach Window is opened when we program as big a gap as possible between the MTR and the TARP. The more *room* you can make between MTR and TARP, the wider the window. For instance, if MTR is 120 and TARP is 400 ms (150 ms), the Wenckebach Window is open—there is a pretty substantial gap between 120 and 150 ms. On the other hand, if the MTR is 140 and TARP is 400 ms (150 ms), the Wenckebach Window is not open as wide—there is not that much gap between 140 and 150 ppm.

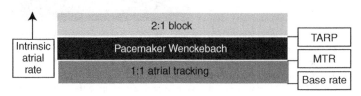

Figure 19.4 Another version of the atrial rate continuum and its effect on upper-rate behavior. Think of pacemaker Wenckebach behavior as the *buffer* to delay 2:1 block as long as possible.

Obviously, clinicians need to make reasonable programming choices. There will be limits to the TARP value—it is not sensible to program an MTR of 100 ppm and a TARP of 100 ms (equivalent to 600 ppm). While that gives you a gigantic Wenckebach Window, the TARP setting there is not workable for reliable pacing at normal rate ranges. However, within reasonable limits, the clinician should set the TARP and MTR such that there is gap between them.

Some clinicians hesitate to program a *Wenckebach Window* because it sounds like trying to set the patient up for Wenckebach pacing. That is never the goal. The objective behind opening the Wenckebach Window is to delay 2:1 block as long as possible. No matter how a pacemaker is programmed, there is a point at which 2:1 block will occur. This is not avoidable and it is the normal and expected behavior of the device to go into 2:1 block at certain high intrinsic atrial rates. The goal of the Wenckebach Window is to delay that point as long as reasonable.

Wenckebach Windows can also be calculated as intervals rather than rates. For instance, if a Wenckebach Window was 110–150 ppm, it could also be described as 545–400 ms, creating a *Wenckebach interval* of 145 ms. These are exactly equivalent; use whichever is more helpful to you for the programming situation.

Upper-rate programming strategies

When programming a dual-chamber pacemaker, the clinician needs to consider how the device will respond when the patient's intrinsic atrial rates exceed the programmed base rate. Of course, some higher-than-base-rate atrial rates are perfectly normal, such as sinus acceleration with activity. On the other hand, many pacemaker patients are susceptible to atrial tachyarrhythmias, which are pathological high intrinsic atrial rates. These rates can get very high, in excess of 200 bpm in some cases, and should not be tracked. Thus, the device clinician has to think ahead to the possibility that the patient may experience high intrinsic atrial rates and the types and conditions of those rates. Complicating this picture is the fact that atrial tachyarrhythmias are not at all unusual in dual-

chamber pacemaker patients and can occur suddenly in pacemaker patients who never had them before. In other words, even if the patient does not seem prone to atrial tachyarrhythmias, it is still a good idea to program upper-rate behaviors to anticipate them.

One way of managing upper-rate behavior is to open the Wenckebach Window. There are other strategies.

For some (but not all) patients, a good upper-rate strategy is to increase the MTR. Increasing the MTR allows the pacemaker to track 1:1 for as long as possible. This can be a good approach for fit patients who tolerate rapid ventricular pacing, but it is not a good choice for a patient with rate-related angina that kicks in around 120 ppm. Thus, programming a high MTR is good for patients without heart failure and who can tolerate high ventricular rate pacing.

For other patients, open the Wenckebach Window as much as you can (separate the MTR and TARP values by as wide a gap as possible).

For patients with known and persistent atrial tachyarrhythmias, there are some other programming strategies and features that will be considered in future chapters.

Programming possibilities (and impossibilities)

Programmers today will not let you program impossible or contradictory values; they typically alert the user that such values are impossible and may suggest alternative values. When programming upper-rate behaviors, clinicians can encounter programmable values that might seem desirable but are impossible. Take a hypothetical example of a dual-chamber pacemaker with a base rate programmed to 70 ppm, an MTR of 120 ppm, a sensed AV delay of 210 ms, and a PVARP of 350 ms. This may seem reasonable, but it is actually a pacing impossibility! Here's why. We know the MTR is 120 ppm. The 2:1 block point is defined by TARP, which is the sensed AV delay plus PVARP converted to rate ($210 + 350 = 560$ ms or about 107 ppm). This is a pacemaker that will go into 2:1 block at 107 ppm but has an MTR of 120 ppm! Those values conflict. The 2:1 block rate is always going to equal or exceed the MTR rate.

In the early days of pacing, clinicians could actually program such values, although the pacemaker obviously could not pace that way. Modern programmers will alert the user to conflicting values, so today's clinicians cannot even try to program a system this way. But it is important for device experts to know why certain programmed values will not work.

Using another example, imagine a dual-chamber pacemaker with these parameter settings: base rate, 60 ppm; PVARP, 300 ms; paced AV delay, 250 ms; sensed AV delay, 200 ms; and MTR, 120 ppm. From this information, it is clear that 2:1 block will occur at 120 ppm (sensed AV delay plus PVARP converted into rate is 200 + 300 = 500 ms or 120 ppm). That happens to be the MTR. When 2:1 block equals the MTR, there is no Wenckebach Window, and the pacemaker will literally transition from 1:1 atrial tracking to 2:1 block. Whenever the MTR and TARP are the same, the Wenckebach Window is closed! (Expressed another way, the Wenckebach Window is the difference between MTR and TARP.) In this example, one way to open the Wenckebach Window—at least a crack—is to change the TARP. TARP cannot be directly programmed, but it can be changed by adjusting the PVARP and/or the sensed AV delay. Using this same example, the clinician could change the PVARP from 300 to 250. That will change the TARP from 500 to 450 ms or 133 ppm. Now, there is a gap between the MTR of 120 ppm and the 2:1 block point (TARP) of 133 ppm, so this programming change created a Wenckebach Window.

Remember that many pacemaker parameters are interconnected. Often, making a change in one parameter will impact other parameters. Sticking with the previous example, perhaps the reason this patient's PVARP was programmed to 300 ms (a relatively long PVARP value) was to prevent retrograde conduction. This particular patient had previous issues with retrograde conduction and PMTs, which were solved pretty neatly by prolonging the PVARP to 300 ms. That worked well, but it closed the Wenckebach Window! Now, the clinician has to consider whether opening the Wenckebach Window back up a little by reprogramming the PVARP to 250 ms is going to affect retrograde conduction. This will depend on the patient's retrograde conduction times.

The point of this exercise is to remind clinicians that programming a pacemaker—like much in clinical practice—is a balancing act. We strive to get optimal benefits for patients, but all of the clinical choices we make have consequences. Retrograde conduction can be wiped out with long PVARPs, but that can adversely impact upper-rate behavior. Upper-rate behaviors can be controlled, but it may set the stage for PMT. Clinicians must be mindful of these ramifications of their programming choices and decide the best programmed parameters for each patient on an individual basis. The reason that pacemakers allow for so many programming choices is that clinicians often need to fine-tune multiple settings to reach the optimal settings for any given patient.

Take another example of a patient prone to PMT with a retrograde conduction interval of 275 ms. To protect this patient from PMT—which he does not tolerate well—the PVARP has been programmed to 325. Since the patient has a paced AV delay of 170 ms and a sensed AV delay of 150 ms, it can be calculated that 2:1 block occurs at around 126 ppm (TARP = 325 + 150 or 475 ms, which is equivalent to about 126 ppm). This is a good strategy to prevent PMT, but notice how a 2:1 block point of 126 ppm limits upper-rate options. With an MTR of 120 ppm, the Wenckebach Window is barely cracked. This patient will experience 2:1 block at rates over 126 bpm, which he may experience during exercise or even during normal everyday activities like carrying groceries or climbing stairs. This presents a real programming dilemma and one that clinicians will encounter in real-world practice. Fortunately, there are few options for clinicians when faced with these programming challenges.

Programming other parameters for upper-rate behavior

The healthy heart will naturally shorten its intrinsic PR period as the sinus-driven rate increases. To imitate this natural shortening of the PR interval at high atrial rate, pacemakers offer what is sometimes called a *rate-responsive* or *rate-adaptive* AV delay. This is actually not a great name because it has nothing to do with *rate response* or sensor-driven pacing. Another manufacturer calls the same feature the *dynamic AV delay*. I think of these as *upper-rate AV delays*. The use of this sort of AV delay parameter means that as the rate increases, the pacemaker will respond with shorter-than-programmed AV delay intervals. This rate-responsive AV delay will go into effect when the patient's atrial rate exceeds a value such as 90 bpm. The rate-responsive AV delay can be programmed to low (1 ms per 1 bpm), medium (2 ms per 1 bpm), or high (3 ms per 1 bpm), that is, from somewhat responsive to maximally responsive. This will automatically shorten the AV delay interval and will also shorten the MSR and MTR. There is a programmable *shortest AV delay* value that can also be programmed to set the limit on how much the pacemaker can shorten the AV delay in response to high atrial rates.

There are also PVARPs and ventricular refractory periods that can be programmed so that these values adjust during periods of atrial tracking. When you program these special features, you can take advantage of a longer sensing window (important to allow optimal intrinsic activity), higher MTR rates, and higher 2:1 block rates.

Mode switching

Mode switching, sometimes called automatic mode switching (AMS) or atrial tachy response, is an algorithm available in dual-chamber pacemakers that essentially turns off atrial tracking during periods of high-rate intrinsic atrial activity. It gets its name from the fact that eliminating tracking changes the mode designation. For instance, mode switching may take DDD pacing and change it to DDI, which in many cases will look functionally just like VVI. (If rate response is programmed on, the mode switch will be from DDDR to DDIR.) The key point of the mode switch is to temporarily disable atrial tracking. Put another way, the goal of mode switching is to prevent the inappropriate tracking of atrial tachyarrhythmias.

Mode switching is available in dual-chamber devices from all manufacturers, and apart from some terminology issues, it works in essentially the same way. To program mode switching, the clinician must set some definitions for the device to use in terms of what constitutes an atrial tachycardia; the clinician programs the rate cutoff. There may

also be mode switch parameters, such as rate, to be programmed. Once these parameters are set up, whenever the device senses an atrial tachycardia, it will switch modes; when the atrial tachycardia resolves, the device switches back to the original mode and originally programmed parameters. This all happens automatically. Some patients are not aware of mode switch episodes, but others may experience uncomfortable or at least noticeable *bumps* during the transition.

While the clinician programs the rate cutoff that defines atrial tachycardia for mode switching, different companies handle this in different ways. Medtronic and Boston Scientific use a rate count criteria and count the mean atrial rate. St. Jude Medical uses something called the filtered atrial rate interval (FARI). This rate is programmed as the detect rate or the atrial tachycardia detection rate (ATDR), depending on the manufacturer of the device. The underlying concept, however, remains the same: the clinician determines what the device will call an atrial tachycardia.

When a device is tracking a high intrinsic atrial rate—say, at 100 bpm—the ventricles are paced to maintain 1:1 AV synchrony with the atria. When the atrial rate go fast enough to trigger a mode switch—say, at 120 bpm—the key programming consideration for the clinician is the mode switch rate. Taking a patient from being paced at or near 120 ppm to the base rate—say, 60 ppm—is a pretty big *bump*! Many devices offer an independently programmable mode switch rate. When programming this mode switch rate, the clinician must consider how fast the patient's rate would be when mode switch starts (that's the atrial tachycardia cutoff rate) and how much of a drop the patient can tolerate. Obviously, the goal is to drive the rate back down to a more normal range, but a good mode switch rate will not make that drop too severe. In the example earlier, a good mode switch rate might be 90 ppm—the rate will come down (from 120 to 90 ppm) but in a tolerable way. This mode switch rate is sometimes called an interim base rate. Boston Scientific devices offer ventricular rate regulation (VRR) to control the ventricular rate following a mode switch. VRR offers a dynamic pacing rate based on the patient's ventricular rate in the presence of atrial fibrillation (AF). The goal of VRR—which is largely automatic—is to minimize the RR interval variations (preventing overly long RR cycles) without increasing the mean pacing rate markedly.

Mode switching is a very useful algorithm, but it is mainly intended for occasional use. In clinical practice, sometimes, patients present with frequent mode switching. This is not optimal device behavior and should be investigated. One cause of frequent mode switching is inappropriate mode switching, which can occur with far-field R-wave oversensing. The device is *tracking* atrial events that are not really there and switching mode! However, it is not unusual to find patients with frequent episodes of appropriate mode switching, most frequently caused by AF. If a patient has frequent episodes of appropriate mode switching and is diagnosed with AF, the physician may decide to prescribe an antiarrhythmic agent or anticoagulation therapy (to help minimize the risk of stroke). The ability of the clinical staff to use diagnostic counters in order to identify a patient having frequent or prolonged episodes of AF should not be underestimated in terms of its clinical and even lifesaving value. If the clinical team notices AF and reports it to the physician and if appropriate therapy, such as anticoagulation therapy, is initiated, stroke may be prevented. The use of diagnostic data to identify AF (especially in patients with no symptoms) should not be trivialized!

The CHADS score is a simple clinical tool to help assess a patients' risk of stroke and if that patient should be put on anticoagulation therapy. CHADS is an acronym for these risk factors: *c*ongestive heart failure, *h*ypertension, *a*ge (>75 years), *d*iabetes, and history of *s*troke. If the patient has any of the first four characteristics, a score of 1 is assigned; a history of stroke counts 2 points. The CHADS score is a fast, easy metric for assessing stroke risk. A patient with AF and a CHADS score of 0 may be able to avoid anticoagulation therapy (although low-dose aspirin might be advised). With a CHADS score of 1, a patient should be on either anticoagulation therapy or a low-dose aspirin regimen. A CHADS score ≥2 demands anticoagulation therapy. Warfarin and the newer drug dabigatran etexilate (Pradaxa®) are commonly used anticoagulation agents.

Patients with frequent episodes of appropriate mode switching should be reviewed for their risk of stroke, as stroke is closely associated with AF.

Conclusion

High intrinsic atrial rates are not at all unusual in pacemaker patients, and the pacing clinician must become comfortable and confident in evaluating device behavior in the presence of high atrial rates. A good consideration is to remember that optimal benefit is derived from 1:1 AV synchrony, but that is not always possible. The least benefit occurs when the patient experiences 2:1 block (and that occurs at the rate identified by TARP). In between these two extremes—best and worst—is a range known as pseudo-Wenckebach or pacemaker Wenckebach. This upper-rate behavior often commences at a 5:4 ratio and then decreases to 4:3, then 3:2, and finally 2:1, which is the same as 2:1 block. As clinicians, our goal is to delay the onset of 2:1 block for as long as is reasonably possible (taking into account what the patient can tolerate well). This delaying tactic is something I call the *Wenckebach Window*. As a rule of thumb, the longer that Wenckebach Window is open, the better, but there are limits. The goal is not to get to pseudo-Wenckebach, but to postpone 2:1 block as long as is reasonably possible. Other parameters that can be adjusted for upper-rate behavior include the AV delay, the PVARP, and the ventricular refractory period. All dual-chamber devices today will automatically switch modes from DDD to DDI (or DDDR to DDIR) in the presence of a programmable atrial tachycardia detection cutoff rate. The automatic mode switch algorithm essentially disables atrial tracking in the presence of atrial tachycardia. This is a useful algorithm, but when patients have frequent mode switch episodes, the clinician should investigate whether or not they are appropriate (they can be caused by oversensing) or if the patient might have AF and should be evaluated for possible anticoagulation therapy.

The nuts and bolts of upper-rate behavior

- Dual-chamber pacemakers have two programmable *speed limits*: the maximum tracking rate or MTR and the maximum sensor rate or MSR.
- Most of the time, the MTR and MSR are programmed to the same rate, typically around 120 ppm. When programming the MTR and the MSR, it is important to consider the highest rates a patient can tolerate well.
- If a pacemaker-mediated tachycardia (PMT) occurs, it will occur at the programmed MTR. If the patient is susceptible to PMTs, consider this when setting the MTR value.
- When the patient's intrinsic atrial rate is at or below the MTR, the pacemaker will pace the ventricles at that rate, for example, 120 ppm. But when the patient's intrinsic atrial rate exceeds the MTR, the pacemaker will revert to ordinary base-rate pacing. This causes an abrupt and often very large drop in rate, for example, from 120 to 60 ppm in a single beat.
- The MTR timing cycle begins with any ventricular event (sensed or paced) and runs to the next ventricular paced event. The MTR will override other timing cycles if it has to in order to maintain the MTR.
- Upper-rate behavior refers to general behaviors of a dual-chamber pacemaker in response to high intrinsic atrial rates, such as atrial tachycardia.
- By far, the optimal dual-chamber pacing behavior is 1:1 AV synchrony or one atrial event for each and every ventricular event. The role of the MTR is to allow 1:1 AV synchrony as long as reasonably possible.
- At very high intrinsic atrial rates, the pacemaker will revert to one of two upper-rate behaviors: pacemaker Wenckebach (also called pseudo-Wenckebach) and 2:1 block (or fixed-ratio block). Pacemaker Wenckebach has a similar appearance to physiological Wenckebach, in that the PR interval progressively shortens until a beat is missed. It may start 5:4 and then progress to 4:3 or 3:2. Fixed-ratio or 2:1 block

occurs when there is one ventricular event for every two atrial events.
- In terms of patient hemodynamics, cardiac output, and well-being, the optimal pacemaker behavior is 1:1 AV synchrony; the least desirable pacemaker behavior is 2:1 block. Between these two is pseudo-Wenckebach. While pseudo-Wenckebach is not the optimal pacing behavior, it can be thought of as a *buffer* to delay 2:1 block as long as possible.
- The total atrial refractory period (TARP) is not directly programmable; it is defined by the sensed AV delay interval plus the postventricular atrial refractory period (PVARP). For instance, if the sensed AV delay is 150 ms and the PVARP is programmed to 250 ms, then TARP is 400 ms (150 + 250 = 400). Changing TARP involves adjusting either the sensed AV delay or the PVARP (or both).
- TARP is an important value to know because it defines the point at which 2:1 block occurs. For instance, if TARP is 400 ms, then 2:1 block will occur at 150 bpm (400 ms converts to a rate of 150 bpm). If the clinician would like to see 2:1 block occur only at rates of 170 bpm, then TARP has to be around 350 ms (170 bpm converts to 353 bpm). This means either the sensed AV delay or the PVARP or both must be shortened.
- When 2:1 block occurs, the pacemaker will pace the ventricle at one-half of the 2:1 block rate. For instance, let's say TARP is 400 ms or 150 bpm. When 2:1 block occurs at 150 bpm, the patient's ventricular rate will be 75 bpm or half of 150 bpm. This rate transition occurs abruptly, from one beat to the next, and some patients find it uncomfortable.
- Pacemaker Wenckebach is usually described as a ratio, such as 5:4, which means 5 atrial events for every 4 ventricular events. Pacemaker Wenckebach will progressively change as the intrinsic atrial rate speeds up from 5:4 to 4:3 to 3:2 and finally 2:1 block.

Continued

Continued

- Pacemaker Wenckebach will always exhibit a clearly discernible pattern, such as 5:4; the ventricular rate will never exceed the programmed MTR; there will be a progressive widening of the AV delay interval until an atrial event falls into the PVARP and is missed; and it will resemble physiologic Wenckebach even though it is a paced rhythm.
- The least desired upper-rate behavior is 2:1 block, which sometimes cannot be avoided. There are limits to how the MTR should be programmed and what are reasonable AV delays and PVARP values.
- Pacing clinicians should try to postpone 2:1 block as long as possible; these efforts might be called the *Wenckebach Window*. The goal of the Wenckebach Window is not to induce pseudo-Wenckebach but to delay 2:1 block as long as reasonably possible.
- Some patients tolerate relatively high MTR values and this may be a good strategy to manage upper-rate behaviors. Patients who can tolerate a high MTR tend to be young and fit. On the other hand, patients with rate-related angina should not be programmed to high MTR values.
- Programmers will not allow clinicians to program conflicting parameter values. However, even when values do not conflict, they influence each other. Any adjustment made to one parameter setting may affect other settings.
- Pacemakers also have a dynamic or rate-responsive AV delay, a function that automatically shortens the AV delay at high intrinsic atrial rates. This mimics the behavior of the healthy heart.
- Mode switching is a function in which the pacemaker turns off atrial tracking in the presence of high intrinsic atrial rates. The clinician can program the atrial tachycardia cutoff rates that define high intrinsic atrial activity. When such rates are exceeded, the pacemaker reverts from DDD or DDDR to DDI or DDIR, respectively. Although the mode is technically DDI or DDIR, it will look like functional VVI or VVIR.
- Mode switching is automatic in the presence of the programmable atrial tachycardia mode switch rate; when the intrinsic atrial rate goes back down, the original mode is restored.
- There may be a programmable mode switch interim pacing rate. For example, let's say the pacemaker was pacing at or near the MTR of 120 ppm. As the intrinsic atrial rate goes to 140 and approaches 150 bpm, the pacemaker paces in pseudo-Wenckebach fashion. If the atrial tachycardia cutoff rate is programmed to 150 bpm, once the intrinsic atrial rate reaches 150 bpm, the pacemaker mode switches by turning off atrial tracking—and pacing at the base rate. If the regular base rate is used, this will cause the pacemaker to go from pacing the ventricle at 120 ppm (MTR) to 60 ppm in a single beat. This transition can be very abrupt and uncomfortable for the patient. A special programmable mode switch rate allows for the pacemaker to decelerate to a more reasonable rate, for example, 90 ppm.
- Mode switching typically occurs when the patient experiences atrial tachyarrhythmias, which can include atrial fibrillation (AF). If such events are brief or occasional, then mode switching provides a good way of managing these episodes. On the other hand, some patients will experience frequent mode switch episodes or stay in a nontracking *switched* mode for prolonged periods of time. When frequent mode switching is observed, the clinician should determine if the patient has AF.
- AF cannot be treated with a pacemaker, although pacemakers have functions like mode switching to help deal with this arrhythmia. AF can be treated with surgical approaches, catheter-based ablations, cardioversion, or drug therapy, but in some cases, it can be a very challenging arrhythmia to manage.
- Patients with AF have a fivefold increased risk of stroke. If a patient has AF, he or she should be considered for anticoagulation therapy.
- Many patients should take anticoagulation therapy to minimize their risk of stroke. A simple tool to assess stroke risk is called

CHADS. CHADS is an acronym that stands for congestive heart failure, hypertension, age (>75 years), diabetes, and history of stroke. For each of the first four conditions the patient has, one point is assigned; the patient is given 2 points if he or she has a history of stroke. With a score of 1, the patient should be considered for either anticoagula-tion therapy or a low-dose aspirin regimen; a CHADS score ≥ 2 means the patient should get anticoagulation therapy. If the AF patient can achieve a CHADS score of 0, it might be possible to avoid or at least delay anticoagu-lation therapy.

- Anticoagulation drugs include warfarin, dabigatran etexilate (Pradaxa®), and others.

Test your knowledge

1 When looking at a rhythm strip showing pacemaker Wenckebach, which of the following would a clinician *not* be likely to see?
  A Clearly discernible atrial pacing spikes
  B A progressive lengthening PR interval
  C A clearly discernible pattern, such as 4:3 or 3:2
  D Something very similar to physiologic Wenckebach

2 What two programmable timing cycles make up TARP?
  A Sensed AV delay plus PVARP
  B Paced AV delay plus PVARP
  C PVARP plus the MTR
  D The VA interval minus PVARP

3 There are two main *speed limits* for dual-chamber pacemakers. What are they?
  A MTR and PVARP
  B MTR and TARP
  C TARP and the mode switch atrial tachycardia cutoff rate
  D MTR and MSR

4 Select from the list below the type of dual-chamber pacemaker behavior that is most optimal for the patient:
  A Pacemaker Wenckebach
  B 1:1 AV synchrony
  C Any fixed-ratio block
  D 2:1 block

5 A dual-chamber pacemaker is programmed to a base rate of 60 ppm with an MTR of 140 ppm and an MSR of 140 ppm. At what intrinsic atrial rate does the pacemaker stop tracking the atrium in 1:1 fashion?
  A 60 bpm.
  B 80 bpm.
  C 140 bpm.
  D It will keep tracking 1:1 at any atrial rate up until mode switching occurs.

6 What is the Wenckebach Window?
  A The duration of time, programmable in minutes, that the patient is in Wenckebach
  B The time after the patient loses 1:1 AV syn-chrony but before 2:1 block occurs
  C The period of time during which atrial tracking is suspended
  D The patient's tolerance level for upper-rate behavior

7 Mr. O'Brien has a dual-chamber pacemaker programmed to a base rate of 70 ppm, an MTR and MSR of 120 ppm, a sensed delay of 150 ms, a paced AV delay of 175 ms, and a PVARP of 250 ms. At approximately what intrinsic atrial rate does 2:1 block occur?
  A 120 bpm
  B 140 bpm
  C 150 bpm
  D 175 bpm

8 Remembering Mr. O'Brien above, imagine that his intrinsic atrial rate is now 140 bpm. What

kind of upper-rate behavior would occur with the device as programmed above?

A 1:1 AV synchrony

B Pseudo-Wenckebach

C 2:1 block

D Mode switching

9 Mode switching changes the mode from DDD or DDDR to DDI or DDIR by essentially doing what?

A Turning on atrial tracking

B Canceling the MTR

C Turning off atrial tracking

D None of the above

10 If a patient has frequent mode switching episodes and these are found to be appropriate, what should the clinician suspect?

A Nothing; frequent mode switching episodes are normal.

B The patient may have atrial fibrillation.

C The MTR is programmed too low.

D The patient has had a myocardial infarction.

CHAPTER 20

Advanced dual-chamber timing

Learning objectives

- Explain what is meant by ventricular-based timing and the key timing clock used in ventricular-based devices.
- Explain atrial-based timing and define its key timing cycle.
- Name a quirk of ventricular-based timing and the pacing state during which it would occur.
- Briefly describe the history of pacemaker timing and name the dominant timing system today
- Name a quirk of atrial-based timing and when specifically it would occur.
- State why clinicians today need to be aware of the distinctions in atrial-based versus ventricular-based timing, even though pacemakers today rely on exclusively atrial-based timing.
- Define how modified atrial-based timing differs from true atrial-based timing.
- Explain briefly why a device might switch from a true atrial-based timing to a modified atrial-based timing.

Introduction

No one is born a pacing expert, and most people who develop an interest in pacing and advance their studies find out the *secret* of cardiac pacing, namely, that pacing can be more complicated than it appears. Take base-rate or lower-rate limit (LRL). It is one of the most fundamental concepts of pacing, one of the main parameters that even newbies know how to program. Most of what was discussed about base rate up to know was useful, helpful, and highly practical—and not entirely true. That statement may be too harsh. The fact of the matter is that the base rate is more complex than was originally presented. Many things in pacing are actually far more intricate and involved than the average real-world clinician needs to know to manage pacemaker patient effectively. That does not mean that we clinicians should not study some of these complexities of pacing. This chapter on advanced dual-chamber timing likely does not contain a lot of information that a clinician would use frequently in everyday practice. These advanced concepts will help you better understand the pacemaker and can be handy in troubleshooting or explaining *quirks* in pacemaker behavior.

Base rate revisited

The base rate, also known as the LRL, is the programmed rate at which the pacemaker will pace in the absence of intrinsic atrial activity. In teaching pacing to beginners, instructors generally say that the base rate is composed of two intervals: the paced AV (PAV) delay and the VA interval. This is true for dual-chamber pacemakers that use something known as ventricular-based timing; such dual-chamber pacemakers could be called ventricular-based pacemakers. However, not all dual-chamber pacemakers use ventricular-based timing systems; some use an atrial-based timing cycle. The type of timing system—ventricular or atrial—is not programmable

The Nuts and Bolts of Implantable Device Therapy Pacemakers, First Edition. Tom Kenny.
© 2015 John Wiley & Sons, Ltd. Published 2015 by John Wiley & Sons, Ltd.

and most pacemakers on the market today rely on atrial-based timing. The important take-away message for clinicians is that each of these timing systems has its own quirks and can result in base-rate variations. Thus, clinicians need to know what to expect in the base rate when the device uses an atrial-based versus a ventricular-based timing system.

Ventricular-based timing

Let's start with a brief review of earlier concepts of dual-chamber pacing:

- The PAV delay is the interval from an atrial paced event until the next paced ventricular event. It is programmable.
- The VA interval is the time from any ventricular event (*sensed or paced*) until the next paced atrial event. The VA interval is sometimes called the atrial escape interval (AEI).
- The VA interval is a fixed timing cycle, not programmable but calculated by subtracting the AV delay from the base-rate interval.

For example, let's say a dual-chamber pacemaker is programmed to a rate of 60 ppm, which translates to an interval of 1000 ms. Let's say the PAV delay in this device is programmed to 200 ms. The pacemaker then calculates and adjusts the VA interval to 800 ms (1000 – 200 = 800).

In a ventricular-based pacemaker, the VA interval is fixed—it does not automatically adjust itself and it times itself from *any ventricular event*, whether intrinsic or paced. Since sensed and paced ventricular events are going to have variations in timing, the device is going to have to make subtle adjustments if it is going to maintain a fixed VA interval. And that is just what the ventricular-based pacemaker does (see **Figure 20.1**).

Because the VA interval remains constant, ventricular-based pacemakers can result in some seemingly unusual base rates. Take, for example, a dual-chamber pacemaker programmed to 60 ppm (1000 ms) with a PAV delay of 200 ms and a sensed AV delay of 150 ms. Just from this information, the pacemaker calculates the VA interval as 800 ms (base rate minus PAV or 1000 – 200). Now let's say that the pacemaker paces the atrium and the beat conducts over the

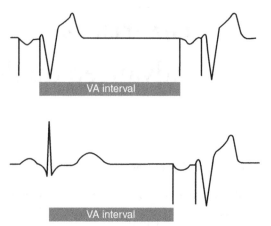

Figure 20.1 In a ventricular-based dual-chamber pacemaker, the VA interval times itself from paced or sensed ventricular events to the next atrial paced event. The VA interval remains constant in ventricular-based systems.

AV node so that the ventricles depolarize on their own—the result is an intrinsic ventricular beat. However, the sensed ventricular event occurs at 150 ms after the atrial pacing spike. (Had the ventricles not beat on their own, the ventricles would have been paced at 200 ms after the atrial spike.) In ventricular-based timing, the VA interval remains constant, so it is 800 ms. Remember that the LRL is composed of the PAV delay plus the VA delay. Using that formula, the base rate would be calculated as 150 ms (AV delay) plus 800 ms (VA delay) or 950 ms. Unfortunately, 950 ms translates to a pacing rate of about 63 ppm! This means that in a ventricular-based pacemaker, clinicians can observe slightly higher-than-base-rate pacing even when the device is functioning appropriately.

When atrial pacing results in intrinsic conduction over the AV node and ventricular sensed events—in other words a pacing state of atrial paced/ventricular sensed events—its higher-than-base-rate atrial pacing will occur in a ventricular-based pacemaker. Note that this is not markedly higher-rate pacing—the difference is usually just a few pulses per minute. However, for clinicians not acquainted with this quirk of ventricular-based timing, it can be extremely perplexing and some clinicians even try to troubleshoot it. There is no need to troubleshoot this particular quirk—it's appropriate behavior when sensed ventricular events control the VA interval timing in ventricular-based devices. But it does mean that a clinician may see a dual-chamber pacemaker pacing the atrium faster than the base rate!

And the problem can worsen when the patient has very rapid intrinsic conduction, which might decrease the AV delay to 100 ms or even lower. Should that happen, the base rate would change from 1000 ms or 60 ppm to 900 ms (100 + 800) or about 67 ppm.

Note that this timing quirk only applies to the pacing state of atrial paced/ventricular sensed events in ventricular-based systems. When the pacing state is atrial paced/ventricular paced events, the base rate will remain at the programmed value. If the patient with a ventricular-based dual-chamber pacemaker is consistently paced in the ventricle, this quirk will not be evident.

Quirks of ventricular-based timing

Pacemaker *quirks* are odd behaviors that sometimes confuse clinicians but which are actually the normal, expected behavior of the device—they are just a little bit counterintuitive. Let's take two dual-chamber pacemaker patients: one has an atrial-based pacemaker (patient A) and one has a ventricular-based pacemaker (patient V). Both patients are constantly in the pacing state of atrial paced/ventricular sensed events. Both devices are programmed the same way: base rate set to 60 ppm, PAV delay 200 ms, sensed AV delay 150 ms, and PVARP 250 ms. In patient A, the base rate of 60 ppm (1000 ms) means the device's main timing cycle of AA is set to 1000 ms. In patient V, the base rate minus the PAV delay can be used to calculate the main timing cycle of VA interval, which is 800 ms (1000 − 200). In both cases, the atrial pacemaker spike captures the atrium and the ventricles contract on their own exactly 150 ms after the atrial spike. Looking at a surface ECG, patient A would be paced at a base rate of 60 ppm, but patient V would be paced at 63 ppm.

Everything in this example is identical except the timing system of the pacemaker. It is easy to see why ventricular-based timing can confuse clinicians!

Atrial-based timing

Realizing that ventricular-based timing had its quirks, engineers at the pacing manufacturers proposed a new, improved atrial-based timing system. Atrial-based timing maintains a fixed AA interval, that is, the timing cycle from one paced atrial event to the next paced atrial event. The AA interval does away with the VA interval altogether; it no longer exists. Timing is made between atrial paced events and that timing cycle is kept constant. This fixed one quirk: the atrial-based timing cycles preserved atrial pacing at the programmed base rate.

This is a very different approach: the pacemaker decided when to pace the atrium based strictly on the last time it paced the atrium. This was a radical switch from ventricular-based timing, where the pacemaker decided when to pace the atrium based on the last time it paced (or sensed) the ventricle. The healthy heart works the same way: the atria control the ventricular activity, not the other way around. Thus, the innovation of atrial-based timing is considered to better mimic normal cardiac behavior than the older system of ventricular-based timing.

The AA interval is not directly programmable as such, but it is very easy to calculate. The AA interval is exactly equal to the base rate. In a dual-chamber pacemaker programmed to 60 ppm, the AA interval is 1000 ms. Thus, a pacing clinician programming the base rate in an atrial-based pacemaker is simultaneously setting the AA interval.

The transition from ventricular-based timing to atrial-based timing occurred roughly in the 1990s. Today, dual-chamber pacemakers all rely on atrial-based timing, but before the 1990s, ventricular-based timing was the rule. Throughout the 1990s, clinicians could count on seeing both atrial-based and ventricular-based pacemakers in the clinic.

Of course, when the patient's pacing state was constantly atrial paced/ventricular paced events, the difference between atrial-based and ventricular-based timing was moot: both devices would pace the patient at the programmed base rate. The main difference occurs when pacing shifts to the state of atrial paced/ventricular sensed events.

Advantages of atrial-based timing

In many instances, the differences observed by clinicians in ventricular-based versus atrial-based pacemakers are subtle and might even seem nitpicky. However, there are some real reasons that atrial-based timing is an improvement over ventricular-based timing.

First of all, atrial-based timing gives clinicians more control over the base rate. If you program a base rate of 60 ppm, you do not have to worry that the pacemaker is going to start pacing at 63 or 65 ppm. While most patients might tolerate a small rate increase like that, the potential pitfall of allowing the base rate creep up occurs by preventing intrinsic atrial activity. For example, let's say the pacemaker is programmed to a base rate of 60 ppm and the patient has an intrinsic sinus rhythm of 62 bpm. Allowing the base rate to creep up even a few pulses can override the patient's intrinsic sinus rate and force atrial pacing.

Second, atrial-based timing is more physiologically intuitive. In the healthy heart, the atria drive the ventricles, not vice versa. Atrial-based timing more closely mimics the natural timing of the healthy heart.

Third, the most vexing aspect of ventricular-based timing, namely, the constant VA interval, was effectively disabled by AA timing. This means that the confusion about above-base-rate pacing excursions is eliminated.

Quirks of atrial-based timing

Of course, no man-made system is ever going to be perfect and that is true of atrial-based timing in dual-chamber pacemakers. This quirk occurs only when a patient transitions from a state of atrial paced/ventricular sensed events to a state of atrial paced/ventricular paced events. This kind of change of pacing state would occur when the patient's conduction over the AV node became blocked. When this shift from atrial pacing/ventricular sensing to atrial pacing/ventricular pacing occurs, atrial-based devices behave differently than ventricular-based devices. In fact, the clinician will likely observe *lower-than-base-rate ventricular pacing for one beat* during this transition.

During atrial paced event/ventricular sensed event pacing, an atrial-based dual-chamber pacemaker

will maintain a constant AA interval that is exactly the same as the base rate. If the patient then transitions to atrial paced/ventricular paced pacing, the AA interval still remains constant—that is a fundamental of atrial-based timing. But now the AV interval (time from atrial event to ventricular event) has lengthened. The AA interval remains constant, but the AV interval portion has lengthened. This pushes out the ventricular pacing portion by the difference between sensed and PAV intervals for one cycle, meaning that the VV interval (time between the last sensed ventricular event and the next paced ventricular event) will actually be longer than the base rate, in other words slower than the base rate. It is easiest to see this on an ECG (see **Figure 20.2**).

Note that this quirk only occurs in atrial-based devices for one beat when the patient switches from atrial pacing/ventricular sensing to atrial pacing/ventricular pacing. However, this one event will look like the pacemaker violated the AA interval (it didn't—the AA interval is preserved) and deviated from the programmed LRL (it didn't—the base rate is timed from atrial events, not ventricular events). Remember that the base rate of a dual-chamber pacemaker is timed from atrial not ventricular events!

True atrial-based timing versus modified atrial-based timing

The late Dr. Seymour Furman, one of the *fathers of pacing*, is credited as having discovered a particular quirk of atrial-based timing and coined two terms that are now firmly entrenched in the pacing lexicon: *true* atrial-based timing versus *modified* atrial-based timing. This quirk occurs when an atrial-based dual-chamber pacemaker encounters a premature ventricular contraction (PVC).

Dual-chamber pacemakers identify PVCs as ventricular events without a preceding atrial event. (Remember, to understand pacing, you have to think like a pacemaker.) When a ventricular-based dual-chamber pacemaker encounters a PVC, the PVC launches a new VA interval. But what happens when an atrial-based device encounters a PVC? As Dr. Furman reported, atrial-based devices not only have quirks, they have different ways of dealing with this situation.

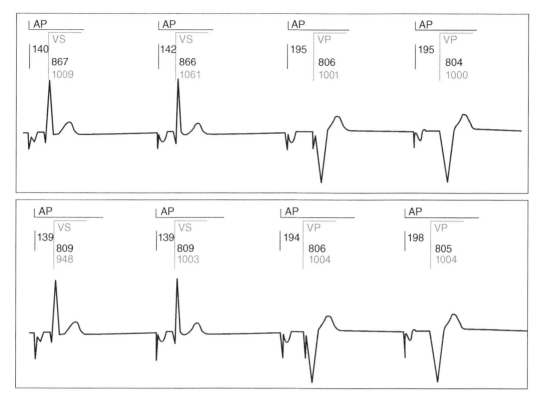

Figure 20.2 The top strip shows an atrial-based device, and the lower strip shows a ventricular-based device. Both devices are programmed to a base rate of 60 ppm (1000 ms) with a paced AV delay of 200 ms. From the second to third complexes, the patient transitions from atrial paced event/ventricular sensed event pacing to atrial paced/ventricular paced activity. The main difference in this change is that the interval from the atrial paced event to the next ventricular event went from being around 140 ms to about 200 ms. That means the AV interval lengthened by about 60 ms. For the ventricular-based device (lower strip), this did not affect timing of the paced AV delay or the VA interval so base rate was maintained—there is no apparent effect of the transition. But on the atrial-based strip above, the interval from the sensed atrial event in complex 2 to the next ventricular event (the paced event in complex 3) is actually extended by those extra 60 ms. Remember that the atrial-based device preserves the AA interval and will alter the timing between ventricular events in order to preserve a fixed AA interval of 1000 ms. The base rate remains unchanged, but if you measure the distance between the second and third ventricular complexes, you can see where that extra 60 ms went!

Some atrial-based dual-chamber pacemakers launch the AA interval when the PVC is detected. As can be seen in **Figure 20.3**, this results in a longer-than-base-rate interval between paced atrial events. This type of prolonged interval between two paced atrial events in the presence of a PVC is known as true atrial-based timing. It only occurs for a single cycle in the presence of a PVC. Of course, if the patient has frequent PVCs, it will occur more often.

True atrial-based timing seems a little unusual because the device launches its AA interval after a PVC, which, after all, is a *ventricular* event. Why should an atrial timing cycle start with a

ventricular event? This was actually an intentional effort by pacemaker engineers to manage the problem of the PVC. Most of the time, when a PVC occurs, the heart's natural response is a pause. The true atrial-based timing approach attempts to mimic the body's natural *pause* by starting the AA interval. True, it lengthens the timing cycle from one paced atrial event to the next, but a PVC in a healthy heart would do the same thing.

Modified atrial-based timing is a little bit different, in that it uses the VA interval! Earlier, it was mentioned that atrial-based devices dispense with the VA interval, but this is the one exception to that rule. When an atrial-based pacemaker using

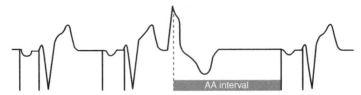

Figure 20.3 When some atrial-based dual-chamber pacemakers sense a PVC (defined by the pacemaker as an event on the ventricular channel not immediately preceded by an atrial event), they launch the AA interval. The AA interval is fixed and corresponds exactly to the base rate. But as the strip below shows, it means the interval between the two paced atrial events is longer than normal, that is, slower than the programmed base rate. Dr. Furman coined the term *true atrial-based timing* for this type of timing cycle.

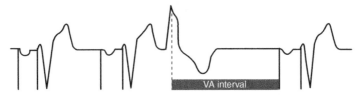

Figure 20.4 Modified atrial based timing will launch the VA interval (rather than the AA interval) in the presence of a PVC. This results in a shorter interval between paced atrial events in the presence of a PVC. Essentially, what is happening is that an atrial-based device reverts to ventricular-based timing in the presence of a PVC!

atrial-based timing encounters a PVC, instead of launching the AA interval (which is exactly equal to the base-rate interval), it launches the VA interval, which is shorter (the VA interval is the base-rate interval minus the PAV delay interval). The bottom line is that modified atrial-based timing better preserves the base rate in the presence of a PVC (see **Figure 20.4**). Another way to think of this is that a device with modified atrial-based timing uses atrial-based timing at all times except in the presence of a PVC when it reverts—for that one cycle—to ventricular-based timing. That is why Dr. Furman called this *modified* atrial-based pacing, because it modifies itself or adapts to PVCs by switching for one cycle to ventricular-based timing.

Most dual-chamber pacemakers today use atrial-based timing but revert to ventricular-based timing in the presence of a PVC. However, some dual-chamber pacemakers have true atrial-based timing and rely on atrial-based timing methodologies for all situations, including PVCs. In true atrial-based timing, the pacemaker relies on the AA timing cycle for all complexes and never uses the VA interval. Right now on the market, Medtronic, St. Jude Medical, Boston Scientific, Biotronik, and Sorin all offer modified atrial-based timing in their dual-chamber pacemakers.

(Biotronik was the last company to switch from true atrial-based timing to modified atrial-based timing.) What this means to clinicians is that in a busy device clinic, clinicians will have to deal with both modified and true atrial-based pacemakers. This quirk between true and modified atrial-based systems only occurs in the presence of a PVC; if the patient never or only very infrequently has PVCs, this difference will not be important.

The real-world importance of understanding timing cycles

Clinicians may wonder why they should bother learning about the nuances of ventricular-based timing when all dual-chamber pacemakers today are atrial-based systems. It would be extremely unusual for a clinician today to encounter a ventricular-based device—unless that clinician is working with a Holter monitor. Holter monitors work on the older ventricular-based timing cycles. It is not at all unusual for a Holter monitor to send up red flags about *pacemaker malfunctions* in terms of violating the base rate—when what is actually happening is that the ventricular-based timing system of the Holter monitor records cardiac activity differently in some instances than the atrial-based timing system of a dual-chamber pacemaker.

Likewise, cardiac monitors use ventricular-based timing. For example, if the pacemaker activity shown in the first strip in Figure 20.2 was captured by a telemetry unit, a clinician might suddenly see that for one beat, the pacemaker paced at 55 ppm instead of the programmed base rate of 60 ppm. This can cause concern that the pacemaker is not working properly, when it is actually the normal and expected behavior of the cardiac monitor. While this kind of lower-than-base-rate pacing only happens for one beat, if the patient is frequently switching from atrial paced/ventricular sensed activity to atrial paced/ventricular paced activity, it will occur each time the transition is made.

Another reason device clinicians need to be mindful about the quirks of both atrial-based and ventricular-based timing (as well as true vs. modified atrial-based timing) is that pacing clinicians are frequently called upon to fix alleged *pacemaker malfunctions*. When clinicians who are not pacing experts deal with pacemakers, they may run into unusual or unexpected pacemaker behaviors and think they are device problems when they are actually just quirks of the timing system. It is not at all unusual for pacing experts to be summoned to fix all sort of *pacemaker problems*, which are actually not problems at all. When troubleshooting a suspected pacemaker problem, the clinician should always remember to think like a pacemaker and consider the possibility that different-from-base-rate pacing may actually owe to timing systems.

Conclusion

All dual-chamber pacemakers today rely on atrial-based timing and most manufacturers use modified atrial-based systems rather than true atrial-based timing. However, clinicians are going to encounter ventricular-based timing in the telemetry unit and with Holter monitors. They may also encounter ventricular-based timing in some very old pacemakers that might still be around. A device clinician needs to understand these timing systems because they have quirks that can sometimes be erroneously perceived as malfunctions. These quirks of the system occur only in very specific situations and thus will not show up for all patients or for any one patient all of the time.

The nuts and bolts of advanced dual-chamber timing

- Ventricular-based timing maintains a constant VA interval, while atrial-based timing maintains a constant AA interval. Both methods will adjust other intervals to preserve a constant VA or AA interval, respectively.
- Ventricular-based timing was invented first but atrial-based pacemakers came on the market in the 1990s. Today, all pacemakers use atrial-based timing. Clinicians may encounter ventricular-based timing systems in Holter monitors, in cardiac monitors, and in very, very old pacemakers.
- When pacemakers pace in the state of atrial paced event/ventricular paced event, both atrial-based and ventricular-based systems behave in the same way. This pacing state will not cause variations in the base rate. But when the pacemaker paces in the state of atrial paced event/ventricular paced event, the ventricular-based system may show faster-than-base-rate pacing.
- A ventricular-based system will pace above the base rate when intrinsic ventricular activity occurs after a paced atrial event. This occurs because the AV delay interval shortens, but the device preserves the VA interval. Since the pacing interval is composed of the AV delay plus the VA interval and since the VA interval remains constant, intrinsic ventricular activity naturally shortens the pacing cycle, resulting in faster-than-base-rate pacing. (The faster base rate will be equal to the difference in the paced AV delay value and the sensed AV delay interval.)
- The faster-than-base-rate pacing seen in ventricular-based systems may be considered a *quirk*. It may be unexpected and can be confusing, but it is not a device malfunction. It is actually the normal behavior of the device.

Continued

Continued

- In the 1990s, pacing engineers addressed the quirks of ventricular-based timing by introducing a new system (atrial-based timing) that preserved the AA interval. Since the atria control pacing in the healthy heart, this new atrial-based system was thought to better mimic physiologic cardiac activity.
- Atrial-based pacing preserves the base rate, which in dual-chamber pacemakers is driven by the atrial channel. This was thought to be the primary advantage of atrial-based timing.
- The AA interval is exactly equal to the base rate. For example, if a dual-chamber pacemaker is programmed to 60 ppm, the AA interval is 1000 ms.
- Atrial-based timing has its own quirks! When a patient changes from the pacing state of atrial paced/ventricular sensed activity to atrial paced/ventricular paced activity (in other words, when the patient stops conducting over the AV node), an atrial-based system will have a lower-than-base rate ventricular rate for one cycle during the transition. This only occurs in this transition. The atrial rate is unaffected. It is only the one cycle from the ventricular sensed event to the next ventricular paced event that is lengthened. However, if the patient transitions in and out of these two states frequently, this slower ventricular rate will occur more often.
- Dr. Seymour Furman is credited with identifying another quirk of atrial-based timing in response to PVCs. He called them *true atrial-based timing* and *modified atrial-based timing*.
- In true atrial-based timing, the dual-chamber pacemaker will start the AA interval in the presence of a PVC. A PVC, as the pacemaker defines it, is a sensed ventricular event without a preceding atrial event. In devices with true atrial-based timing, this launches the AA interval. The thought behind this rather counterintuitive idea is that the healthy heart normally experiences a short pause following a PVC and launching the AA interval is thought to help preserve that pause. Devices from Biotronik use true atrial-based timing.
- In modified atrial-based timing, the dual chamber pacemaker reverts to ventricular-based timing in the presence of a PVC. When a PVC is sensed, the pacemaker launches the VA interval. Normally, an atrial-based pacemaker does not use the VA interval, except in this one case. Devices from all manufacturers today use modified atrial-based timing.
- Understanding these advanced dual-chamber timing cycles will help clinicians troubleshoot alleged device problems (which may not be problems at all) and to reconcile activity observed on the Holter or cardiac monitors that may suggest device problems (but which may be related to timing mechanisms).

Test your knowledge

1 The above ECG comes from a dual-chamber pacemaker programmed to a base rate of 60 ppm, a paced AV delay of 200 ms, a sensed AV delay of 150 ms, and a PVARP of 250 ms. Knowing that information, what kind of timing does this pacemaker use?

A Modified atrial-based timing.

B True atrial-based timing.

C Ventricular-based timing.

D There is not enough information to tell.

2 In atrial-based timing systems, what is the *big clock* that must remain constant?

A The AA interval

B The AV delay interval

C The VA interval

D None of the above

3 Mr. Jefferson just got a new pacemaker that was programmed to a base rate of 60 ppm, paced AV delay of 175 ms, sensed AV delay of 150 ms, and PVARP of 250 ms. Because it is a brand-new device, what can be said about its timing system?

A It is ventricular based.

B It is atrial based.

C It is programmable and can be set to either atrial or ventricular timing.

D It could be either atrial or ventricular and it is not programmable.

4 Using the above example, what would Mr. Jefferson's AA interval be?

A 825 ms.

B 850 ms.

C 1000 ms.

D There is not enough information to know.

5 Atrial-based pacing has a quirk that occurs for one cycle when a patient transitions from atrial paced event/ventricular sensed event pacing to atrial paced/ventricular paced activity. What happens?

A The ventricular pacing rate is above the base rate for one cycle.

B The atrial pacing rate is above the base rate for one cycle.

C The ventricular pacing rate is below the base rate for one cycle.

D The atrial pacing rate is below the base rate for one cycle.

6 Ventricular-based pacing has a quirk that occurs when the patient is in the pacing state of atrial pacing/ventricular sensing. What happens?

A The pacemaker paces faster than the base rate.

B The pacemaker paces slower than the base rate.

C The pacemaker turns off atrial tracking temporarily.

D The pacemaker extends the VA interval to preserve base-rate pacing.

7 Which of the following might be considered the best reason to think that atrial-based

timing is superior to ventricular-based timing for dual-chamber pacing?

A Atrial-based timing uses less energy and preserves battery life.

B Atrial-based timing is more physiological (the atria drive the pacing rate).

C Ventricular-based pacing could force excessive and unnecessary ventricular pacing.

D Atrial-based timing has no quirks at all.

8 The difference between the so-called true atrial-based timing and modified atrial-based timing occurs when an atrial-based dual-chamber pacemaker encounters what type of event?

A Transition from ventricular sensing to ventricular pacing in the presence of atrial pacing

B Ventricular conduction

C PAC

D PVC

9 What is the main distinction between *true atrial-based timing* and *modified atrial*-based *timing*?

A Modified atrial-based timing uses a variable AA interval.

B Modified atrial-based timing reverts to ventricular-based timing in one situation.

C Modified atrial-based timing allows the clinician to program an interim AA interval.

D Modified atrial-based timing mode switches in the presence of a PAC.

10 In a dual-chamber pacemaker with modified atrial-based timing, what does the device do when it encounters a PVC?

A Nothing; it ignores all PVCs.

B It initiates the AA interval.

C It initiates the VA interval.

D It initiates the PVC detection window.

CHAPTER 21

21

CHAPTER 21

Rate-responsive pacing

Learning objectives

- Define chronotropic incompetence and name some common symptoms of this condition.
- Explain the relationship between metabolic demand and heart rate.
- Briefly state the three stages of CI.
- Define key terms associated with normal exercise physiology: tidal volume, minute ventilation, cardiac output, anaerobic threshold, and metabolic equivalent (MET).
- Explain how one might use METs for various levels of activity.
- Define minute ventilation and explain how it differs during rest and exertion.
- Describe at least three different types of sensors and explain how they work.
- Name the kind of sensor used in the first commercially available rate-responsive pacemaker.
- State why a PASSIVE setting for rate response might be used.
- Name three or four of the main types of rate-responsive parameters and what they control.

Introduction

One of the most common cardiac disorders present in pacemaker patients is chronotropic incompetence (CI) or the inability of the heart to increase and decrease its rate appropriately in response to workload. CI with symptoms is a class I pacemaker indication all by itself, but it is not unusual to see patients with other pacemaker indications present with CI or develop it over time. CI is a progressive

disorder and it presents a real challenge to patients struggling with a heart rate that won't keep up with them! Pacemakers offer an important treatment option for CI (in fact, it's the only effective treatment, period): rate response. Known as rate-responsive, rate-adaptive, rate-modulated, or sensor-driven pacing, this device's features allow some kind of sensor to help the pacemaker know when to pace faster in response to workload. Rate-responsive parameter settings then allow the clinician to regulate how quickly and how aggressively this rate support works. Today, every pacemaker is equipped with a rate-responsive sensor, but in many cases, it is never turned on. This number is probably much too low! Many patients can benefit from rate response and clinicians should become comfortable learning how to turn on and adjust rate-responsive pacemaker settings.

Chronic incompetence (CI)

CI can be defined as the inability of the heart to regulate its rate appropriately to respond to physiologic stress. That *stress* might occur with exercise or exertion, with high metabolic demand, or with emotional stress or fever. CI is actually in and of itself an indication for cardiac pacing (class I). There are a few important symptoms that suggest CI:
- An inability to ever achieve maximum heart rate (MHR), even when exercising
- Being able to achieve the MHR during exercise but only after a long delay
- Difficulty in heart rate recovery following exertion and/or MHR
- Unstable cardiac rate during exercise

The Nuts and Bolts of Implantable Device Therapy Pacemakers, First Edition. Tom Kenny.
© 2015 John Wiley & Sons, Ltd. Published 2015 by John Wiley & Sons, Ltd.

Patients with CI may present at the clinic saying they have difficulty with exercise (which may include such things as walking across a parking lot or climbing stairs at the house), suffer from loss of breath or fatigue much earlier than they should, or have trouble with their heart rate after exertion (i.e., their heart rate does not return to normal quickly and continues to beat rapidly long after the exercise is over). Many patients do not know about CI and will attribute their symptoms to their age and overall fitness level or just complain that they get tired more easily than they ever did before or that they are light-headed with exercise.

While it is common for clinicians to think of CI in terms of being unable to accelerate the heart rate appropriately during exercise, it may also occur when the patient cannot maintain an adequately rapid rate during exertion or if the heart does not decelerate appropriately after exercise. A handy way to think of CI involves the three stages of CI:

1 The inability to increase the rate appropriately

2 The inability to maintain an accelerated rate appropriate

3 The inability to decelerate the rate appropriately

Most people with CI have all three stages, but it is possible to have one or two of these without having all three. It is also possible for some people to have all three stages of CI but that one stage is more severe than the others. Some typical patterns from these stages of CI are shown in **Figure 21.1**.

Symptomatic CI is a class I pacing indication. For the pacing guidelines, CI is defined as failing to achieve the so-called MHR. MHR is defined by this formula:

$$80\% \times (220 - age)$$

For instance, in a 60-year-old person, the MHR would be 128 bpm (80% of 160). Keep in mind that this formula is a rule-of-thumb value rather than an exact number. Another definition of CI is any MHR during maximal exercise that is under 120 bpm. In other words, if a maximally exercising patient has a heart rate that does not go above 120 bpm, that patient is chronotropically incompetent. The first rule of thumb relies on the patient's age, but the second definition is independent of age. From these definitions, it is clear that the primary stage of CI used to diagnose CI involves the patient's ability to accelerate cardiac rate appropriately. This is not the full picture of CI, but it may be the most clinically relevant.

CI may be caused by any number of conditions or the interplay of two or more conditions shown below:

- Age-related sinus node dysfunction
- Secondary CI to other cardiac diseases
- Side effect of medication
- Autonomic dysfunction
- Endocrine–metabolic disease

By far, the most common cause of CI is unavoidable: age. It appears that as we age, our cardiac conduction system ages along with us and can no longer respond as well or quickly to changes in

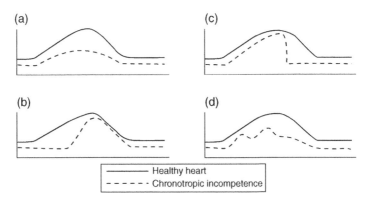

Figure 21.1 Some stages of CI. The healthy heart is shown in the solid line and the CI patient's rate is shown with the broken line. (a) and (b) show two different manifestations of stage 1 CI, the inability to accelerate the rate appropriately. (c) shows stage 3 CI, the inability to decelerate properly. (d) shows stage 2 CI, the inability to maintain an accelerated rate appropriately.

metabolic demand. It is also important to note that many cardiac medications, such as beta-blockers or calcium-channel blockers, can cause CI because they slow cardiac conduction overall.

CI is prevalent in the pacemaker population and is particularly prevalent among pacemaker patients who also have atrial fibrillation. Although symptomatic CI is a class I pacemaker indication in and of itself, many patients who get pacemakers for other indications also have symptomatic CI.

CI is a progressive disorder. It can develop in patients who did not have it previously, including pacemaker patients, and it can worsen markedly over a short period of time. Thus, many pacemaker patients have CI when their pacemaker is first implanted and many more will develop CI after their pacemaker is implanted. Moreover, relatively mild CI usually worsens to more severe forms. For that reason, pacemaker clinicians need to be aware how to optimally manage CI.

Determining heart rate needs in pacemaker patients

The average person (without a pacemaker) under age 65 elevates his or her heart rate over 90 bpm 178 times per day; it is not much different with older people who experience heart rates over 90 bpm 151 times a day [1]. Even to clinicians, this number is surprising and far exceeds what most of us would have ever guessed. The ramifications of this finding are profound. If pacemakers attempt to imitate the behavior of the healthy heart, this suggests that pacemakers ought to be helping patients raise the heart rates above 90 bpm many times every single day!

When programming rate response for a pacemaker patient, there are a number of considerations to take into account. First of all, during the so-called activities of daily living (ADL), the heart rate goes up for a short period of time but does not achieve the maximal rate. Thus, most patients need to be able to have submaximal rate accelerations for short periods of time many times a day. This type of submaximal pacing for ADL may vary slightly between younger and older patients (younger patients may need more if they are more active). Sedentary patients need more aggressive submaximal rate support. Women tend overall not to need as much rate response as men, likely because they are less likely to have sinus node dysfunction. However, each patient needs to be evaluated individually based on his or her overall fitness, age, and lifestyle.

The most frequent type and duration of exercise for a pacemaker patient is walking for about 5 min. They may repeat this activity many times a day, but the actual exercise does not last very long. This tells the pacemaker clinician a few things in terms of setting up rate response, namely, rate response must be quick. If a 75-year-old pacemaker patient decides to go out for a 10 min walk, his rate response needs to kick in quickly. If the rate response takes 5 min to activate, this does not help him! Moreover, the pacemaker patient might be cooling down just as the rate response gets going. Thus, one of the most important attributes of any rate-responsive pacemaker is that rate response is quick. The sensor in the device must detect and respond to patient activity as rapidly as possible.

To be fair, not every patient exercises for short spurts. Marathon runners and other elite athletes, for example, exercise for hours at a time. But let's face it; how many elite athletes have pacemakers? There may be some, but this is not the *typical pacemaker patient*. If a marathon runner gets a pacemaker, his rate response may need some special tweaking!

Normal exercise physiology

In order to understand CI, it is necessary to take a step backward and review normal exercise physiology with a healthy heart. When discussing normal exercise physiology, clinicians use a variety of specific terms that are useful to us in rate-responsive pacing. This vocabulary includes the term *tidal volume*, which refers to the volume of air that a person inhales and exhales during one normal respiratory cycle or breath. The respiratory rate refers to how many respiratory cycles occur in 1 min. Minute ventilation (MV) is tidal volume times respiratory rate; in other words, MV tells us the volume of air inhaled and exhaled in 1 min. Another way of thinking of MV is depth times rate of respiration.

The point of these terms is clear to anyone who has ever been to a gym or jumped on a treadmill. As a person exercises, he or she tends to inhale and exhale more deeply (increasing tidal volume) and breathe more rapidly (respiratory rate increases); as the tidal volume and respiratory rate increase, so does MV.

So far, we have focused on the pulmonary side of the equation, that is, the work that the lungs are doing. Let's move over to the cardiac side, since the heart and lungs work so closely together. Stroke volume refers to how much blood the heart pumps out during one cardiac cycle. The heart rate is how many times the heart beats during 1 min. Cardiac output is stroke volume times heart rate. Looking at it another way, the tidal volume and the stroke volume are similar (air vs. blood, lungs vs. heart); the respiratory rate and heart rate are similar (breaths vs. beats); and MV and cardiac output are similar (lungs vs. heart).

As we exercise, our respiratory and heart rates increase, our tidal volume and stroke volume increase, and our MV and cardiac output go up. As long as the body can get enough oxygen, it can keep exercising comfortably. Exercise demands oxygen. But if at some point, the body cannot get the oxygen it needs to sustain exercise, it produces fatigue and other symptoms. This point is called the anaerobic threshold. Anaerobic means *without oxygen*.

When a healthy person exercises, stroke volume (how much blood is ejected per cardiac cycle) plays an important role at the lower end of exercise levels. As exercise intensity and duration increase, stroke volume becomes less important than heart rate. Thus, cardiac output is governed by stroke volume at lower levels of exercise and heart rate at higher exercise levels. In fact, faster heart rates can increase cardiac output as much as 300%, while changes in stroke volume can increase cardiac output by about 50%. This is the reason that pacemakers address CI with *rate* response, that is, faster rates have a greater impact on cardiac output.

Metabolic equivalents

The easiest way to think of metabolic equivalents or METs is as a unit of exercise or work. Think of rest as being 1.0 MET and shoveling as 9.0 METs. Between those extremes, driving might count as 1.5 MET, while walking at 4 mph (15 min mile) counts as 5 or 6 METs. Understanding METs helps the clinician to quantify exertion levels in a way that maps onto rate response (see **Figure 21.2**). Shoveling requires more metabolic response than walking a 15 min mile and both place greater metabolic demand on the body than driving a car. In evaluating METs, it will be evident that even seemingly low levels of activity like driving, shopping, and strolling (30 min mile) actually place a metabolic demand on the body. Regardless of age, all pacemaker patients can benefit from elevated pacing rates during these moderate activities or ADLs.

The range of METs that a patient achieves depends on their overall fitness level. Athletes, for instance, can exercise at a range of 14–23 METs. Very active patients (who are not athletes) exercise at a range of 11–15 METs. Most pacemaker patients can be classified as sedentary people, and the sedentary tend to exercise at around 8–11 METs. Of particular concern here—and we will discuss this in more detail later—are congestive heart failure patients whose exercise range is <5 METs. Thus, the more fit a person is, the harder that person can work!

Minute ventilation (MV)

MV as defined earlier is the respiratory rate times the tidal volume, and it refers to how much air is moved in and out of the body during 1 min. A normal healthy person takes about 10–16 breaths per minute at rest (average 12), which increases to 20–60 breaths per minute during exercise. Obviously, the greater the exercise or METs, the faster the respiratory rate. Tidal volumes or the depth of inhalation is about half to 1 l per breath at rest and 2–5 l per breath during exercise. Thus, in a normal person, exercise can result in about a fivefold increase in both respiratory rate (from about 12 to 60 breaths per minute) and tidal volume (from about 1 to 5 l per breath). These are pretty big changes!

MV and heart rate are very closely correlated in healthy individuals. The correlation is so direct that knowing a healthy patient's MV allows the heart rate to be predicted with good accuracy. Moreover, there is a direct proportional relationship between heart rate, MV rate, and METs in healthy people. As one goes up, the others go up,

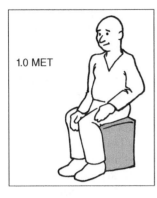
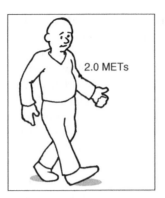
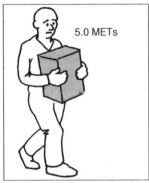
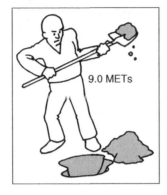

Figure 21.2 METs vary depending on workload. The more work, the higher the METs and the greater cardiac response required.

and they increase to the same degree and following the same pattern (see **Figure 21.3**).

Healthy people are able to increase their ability to do work, also known as their *functional capacity*, by increasing their heart rate in proportion to the workload. Of course, this only works up to a certain point. We have all observed that when we go for a jog, climb some stairs, or unload groceries from the car, our heart rate increases to help us get the work done. While a healthy person can increase functional capacity in response to workload, patients with cardiac disease are more limited in this ability.

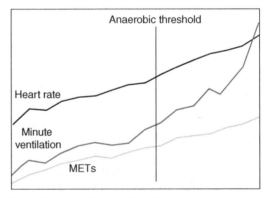

Figure 21.3 In healthy and chronotropically competent people, the heart rate, the minute ventilation rate, and METs are correlated and proportional to each other. This has important implications to pacing, which attempts to mimic the healthy heart. The anaerobic threshold, indicated here with a vertical line, is the point at which the body's needs for oxygen exceed its ability to take it in. All people, including the very fit, have an anaerobic threshold or the point at which exercise is no longer possible.

Healthy chronotropic response: a review

Picking up all of the information covered so far, healthy chronotropic response occurs when a person's heart rate and cardiac output increase with activity or workload. Healthy chronotropic response is immediate; the heart should respond to exercise within no more than 10 s after the onset of activity. The heart rate increase should be proportional

and be reliably maintained over the course of the activity. For example, walking at an average speed should raise the healthy heart to a rate of 90 or

100 bpm. As the activity intensifies, the cardiac output is less affected by stroke volume and much more affected by rate. Thus, rate increase is crucial with greater workloads. When the exertion ceases, the heart rate should lag about 5 or 10 s before it decelerates back to the resting state.

This is how rate response should work—it should mimic the healthy heart.

Diagnosing CI in pacemaker patients

Earlier, it was discussed that CI could be diagnosed based on patient symptoms. A treadmill or stress test might be used to get further information (a patient with CI will not show appropriate rate increases during the treadmill test). In some instances, a monitor or implantable loop recorder might be used to gather data. If the patient has an implanted pacemaker, the pacemaker itself can be a great diagnostic tool to help find evidence of potential CI. In fact, if the patient already has a pacemaker, device diagnostics are an excellent tool for CI diagnosis.

Histograms
Histograms are data reports available from the pacemaker that can show how fast the pacemaker has paced (recording every single beat since the last follow-up) and how much intrinsic versus paced

activity as occurred. Think of histograms as big, global reports that provide percentages at various rate ranges or percentages paced. Some histograms are designed to show trends over time (see **Figure 21.4**). The histogram of a CI patient will show lots of lower-rate activity and little-to-no activity at rates above about 70 or 80 ppm.

Counters
Likewise, the counters can give evidence of CI. Therapy history or diagnostics also offer counters that report the percentage of time the patient spends in various pacing states. For instance, the pacemaker might report that a patient had 70% atrial paced/ventricular sensed activity, 18% atrial paced/ventricular sensed activity, and so on. If there is a lot of atrial pacing (which would occur at the base rate in a nonrate-responsive mode), it suggests a need for rate response because it means the sinus is not able to drive the rate higher in response to activity.

Trends
A trending plot or trend may be available in a pacemaker that gives an overview of pacing behavior. Some devices also offer a sensor-indicated rate even if rate response is not active. This shows what the pacing rate would have been if the sensor had been turned on. If there is a marked deviation between what the pacemaker without rate response

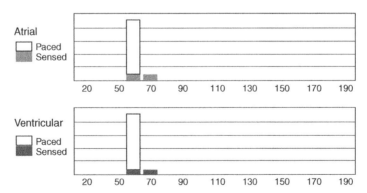

Figure 21.4 This rate histogram from a pacemaker patient shows the atrial channel above and the ventricular channel below. This patient spent the majority of time being paced in the atrium at around 60 ppm and being paced in the ventricle at around the same rate. There was a small amount of intrinsic activity in atria and ventricles at around 70 bpm but nothing faster than that. Since there is almost no activity above 60 ppm (and literally nothing above 80 ppm), this patient should be considered chronotropically incompetent, since even a sedentary patient should have rate excursions above 70 ppm several times a day. The only exception to this would be a very sedentary patient, such as a person who is chair bound or bed bound.

did and what it would have done if the sensor had been able to control the pacing rate, then the patient has CI.

Managing pacemaker patients with CI

Virtually all dual-chamber pacemakers today offer rate response and most single-chamber pacemakers do as well. If a patient has or is suspected to have CI, the best strategy is to turn on rate response. In that respect, managing a pacemaker patient with CI is easy. Understanding exactly how to program rate response for that individual patient is a little more complex, and we will go over that in the next section.

While most CI pacemaker patients report feeling better when rate response is turned on, some patients paradoxically will complain that rate response makes them feel worse. This can occur in heart failure patients. Remember that the longest period of the cardiac cycle is diastole, which is crucial to adequate filling of the heart with blood. With rate response on, the patient is subjected to shorter cardiac cycles, and as the cardiac cycle shortens, diastole is proportionally the most affected. Thus, some heart failure patients can get symptomatic by this abbreviated diastolic period. Thus, some heart failure patients do not tolerate rate response. Since they are often sedentary to very sedentary to begin with, rate response can often be successfully programmed off for such patients.

Another patient that may not tolerate rate response is the coronary artery disease (CAD) patient with rate-related angina. These patients may suffer moderate to severe symptoms with accelerated pacing rates. To understand this, recognize that diastole (the longest component of the cardiac cycle) is also the time during which coronary arteries are perfused. When the rate increases, the cardiac cycle shortens and this shortens the perfusion period with it. Thus, at faster rates, certain CAD patients do not get the perfusion they need and angina occurs. Patients with ischemic heart disease may not tolerate pacing at higher rates. When treating an ischemic heart disease pacemaker patient, use rate response carefully, cautiously, and under clinical supervision. It may be turned on, but settings should be kept low

(not aggressive) until it is known how the patient tolerates higher-rate pacing. Many such patients benefit from a certain degree of rate response. Remember the old adage: start low and go slow!

This brings me to a very important point. A clinician can get too focused on histograms and pacemaker behavior and not do the right thing for the patient. For instance, the histogram may indicate that the patient has CI and needs rate response. But the patient may have heart failure or CAD and be highly symptomatic even though his CI (taken in isolation) would have benefited from rate response. Even though we like to think of ourselves as pacing experts, we should always be *pacemaker patient* experts and focus on what is good for the patient, not what the device alone tells us. A patient may indeed need rate response according to the device diagnostics, but if it brings him to the emergency room with an acute myocardial infarction, we made the wrong programming choices!

That being said, such patients are relatively rare. Most pacemaker patients with CI can and do benefit from rate response. But as responsible, diligent clinicians, we need to be mindful that there is no *always* in cardiac pacing, and we should be aware that some patients simply do not benefit from rate response.

Rate response in pacemakers

Rate-responsive pacing goes by many names: rate-adaptive pacing, rate-modulated pacing, and even sensor-driven pacing. There are several different types of rate-responsive sensors. The sensor controls the atrial channel in a dual-chamber pacemaker (remember that the atrial chamber controls the rate in a dual-chamber device), and the sensor controls the ventricular channel in a single-chamber ventricular pacemaker. When the sensor is controlling the rate—for instance, the patient is exercising and the sensor is accelerating the pacing rate—that rate is known as the *sensor-indicated rate*. (*Sensor-driven pacing* is the term used to refer to the rate-responsive feature in general; when that features is actively controlling the rate, the rate is called sensor-indicated rate.) The speed limit for the sensor-indicated rate is the maximum sensor rate or MSR, which has been mentioned in earlier chapters.

For example, imagine a dual-chamber pacemaker programmed to a base rate of 60 ppm, an MSR of 120 ppm, and rate response turned on. If the ECG shows consistent atrial paced/ventricular paced activity at around 90 ppm, that would reflect the *sensor-indicated rate*. That is sensor-driven pacing in action.

The optimal sensor

The very best sensor a person can have is a healthy sinus node. However, patients with CI no longer have a functional sinus node and must rely on some other systems to help regulate heart rate. Pacemakers can help patients with CI by using sensors to help adjust the heart rate to better meet the patient's metabolic demand.

The history of sensor-driven pacing has been dominated by the search for the ideal sensor. Ideally, a sensor would be sensitive to changes in metabolic demand that occur at a range of activities, starting with sleep or rest, at one extreme, to exertion and heavy exercise at the other extreme. The ideal sensor must be able to respond to changes in metabolic demand quickly but also proportionately—in other words, it has to be fast but also only as aggressive as necessary. The ideal sensor also had to accommodate a smooth rate deceleration, supporting the pacing rate as it came back down to normal. While many pacemaker patients are geriatric and sedentary, some pacemaker patients are children, teenagers, and young adults; some pacemaker patients are fit, active, and even athletic. Since it was never clear which pacemaker would be inserted into which patient, the sensor had to accommodate a wide range of patient lifestyles. The ideal sensor would have to adjust itself automatically to meet patient's needs. And there are also some clinical considerations. Doctors and nurses want a sensor that is easy to adjust and one that does not require excessive amounts of time to program and monitor. One other key attribute of the perfect sensor: it should be physiologic. This is one of the key shortfalls of modern sensor technology. A physiologic sensor would rely on the body's own systems to help adjust rate. Instead, many sensors today use external (nonbody) cues to adjust the rate.

The perfect sensor would also work well right out of the box and not require the use of special leads or adapters. In the early days of rate-responsive pacing, pacing engineers developed a rate-responsive device that used blood temperature as a physiologic sensor. In order to measure blood temperature, the device required a special lead with a tiny thermistor (a thermometer-like component). The concept behind blood temperature as a sensor was very sound; there is a good and tightly proportional correlation between blood temperature and workload. While this approach sounds good, there was a way to fool this kind of sensor—temperature changes such as being in a hot tub, taking a hot shower, or being in a hot environment like a sauna. The blood-sensing system was commercialized by Cook Medical in a device known as the Kelvin pacemaker, but it never gained acceptance. This device is a good example of how pacing engineers can sometimes come up with something that looks great on the drawing board but does not actually work well in real life.

Activity sensors

The first commercially released rate-responsive pacemaker came from Medtronic (Activitrax®) and used what is called an activity sensor. An activity sensor is a piezoelectric crystal that responded to muscle vibrations. The concept was that the patient's metabolic demand increased with activity, and activity could be associated with vibrations. A patient asleep or sitting in a chair does not create much in the way of muscle vibrations, but as the patient gets up and walks, their muscles create vibrations that are then sensed by the piezoelectric crystal and interpreted as activity. If that patient starts to walk quickly, climb a ladder, or unload packages from the car, the vibrations increase.

The activity sensor was composed of a piezoelectric crystal (which is a component also found in microphones) bonded to the inside of the anterior face of the pulse generator. Even very subtle vibrations could be picked up by the crystal that then relayed them to the pacemaker circuitry where they were interpreted as activity levels.

The Activitrax pacemaker and its activity sensor worked very well and offered some key advantages. First, it was extremely simple and easy to adjust and required no special hardware. Second, it worked well in most situations to keep the sensor-indicated rate at the right levels. But it was not perfect. Like all other sensors, the activity sensor had some limitations. Tapping or putting pressure on the implant site could fool the sensor, which was bonded to the inside front of the pulse generator. Any environment with a lot of vibrations (such as being in a helicopter, using heavy equipment, riding on a train) could fool the sensor. Certain medical procedures, such as lithotripsy (an ultrasound procedure used to help break up kidney stones), misled the sensor. By far, the best (and most cited) example of the shortcoming of the activity sensor involved patients going up and down stairs. From a workload perspective, a person does more work climbing up stairs than coming down stairs. However, walking downstairs created far more vibrations because each footfall *slammed* into the step. Going upstairs created only slight vibrations, since people tend to walk more softly on the balls of their feet going upstairs. The result is that an activity sensor will have a much faster sensor-indicated rate for the person going downstairs than the same person going upstairs.

Thus, the activity sensor had many advantages, but it was not perfect. Pacing engineers continued to look for better technologies.

Accelerometer

The next major innovation in sensor technology still used the same piezoelectric crystal, but in a different way. Accelerometers are piezoelectric crystals that respond to motion or acceleration across a plane. Instead of attaching the sensor to the inside of the pulse generator can, the accelerometer was affixed within the pulse generator to the circuit board in such a way that it acted like a little diving board inside the can. When the patient moved front to back (accelerated), the *diving board* moved, and the pacemaker circuitry could interpret this motion to help adjust the pacing rate. The accelerometer preserved some of the advantages of the old activity sensor: it was simple, it responded quickly, it was highly effective in most situations, and no special lead was required. It also offered a major advantage over the old activity sensor: it was not as easily fooled by pressure or tapping on the device. In fact, many of the things that could fool activity sensor (e.g., going up and down stairs) could be better interpreted by the accelerometer.

Accelerometers were sensitive to changes in the anterior–posterior plane. (By contrast, activity sensors were sensitive to up-and-down motion or footfall.) Since the most frequent activity of the average pacemaker patient is walking, the accelerometer is poised to work well for that kind of activity (which creates anterior–posterior motion).

Of course, accelerometers also have their shortfalls. A person in a rocking chair can easily *fool* the accelerometer because there is motion even though there is little actual work. Like activity sensors, accelerometers were not particularly sensitive to things like lifting heavy packages, stress, emotion, or walking on an incline. Some things that did not seem like they would work actually did. For instance, it was thought that exercise on a stationary bicycle would *fool* the accelerometer because although the patient was exercising, he was remaining still. In actual practice, accelerometers work reasonably well for people who exercise on a stationary bicycle. The reason is that when a person moves his legs to pedal the bicycle, it causes movement in the shoulder area. This movement is not huge, but it is persistent, and it suffices to cause the accelerometer to increase the pacing rate. Another concern with accelerometers was that they would misinterpret motion when people are riding in cars, planes, or other vehicles. This is actually not a problem because the accelerometer is set to look for only motion in a certain frequency range (around 1 Hz). One hertz is a typical frequency range for walking.

By far, the best advantage offered by accelerometer technology (besides simplicity, reliability, and ease of use) is that it responds quickly. Like the activity sensor, it can be fooled. But the main drawback to accelerometers was that they caused sensor-indicated rates that were not necessarily proportional to workload. Accelerometers, like activity sensor, could only measure metabolic demand indirectly and that was imprecise.

As is typical with cardiac pacing, technology drives practice. The accelerometer was imperfect, but it worked better than the older activity sensor, which gradually faded from use. Accelerometers are still widely used today. One reason may be that accelerometers are far more effective at lower levels of exercise than higher levels, and most pacemaker patients tend to need rate support in that range.

Minute ventilation (MV)

The MV sensor was first introduced by a company known as Telectronics, since acquired by St. Jude Medical. Remembering that MV is the respiratory rate times the tidal volume, this sensor uses respiration as a measure of metabolic demand. Changes in MV correspond well to METs; the response is tightly proportional. The higher the MET value, the greater the MV value.

In very simple terms, in a healthy person, there is a direct, linear relationship between increases in heart rate and increases in MV up to the anaerobic threshold. Once the anaerobic threshold is reached (the point at which the patient cannot get sufficient oxygen to support his metabolic demand), MV has a curvilinear relationship to heart rate. If the patient continues to work beyond his anaerobic threshold, MV tends to increase more rapidly than heart rate.

Because the MV sensor relies on the body's own system to help adjust the pacing rate, the FDA allowed the MV sensor to be labeled as a *physiologic sensor*. According to FDA labeling, it is the only sensor on the market today that can claim to restore chronotropic competence.

The first challenge of the MV sensor was to find a way to reliably measure MV (depth times rate of breathing). It solved this challenge by measuring transthoracic impedance or the change in resistance (impedance) across (trans) the chest cavity (thoracic). The MV system does not require a *special* lead but it does require that the pacing lead be bipolar. The MV sensor is located in the pulse generator and it sends out a low-level current pulse to the lead's ring electrode. This pulse output is much too small to capture the heart. A circuit is formed between an indifferent electrode located in the pulse generator and the ring electrode on the bipolar lead. The voltage signal is measured between the lead tip and the indifferent electrode in the header. There will be a slight difference between these two voltage measurements, and it is their difference that is used to measure transthoracic impedance. Note that transthoracic impedance changes constantly; it changes with respiration rate and tidal volume and it changes with inspiration versus expiration. These constantly changing signals are what the pacemaker uses to determine the sensor-indicated rate. One important point is that the transthoracic circuit (ring electrode to indifferent electrode in the pulse generator) is entirely distinct and independent of the pacing and sensing circuits.

The MV sensor offers some important advantages. It is a physiologic sensor and works particularly well at higher levels of intense activity (a shortfall for activity sensors and accelerometers). It provides a more proportional rate response, which can be very important for active patients. On the other hand, the MV sensor is not perfect. It is much slower to respond to changes in exertion than the activity sensor or accelerometer. And, like other sensors, MV sensors can be fooled. Vigorous arm movements, for example, can *trick* the sensor into rate response (see **Table 21.1** for a comparison of these three sensors).

Table 21.1 Key points of comparison among activity sensors, accelerometers, and MV sensors

Sensor type	Advantages	Disadvantages
Activity	Quick response	Can be fooled by vibrations
	Good at detecting low workload	
	Excellent for short bursts of submaximal activity	Not proportional to workload
	Simple	Not particularly good at high levels of exertion
	No special lead	Not physiologic
Accelerometer	Quick response	Can be fooled by motion in a plane (rocking chair)
	Good at detecting low workload	Not proportional to workload
	Excellent for short bursts of submaximal activity	Not particularly good at high levels of exertion
	Simple	Not physiologic
	No special lead	
MV sensor	Very good at detecting and responding to intense workloads	Slower to respond
	Proportional to workload	Requires a bipolar lead

Blended sensors

Pacing engineers had invented several very good sensors but no perfect sensor, so the next innovation sought to blend the advantages of the accelerometer (rapid response) with the MV sensor (proportional response). The result was the blended sensor, sometimes called a dual sensor system or integrated sensors. A blended sensor uses both an accelerometer and transthoracic impedance (MV) to gather the input necessary to change the sensor-indicated rate in response to workload (see **Figure 21.5**).

The blended sensor has a special algorithm that makes it work well. When the accelerometer indicates that the patient should be paced at a rate faster than the MV sensor indicates, the pacemaker takes both inputs and *blends* them to reach an interim rate. Thus, it does not accelerate as fast as an accelerometer, but it accelerates faster than a regular MV sensor. However, once the MV sensor determines that the patient's sensor-indicated rate should be faster than the sensor-indicated rate determined by the accelerometer, then MV takes over and there is no more blending. This allows the MV sensor to do what it does best, namely, respond to higher-intensity workloads. A good way to think of the blended sensor is that neither of the two sensors has total control—the accelerometer is more in control at the lower end of activity, while the MV sensor is in charge at the higher levels.

Pacemakers with blended sensors can also be programmed to operate with a single sensor, so a blended sensor device offers the clinician the choice of accelerometer only, MV sensor only, or the blended sensor. There may be situations where patients would benefit more from one type of sensor than another. For instance, a very old, sedentary patient may only ever require an accelerometer.

The advantages of the blended sensor system are many. It is physiologic (MV is a physiologic sensor), it is prompt to respond (accelerometers respond rapidly), and it provides proportional rate response. A blended sensor does require a bipolar pacing lead but not a *special* or proprietary lead; any bipolar lead will work. One of the drawbacks to the blended sensor is that they are little more complex to learn and operate.

Closed-loop stimulation

The closed-loop stimulation (CLS) system is only available from Biotronik. CLS is a unique sensor, and there are clinicians who opt for CLS devices because of this rate-responsive sensor technology.

The CLS system looks for changes in cardiac contractility (inotropy) to measure workload. Like an MV sensor, the CLS system requires a bipolar lead but any bipolar lead will work. It uses the lead and an electrode in the pulse generator can to measure changes in cardiac contractility. Contractility is one of the parameters that has a direct effect on cardiac function, so measuring it rather than respiration or movement is thought to provide a more direct and accurate form of rate response.

The right ventricular lead's tip electrode is used to measure an impedance signal from a small area

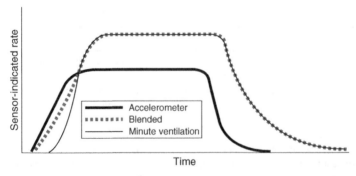

Figure 21.5 A simple diagram of a blended sensor taking input from an accelerometer (notice rapid onset of rate response) and minute ventilation (MV) sensor (notice higher rates in response to exertion). The goal of the blended sensor system is to merge the advantages of the accelerometer with MV. If the accelerometer indicates a rate faster than the rate indicated by MV, the sensor inputs are combined to achieve the sensor-indicated rate. If the MV sensor indicates a faster rate than the accelerometer, then the sensor switches to be 100% MV—in other words, if MV indicates a rate above the rate indicated by the accelerometer, *MV rules*.

of tissue inside the right ventricle at or near the point of lead-to-myocardium interface. This localized *intracardiac impedance signal* provides an assessment of cardiac contraction by measuring myocardial wall motion changes. These multiple changes in impedance allow the pacemaker to evaluate cardiac contractility and then adjust the pacing rate accordingly.

CLS works by using this impedance data to first create a reference curve for one entire cardiac contraction, which reflects the contraction dynamics for a given patient at rest. This can be thought of a patient-individualized baseline for one cardiac contraction, created from multiple measures. CLS then works by constantly comparing current impedance values for particular phases of the cardiac contraction against the reference baseline. When the current impedance values differ substantially from the reference values, a change in contractility is noted, which signals the device to adjust the sensor-indicated rate. The rate response is proportional to the change in impedance (current values vs. reference values); the greater the difference, the more rate support.

The advantage of the CLS sensor system is rate response highly proportional to the level of exercise. In testing, CLS sensor provides rate support similar to normal sinus rate response in healthy patients. CLS requires no special lead and is relatively simple to program and set up. Another key advantage of CLS sensors is that they work well for a wide range of patients, from the frail and bedbound to the very active. Because CLS looks at cardiac contractility, it can even respond to emotional stress, something that activity sensors and accelerometers cannot. Another major advantage of the CLS sensor is that it is the only commercially available sensor that has proven in clinic trials to be responsive to emotional stress.

Other sensors

The main sensors in use in cardiac pacing today are the accelerometer, the MV sensor, blended sensors, and CLS. Older sensor technology included a piezoelectric activity sensor, a blood temperature (thermistor) sensor, and a QT sensor. There is also a combined sensor of QT plus activity sensor.

The QT interval sensor works by measuring the duration between the ventricular pacing spike (the Q) and the evoked T-wave. The concept behind QT interval sensors is that the QT interval will shorten with exercise. The main drawback of this type of sensor—which is rarely used today—is that it only works when the pacemaker is pacing.

While these may be of historical interest, they would only very rarely be seen in clinical practice today. Sensor technology likely to be encountered in clinical practice today is summarized in **Table 21.2**.

Programming rate response

Rate response adds new parameters to the pacemaker and increases the complexity of the device. For this reason, some clinicians may avoid the use of rate response. Another challenger in optimizing rate response in the device clinic is the fact that programmable parameters for rate-responsive pacemakers vary substantially among manufacturers. Thus, a clinician may feel quite confident programming Medtronic-style rate response but be confused when dealing with St. Jude Medical settings. The best way to learn about rate-responsive devices is to dig in depth in the manuals for the leading devices of all manufacturers. For now, this will be a general overview—bear in mind that the specifics can vary by manufacturer and even among devices by the same manufacturer.

Table 21.2 Sensor technology in use today by major pacemaker manufacturers

Company	Accelerometer	Minute ventilation	Blended	Closed-loop stimulation
Medtronic	Yes	Yes	Yes	No
St. Jude Medical	Yes	No	No	No
Boston Scientific	Yes	Yes	Yes	No
Biotronik	No	No	No	Yes
Sorin	Yes	Yes	Yes	No

Turning rate response on

The very first parameter the clinician must address is whether or not to turn rate response on. All devices today offer rate response, but it is usually turned off in the device when it comes out of the box and is not activated until the clinician turns it on. As soon as rate response is turned on, the device adds an R to the fourth position of its mode designation, that is, it goes from a DDD to a DDDR system or VVI to VVIR, and so on.

So when should the clinician make the decision to turn on rate response? Rate response should be turned on if the patient is found to have CI and can tolerate rate response. But turning on rate response is not enough—the clinician needs to decide how to program the other settings.

In real-world clinical practice, only about 50% of pacemakers have rate response turned on. Based on what we know about CI, this number is probably too low. But there may be many reasons that clinicians avoid activating rate response: the patient may not tolerate it, the patient's CI may not have been diagnosed, or the clinician does not think it is necessary. In some cases, clinicians may want to keep the pacing system as simple as possible and they do not activate rate response because it adds many new parameters and more complexity to the device.

In some devices, rate response can be turned to a setting called PASSIVE. PASSIVE rate response does not provide rate response to the patient but it does record in its diagnostics what the device would have done had rate response been activated. In other words, the clinicians can *test-drive* rate response before it is activated. The PASSIVE setting offers a way to evaluate rate response in a patient without having to turn it on. The clinician who uses the feature will program the PASSIVE feature on and then—after a given period of time—download the patient's diagnostics to assess what the sensor would have done and if this would have been better for the patient than his or her actual rates. Since the PASSIVE setting does not affect pacing rates and uses very little energy, it is highly recommended that it be utilized in all patients (unless you know for sure that rate response should be turned on—in that case, turn it on!).

PASSIVE mode can also be used to evaluate the type of sensor (for instance, should the clinician select the accelerometer sensor, the MV sensor, or the blended sensor) or specific sensor settings (for instance, the sensor can be programmed to very aggressive settings and tested in PASSIVE before those settings are made active and would influence the patient's actual pacing rate). Thus, PASSIVE settings offer the clinician a lot of good options to see "what if?" for rate response settings in a given patient (see **Figure 21.6**).

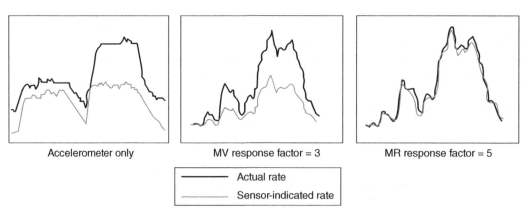

Accelerometer only   MV response factor = 3   MR response factor = 5

———— Actual rate
———— Sensor-indicated rate

Figure 21.6 The PASSIVE setting can show what the sensor-indicated rate would have been in a patient before rate response is actually activated. This feature allows clinicians to verify the appropriateness of rate response in a given patient and can also be used to see if a specific sensor type or sensor settings are more appropriate for a given patient. In the three trending plots below, rates were captured for what the pacemaker would have done with an accelerometer sensor only, an MV sensor only, or the blended sensor. Note that the accelerometer deviated from the patient's actual rate at the higher end of exercise intensity. MV at a setting of 3 did not provide adequate rate support for this patient. On the other hand, MV at a setting of 5 provided almost perfect rate response.

Optimizing rate response

The difference between manufacturers is probably most evident to clinicians when it comes to programming the various parameters in order to optimize rate response. There are some commonalities of course and there are common concepts, which will be discussed here.

The first parameter associated with rate response that needs to be programmed once the device is made rate response is the MSR. The MSR was discussed earlier and presented as the *speed limit* for the sensor, setting the absolute maximum rate the pacemaker would pace in response to sensor input. When selecting a value for the MSR, it is important to consider how much rate support the patient is likely to need and how fast a rate the patient can tolerate. A little old lady who becomes symptomatic at rates above 100 ppm should have a low MSR, while a fit patient who exercises a lot may need a higher MSR, such as 140 ppm. Very often (but not always), the MSR value is the same as the maximum tracking rate (MTR), the fastest rate at which the dual-chamber pacemaker will pace the ventricles in response to intrinsic atrial activity (atrial tracking).

The device may also require the clinician to set an activity threshold, which basically determines how sensitive the device is to activity. For instance, if the clinician wants rate response to kick in when the patient is only slightly active, a low threshold is appropriate (see **Figure 21.7**).

Another rate-responsive parameter is slope, also called the response factor. This determines how aggressive rate response is in ramping up in response to activity. For patients who are very active and need a lot of rate support during intense exercise, aggressive rate response may be appropriate. The slope may be programmable (for instance, from 1 to 16 in some devices). Slope determines the pacing rate that is actually achieved for a given level of activity. For instance, a patient is walking briskly. At a low slope value, that may cause the device to pace at 90 ppm, but at a very high slope value, it may trigger a pacing rate of 120 ppm. Slope is a parameter that confuses many clinicians, so here is an easy way to think about it. Imagine three DDDR pacemaker patients with exactly the same devices at exactly the same parameter settings doing exactly the same thing—doing a power walk. If you changed only the slope on these patients—for instance, the slopes are now programmed to 1, 8, and 16—you will see three entirely different actual pacing rates (likely something in the neighborhood of 90, 110, and 120 ppm). Another consideration to bear in mind when setting the slope value is that the higher the slope value, the faster the patient will achieve MSR.

Pacemakers may also allow the clinician to set the acceleration time, sometimes called the reaction time, and its counterpart, the deceleration time or recovery time. This helps adjust how rapidly rate response ramps up and ramps back down. Basically, these rates determine how fast the patient will hit the MSR (at one end) or return back to the base rate (at the other end).

A brief summary of these key parameters appears in **Table 21.3**.

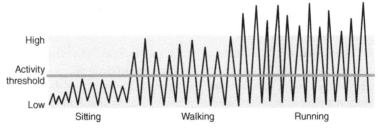

Figure 21.7 The activity threshold determines the point at which signals from the system reach the point to trigger a change in sensor-indicated rate. Note that at lower levels of activity, signals may still be perceived. The threshold simply determines the point at which these signals are large enough to trigger rate response. The threshold shown below is an adjustable value and can be moved up or down depending on when the clinician thinks it appropriate to initiate rate response.

Table 21.3 Some of the main parameters and their function involved in rate-responsive pacing

Parameter (and alternate names)	What it does
Lower rate limit, LRL, base rate	How fast the pacemaker will pace in response to an absence of sensed activity
Maximum sensor rate, MSR	The fastest rate the pacemaker will pace in response to sensor input
Threshold	The point at which signals to the sensor will trigger rate response
Reaction time	How fast the sensor-indicated rate will drive toward the MSR
Recovery time	How fast the sensor-indicated rate will drive toward the LRL
Slope	How fast the patient will be paced in response to activity

AUTO

Most devices offer a timesaving feature for programming rate-responsive settings: the automatic or AUTO feature. In many cases, the clinician can simply program Auto Threshold, Auto Slope, or other automatic values and allow the pacemaker to automatically set and adjust these parameter settings. Automatic values are based on the pacemaker's information about the patient's activity levels, and they are designed to be appropriate for most patients. For most patients, setting AUTO values is the smart thing to do. It saves time and it offers good, individualized settings. Some of the times that clinicians should tweak or fine-tune rate-responsive parameters are these:

- For unusual patients, such as the pacemaker patient who happens to be a mountain climber
- For patients who have trouble tolerating certain rate-responsive settings (for instance, you can program rate response to make it very mild for patients who do not tolerate higher-rate pacing)
- When the doctor or clinician believes that rate response can be optimized in some way

- In most other cases, AUTO settings work well and save time for the clinician.

Conclusion

Rate-responsive pacing is a very beneficial feature that probably should be used more frequently than it is. This type of pacing allows the pacemaker to accommodate the normal types of rate accelerations that would be typical of the healthy heart during routine everyday situations. All pacemakers today offer rate response, but the sensor technology they use and how rate response is programmed or fine-tuned can differ. The optimal sensor remains the healthy sinus node, but when a patient has CI, that is no longer an option. The most commonly used sensors today are accelerometers (acceleration or anterior–posterior motion), MV (measured as transthoracic impedance), blended sensors (using inputs from both accelerometers and MV), and CLS, available only in Biotronik devices. Rate response is a very beneficial feature and pacing clinicians should become familiar with its use and learn how to adjust it to meet the individual needs of pacing patients.

The nuts and bolts of rate-responsive pacing

- Chronotropic incompetence (CI) is the inability of the heart to regulate its rate in response to physiologic stress. CI is a progressive disorder.
- CI may provoke symptoms, such as the inability to achieve the maximal heart rate (even when exercising), achieving the maximal heart rate during exercise but only after a protracted period of time, difficulty recovering from exertion (rate deceleration), or unstable heart rates

  during exertion. Note that CI may occur during rate acceleration, maintenance of a high rate, or deceleration of the rate back to normal following exertion. Patients with CI may report feeling overly tired, unable to do all of the physical things they used to do, or getting light-headed or unwell during exertion.
- CI with symptoms is a class I pacemaker indication.

- The maximum heart rate can be calculated as 80% × (220 − age). Some physicians feel that any patient who cannot achieve a heart rate above 120 bpm (regardless of age) has CI.
- The main causes of CI include age-related sinus node dysfunction, cardiac diseases, side effects of medication, autonomic dysfunction, and endocrine–metabolic disorders. Note that some cardiac medications, such as beta-blockers, may cause CI.
- Elderly people get their heart rates over 90 bpm more than 150 times a day. The need for rate response is surprising!
- Pacemaker patients mainly need rate response to manage their *activities of daily living* or ADL, which is a lower level of activity. The most common exertion performed by pacemaker patients is walking. While there are marathon runners, mountain climbers, and athletes with pacemakers, these are not the typical patients.
- The respiratory system and the cardiac system work together during exercise. Tidal volume refers to how much air we breathe in and out during inspiration and expiration. Respiratory rate refers to how many breaths we take per minute. Tidal volume times respiratory rate equals minute ventilation (MV).
- The amount of blood that the heart ejects during one cardiac cycle is the stroke volume. Stroke volume times the heart rate equals the cardiac output.
- When a person exercises, cardiac output is far more impacted by increased heart rate than increased stroke volume. Faster heart rates can increase cardiac output by 300%, but greater stroke volume can increase cardiac output only by about 50%. Thus, the pacemaker can influence cardiac output by adjusting rate in response to workload.
- Metabolic equivalents (METs) are units of work. Walking is about 1.0 MET, and shoveling snow would be 9.0 METs. Sedentary people exercise at around the range of 8–11 METs, while athletes might exercise at a range of 14–23 METs.
- METs can be closely correlated to MV.
- CI can be diagnosed in pacemaker patients using histograms showing cardiac activity and rate ranges. Counters and trends may also be useful.
- Not all pacemaker patients will tolerate rate response. Patients with rate-related angina, for example, may not do well with rate response. Some patients may have CI but not need rate response, for instance, those with very limited mobility.
- Rate-responsive pacing can also be called rate-adaptive pacing, rate-modulated pacing, or sensor-driven pacing. The pacing rate under rate response is called the sensor-indicated rate.
- The optimal sensor is one that is simple and easy to use, does not require a special lead, responds quickly, and is proportional to the degree of work. Unfortunately, the optimal sensor has yet to be found! No sensor available today is perfect, but all of them work very well.
- The world's first rate-responsive sensor was a piezoelectric activity sensor in the Activitrax pacemaker from Medtronic. It sensed vibrations.
- The next innovation in sensor technology was the accelerometer. It also used a piezoelectric crystal but it measured movement or acceleration in the anterior–posterior plane.
- Activity and accelerometer sensors could be fooled. For instance, an activity sensor would accelerate the pacing rate if the pacemaker can was tapped. An accelerometer could be fooled by a rocking chair. Both of these sensors had a quick onset of action and worked particularly well at low levels of activity.
- MV sensors measure transthoracic impedance to gauge MV. This sensor is very proportional to workload but it has a slower onset of action than the accelerometer or activity sensor. An MV sensor can be fooled by big arm movements.
- The only sensor that can be labeled physiologic according to the FDA is the MV sensor.
- The closed-loop stimulation (CLS) sensor is available only from Biotronik and it measures cardiac contractility. It offers proportional response to activity and can respond to emotional stress as well as physical exertion.

Continued

Continued

- The blended sensor uses input from two sensors (e.g., the MV sensor and an accelerometer) to offer rate response. The goal of a blended sensor is to use the advantages of different sensors. For example, this type of blended sensor offers the rapid onset of an accelerometer with the better performance at intense exercise of an MV sensor.
- Devices with blended sensors allow the clinician to program the sensors individually or together.
- Many devices offer a PASSIVE rate response setting that allows the clinician to see what the sensor-indicated rate would be before rate response is turned on. The PASSIVE mode can also be used to *test-drive* certain rate-responsive parameter settings.
- Other sensor technologies are not used much today: the QT interval and blood temperature are among those.
- There are several rate-responsive parameters that can be used to fine-tune rate response.

- Alternately, the clinician can use AUTO settings to allow the device to optimize rate response for a given patient.
- The maximum sensor rate (MSR) defines the fastest rate at which the pacemaker will pace in response to sensor input. It is often programmed to the same value as the maximum tracking rate, but it is independently programmable.
- Threshold is the sensor input level that triggers rate response. It can be adjusted.
- Reaction and recovery time govern how rapidly rate response ramps up to the MSR and decelerates back to the base rate. This is also programmable.
- Slope often confuses clinicians, but it is a programmable parameter that can adjust how fast the patient will be paced during rate response. In other words, for a patient doing a power walk, the clinician can determine how fast the rate-responsive rate for that level of activity should be.

Test your knowledge

1 Using the above histogram, what can you say about this dual-chamber pacemaker patient?
   A He is chronotropically incompetent.
   B He is chronotropically competent.
   C He does not need a pacemaker.
   D He has sick sinus syndrome.

2 Using the same histogram above, what does this mean in terms of whether or not the patient needs rate response?
   A He clearly needs rate response right now; turn on rate response at once!
   B He would probably benefit from rate response right now.
   C He doesn't need rate response right now, but he might in the future.
   D He doesn't need rate response now, and he most likely never will.

3 Which of the following has the most effect on cardiac output?
   A Stroke volume
   B Minute ventilation

   C Heart rate
   D Respiratory rate

4 Name two components used to calculate minute ventilation.
   A Respiratory rate times transthoracic impedance
   B Heart rate times respiratory rate
   C Cardiac contractility times heart rate
   D Respiratory rate times tidal volume

5 How does an MV sensor measure minute ventilation?
   A Transthoracic impedance
   B Cardiac contractility
   C Vibrations
   D Blood temperature

6 In many pacemakers, rate response is never turned on. Why is this sometimes the case?
   A Rate response adds complexity to the device (more parameters to program).

B Some patients do not tolerate rate response (for instance, patients with rate-related angina).

C Some patients do not need rate response (for instance, bedbound patients).

D Any of the above.

7 A 21-year-old very active male patient gets a pacemaker. What should be the clinician's first thought regarding rate response?

A Rate response should be programmed off.

B Rate response should be programmed on.

C He should be tested on a treadmill for CI before rate response decisions are made.

D It is unlikely this patient will ever need rate response.

8 Which feature would be most helpful for the clinician who would like to test rate response before programming it on and why?

A Histograms can show whether the patient is able to achieve appropriately high rates.

B SLOPE would adjust how aggressive pacing should be and determine the need for rate response.

C The AUTO feature would automatically program the right settings.

D The PASSIVE setting would show the sensor-indicated rates without actually pacing the patient at that rate.

9 Mr. Peterson has a DDDR pacemaker but he has been complaining of having a racing heart long after his exercise is over. Which parameter should be checked and possibly adjusted to help with this problem?

A Slope

B Recovery time

C Reaction time

D Threshold

10 Give an example of a blended sensor widely available in pacemakers today.

A Minute ventilation and accelerometer

B Minute ventilation and closed loop stimulation

C QT interval and closed-loop stimulation

D Activity sensor and blood temperature sensor (thermistor)

Reference

1 Manulli, M., Birchfield, D., Yakinov, K. *et al.* (1996) Do elderly pacemaker patients need rate adaptation—implications of daily heart rate behavior in normal adults. *PACE* **19** (pt 11), 681 (abstract)

CHAPTER 22

Special features

Learning objectives

- Describe the role of the dynamic AV delay and when it would be most appropriately used.
- Explain the objective to prolonging the AV delay in certain patients.
- Briefly explain how auto sensitivity works and describe a type of pacemaker patient who might benefit from this feature.
- Name the potential benefits of automatic capture algorithms and why they would be used.
- Describe a type of patient who would benefit from an automatic algorithm controlling the PVARP.
- State briefly how a mode switching algorithm works and what sort of patient would benefit from this feature.
- Explain how the *dispersion of refractoriness* relates to atrial overdrive pacing.
- State the main difference in rate hysteresis for single-chamber versus dual-chamber devices.
- Describe the search feature in rate hysteresis and why it can help intrinsic activity emerge.
- Name a situation in which rate smoothing would be beneficial and how it is programmed.

Introduction

There are several pacemaker manufacturers, all of which offer important and useful feature to manage specific challenges in pacing. For the purposes of

this book, special features related to capture will be treated in the next chapter. All of the other special features are included here. The best way to think of special features is to consider when these would best be used and the ideal patient for such features. Not all special features are appropriate for all patients. In fact, some of these special features should only ever be used for a small subset of patients. Despite the fact that these are not the mainstays of cardiac pacing, it is important for clinicians to know that these features exist and what they generally are intended to accomplish.

Features related to the AV delay

shorter AV delays

The AV delay has been discussed throughout this book, along with the fact that in the healthy heart, the natural PR interval shortens as the heart rate increases. To review this concept, imagine a pacemaker patient with a pacing interval programmed to 1000 ms (60 ppm). This patient has a sensed AV delay programmed to 200 ms. Thus, the AV delay takes up 20% of the whole cycle. Now, imagine that the patient's heart rate has increased to 100 ppm for a pacing interval of 600 ms. Allowing the sensed AV delay to stay 200 ms now means that the AV delay is more than one-third of the whole cycle! This would be disproportional and throw off the cardiac cycle by allowing a relatively long AV delay. Thus, pacemakers have found special features that allow them to better mimic this natural behavior by allowing the AV delay in the pacemaker to shorten with increasing rates. These features are called by different names by different companies (see **Table 22.1**).

The Nuts and Bolts of Implantable Device Therapy Pacemakers, First Edition. Tom Kenny.
© 2015 John Wiley & Sons, Ltd. Published 2015 by John Wiley & Sons, Ltd.

Table 22.1 All pacemaker companies offer special features that shorten the sensed AV delay automatically as the heart rate increases, but their names differ by manufacturer

Company	Name of feature
Biotronik	Dynamic AV delay
Boston Scientific	Dynamic AV delay
Sorin	AV delay
Medtronic	Rate-adaptive AV delay™
St. Jude Medical	Rate-responsive AV delay

Note that two manufacturers call this feature a name that may cause a clinician to think of sensor-driven pacing; this is not the case. These features are used to adjust the AV delay in response to higher pacing rates, which may be caused by atrial tracking (high intrinsic atrial rates) or by sensor-indicated rates.

Every pacing company offers this feature and they all are designed to achieve the same goal; however, the algorithms are different. Some shorten the AV delay by a specific number of milliseconds for every 1 bpm increase in rate. Some may only shorten the AV delay after a specific point. Others shorten the AV delay by a percentage value. Note that this feature applies to atrial tracking (DDD and VDD modes) and affects the sensed AV delay when rate response is either off or not in effect. When rate response is controlling the heart rate, this feature may also apply to the paced AV delay (at sensor-indicated rates) in DDDR and VDDR modes. This feature is only available in pacing states where the pacemaker paces the ventricle above the base rate (atrial sensing/ventricular pacing or atrial pacing/ventricular pacing states, the latter only occurring with sensor-driven pacing).

This automatic shortening of the sensed AV delay during atrial tracking works well in patients with heart block (any degree) and probably should not be used in pacemaker patients with normal conduction. A consideration in the use of this feature is that shortening the sensed AV delay likely increases the probability of right ventricular pacing. Thus, if the patient has the ability to conduct intrinsically, it is preferable in most cases to preserve the intact intrinsic conduction (and avoid unnecessary right ventricular pacing) than it is to shorten the AV delay. This is a bit of a balancing act (mimicking healthy cardiac behavior vs.

unnecessary right ventricular pacing), but that is the reasoning behind avoiding the use of this feature in individuals with normal conduction.

This feature can apply to the sensed AV delay or the paced AV delay. If these are programmed to different values, bear in mind that the decrements to the AV delay are applied systematically so that the sensed AV delay will never be as short as the paced AV delay. This is because the point at which they start to adapt is different.

Since any pacemaker features interlock and impact other features, it is useful to think of how this feature affects TARP. Recall that TARP is a calculated value made up of the paced AV delay plus the PVARP and that it defines the point at which 2:1 block occurs. As an example, let's take a patient with a paced AV delay of 200 ms and a PVARP programmed to 300 ms. This patient has a TARP of 500 ms, which means that 2:1 block will occur at 120 bpm (500 ms *translates* to 120 bpm). Leaving the PVARP at 300 ms, the clinician now programs a sensed AV delay of 150 ms (shorter than the paced AV delay), and dynamic AV delay. This particular feature allows the sensed AV delay to get as short as 100 ms. With this particular scenario, the TARP now changes (even though PVARP stays the same). At the shortest value of the sensed AV delay, TARP would be 400 ms (100 + 300 ms), which means 2:1 block would not occur until 150 bpm. This shows a good way that the clinician can *open the Wenckebach Window* on upper-rate behavior by using this special feature. Thus, dynamic AV delays offer better upper-rate behaviors. In fact, its main purpose is to delay 2:1 block.

Longer AV delays

Other special features are designed to prolong the AV delay in an effort to encourage intrinsic ventricular activity and, in so doing, reduce right ventricular pacing. All manufacturers offer these features, but they have different names and different algorithms by company (see **Table 22.2**).

All of these special features extend the AV delay with the goal of encouraging intrinsic conduction and, in so doing, decreasing the likelihood of right ventricular pacing. Thus, these are the counterpoint to the dynamic AV delays that shorten as rate increases. Here, the AV delays extend to give the ventricles maximum opportunity to depolarize and contract on their own.

Table 22.2 All pacemaker manufacturers offer at least one feature designed to discourage right ventricular pacing by prolonging the AV delay

Company	Name of features
Biotronik	AV hysteresis
Boston Scientific	AV Search Hysteresis™
	RythmIQ™
Sorin	DDD/Automatic Mode Conversion (AMC)
	SafeR™
Medtronic	AV Search™
	Managed Ventricular Pacing™ or MVP™
St. Jude Medical	AutoIntrinsic Conduction Search™ (AICS)
	Ventricular Intrinsic Preference (VIP)

Some of these names use the term *hysteresis*, which refers to a prolonged pacing interval; AV hysteresis should thus be thought of as a prolonged AV interval.

The optimal candidates for this feature are patients with intermittent first- or second-degree AV block; it is not a good feature for patients with complete or third-degree heart block (because the patient does not have the ability to conduct and no amount of AV delay is going to avoid ventricular pacing).

In the case of this special feature, there are some interesting variations among the manufacturers' algorithms. The DDD/AMC and SafeR™ features from Sorin and the MVP™ from Medtronic offer a similar approach and it differs from what the other features offer. In this feature, the dual-chamber pacemaker works as a functional AAI or AAIR pacemaker. An AAI or AAIR device paces and senses in the atrium but does not pace the ventricle. Assuming the patient had intermittent lower-degree AV block, as long as the patient's conduction was intact, the functional single-chamber atrial pacing mode would remain. This would result in two main pacing state activity patterns: either sensed atrial activity/sensed ventricular activity (no pacing) or paced atrial activity/sensed ventricular activity (atrial pacing conducting over the AV node to the ventricles). This would work well, but if the patient's intermittent AV block set in, the pacemaker would switch modes and go to DDD or

DDDR, allowing it to pace the ventricle. The device would stay in DDD or DDDR mode until a periodic check confirmed that AV conduction had been restored; at that point, the pacemaker would switch back to functional AAI or AAIR pacing until conduction was lost again. Thus, these features could be thought of as function AAI or AAIR pacing with ventricular backup.

AAI or AAIR mode is actually an excellent pacing mode for patients with intact conduction because it allows for intrinsic conduction and therefore avoids right ventricular pacing. The main drawback to implanting atrial single-chamber pacemakers is that most physicians hesitate to leave a patient completely without ventricular pacing support. If the patient has intermittent AV conduction—even very infrequently—there are going to be times when ventricular pacing is a necessity. This feature offers a solution in that it allows as much single-chamber atrial pacing as possible but provides ventricular pacing when needed.

When discussing these features, be aware of yet another terminology pitfall—the use of the term *mode switching*. Mode switching, as discussed earlier in this book in upper-rate behaviors, is an algorithm that turns off atrial tracking in the presence of high intrinsic atrial rates and thus switches the pacing mode. These features may also change the pacing mode, and they are sometimes also called *mode switching*. Do not mix up these types of mode switches. The classic *mode switching* involves turning off atrial tracking in the presence of atrial tachyarrhythmias (AT); this is the older term and is very widely used. For the sake of terminology, I prefer to call this behavior *switching modes* or mode conversion and the older feature *mode switching*.

Another terminology pitfall occurs with MVP™ from Medtronic, which is the special feature described earlier. In Medtronic's terminology—and on their programmer—MVP is called a mode. To activate MVP, the clinician has to go to the *mode* section and program the *MVP mode*. Technically, MVP is not a pacing mode at all; it's a feature. But clinicians will hear it called a mode. Do not let this confuse you—MVP is simply a feature that is programmed from the mode page of the programmer.

AV Search Hysteresis is another algorithm aimed at encouraging AV conduction and thereby

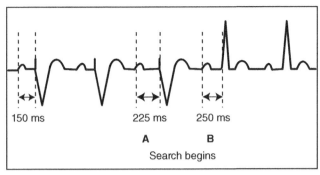

AV delay = 150 ms
AV increase = 50%
AV search interval = 32 cycles

Figure 22.1 This is an example of AV Search Hysteresis from Boston Scientific. In this case, the sensed AV delay is programmed to 150 ms. In every 32 beats, it is increased by 50% (50% of 150 = 75), resulting a new AV delay of 225 ms. This longer AV delay will be used for 32 cycles. The first time it is used, the pacemaker paces the ventricle at 225 ms (see A). The second time this longer AV delay is used, intrinsic conduction occurs at 200 ms (see B). This new, longer AV delay will be used until ventricular pacing occurs, at which time the originally programmed value of 150 ms is restored. After the next 32 cycles, the AV delay will be extended to 225 ms again. Note that on an electrogram with markers, an HY would appear indicating hysteresis.

reducing ventricular pacing. At programmable intervals, the AV delay automatically increases so it can *search* for intrinsic conduction. A better way of describing this is that the AV delay is periodically extended so it can *wait for* any intrinsic conduction that might occur. If intrinsic ventricular activity occurs, the AV delay remains lengthened to allow as much of this intrinsic conduction as possible. On the other hand, if the AV delay waits for intrinsic conduction and none occurs, it paces the ventricle and resumes the shorter AV delay until the next *search cycle* occurs. This type of feature is available in several different pacemakers and is available in DDD, DDDR, VDD, and VDDR modes. The AV delay increase during these search cycles increased either by a fixed millisecond value or by a percentage value (see **Figure 22.1**).

Clinician considerations

Pacing clinicians see lots of different devices every single day and they are not the only healthcare professionals involved in the care of these patients or programming their devices. As a result of this, clinicians must be mindful that many of the dual-chamber pacemaker patients at the clinic may have certain special features turned on. As a result, the AV delay value seen on the ECG may not necessarily match the programmed value of the AV delay

as stated in the parameter settings. Just as clinicians can often see different-than-base-rate pacing in a pacemaker patient that is not inappropriate, it is also possible to see shorter- or longer-than-programmed AV delay intervals!

Features related to sensitivity and pacemaker output

Automatic sensing

Pacemakers today all offer automatic sensing, that is, the device itself is able to monitor and measure intrinsic activity and self-program itself to appropriate sensing values. Pacing clinicians should know how to do this manually, but this is no longer a clinical necessity. Automatic sensitivity settings save clinical time and may protect patients because changes in sensing thresholds will be noted by the device and settings adjusted appropriately without the need for an in-office follow-up visit (see **Table 22.3**). Although these algorithms have different names, they all function in essentially the same way:

• The intrinsic signal is measured.
• The sensitivity setting is adjusted accordingly.

Automatic sensing is a practical feature that can be used in just about any pacemaker patient. While clinicians will want to program this on for most

Table 22.3 All pacemaker manufacturers offer automatic sensitivity setting that measures intrinsic atrial and/or ventricular signals and adjusts the sensitivity setting appropriately and automatically

Company	Name of feature
Biotronik	Auto Sensitivity Control
Boston Scientific	Auto Sense
Sorin	Auto Sense
Medtronic	Sensing Assurance™
St. Jude Medical	Sensibility™

patients, they should bear in mind that (like any special feature) automatic sensing does have its drawbacks. For one thing, it can be *fooled* by premature ventricular contractions (PVCs), which often have substantially larger-amplitude signals than regular cardiac activity. A PVC may cause automatic sensing to readjust to this large signal and subsequently miss later more normal-amplitude signals. Thus, clinicians may want to avoid this algorithm in patients who experience a great deal of PVCs. For such patients, the clinician can program *fixed sensitivity* and manually assess waveforms and set a fixed sensitivity setting.

While all companies offer this important feature and it is conceptually the same in all devices, there are the usual nuances among companies in terms of how it is programmed and, in particular, how often it checks intrinsic signals to adjust sensitivity values. Note that auto sensitivity features can only measure intrinsic signals when the device is sensing—if the device paces constantly, there will be no intrinsic activity to measure. Thus, pacemaker-dependent patients or patients who are paced very frequently do not need this feature, since their devices do not do much, if any, sensing.

Auto sensitivity is available in single-chamber and dual-chamber pacemakers.

Pacemaker outputs

The pacemaker pulse is defined by two parameters: the pulse amplitude (how big the waveform is) and the pulse width or pulse duration (how long the signal lasts). A pacemaker patient has a measurable capture threshold, that is, the size the output pulse must be in order to reliably capture the heart. The capture threshold is defined by those same two

parameters: pulse amplitude and pulse width. Once the clinician knows the patient's capture threshold, programming the output pulse involves a bit of a balancing act. On the one hand, the clinician wants to be sure to program the pacemaker's output to be more than sufficient to reliably capture the heart. After all, capture is what pacing is all about and the clinician wants to eliminate any margin for error. It is well known that capture thresholds fluctuate throughout the course of the day and with certain activities, medications, disease progression, and other factors, so there has to be some *cushion* built into the pacemaker output to allow for these variations. On the other hand, the pacemaker is run on a battery that has a finite capacity; the less energy that is wasted, the longer the device will last. Thus, clinicians constantly face the tug-of-war between programming sufficiently generous safety margins for the output pulse (to assure reliable capture) and energy-efficient output parameters (to assure longer device life and fewer replacement surgeries for the patient).

The patient's capture threshold values are lowest at implant, then increase markedly, and finally decrease to a plateau in about 6–8 weeks. This *acute-to-chronic* phase is characterized by very high thresholds; it is smart to program the device to relatively high output settings to accommodate this transition. The patient's *real* or chronic thresholds do not level off until about 6–8 weeks and then will remain at or near those levels for the life of the device, barring any unusual events (such as disease progression or medications that may alter the thresholds). Keep the *acute-to-chronic* threshold transitions in mind when thinking about device follow-up. The pacemaker is programmed at implant and the output values (pulse amplitude and pulse width) are set. If the patient stays overnight at the hospital, the device may be checked before discharge. Even if there is a predischarge check, it will not be a real *follow-up* with reassessment of device thresholds. Normally, the patient goes home and comes back to the clinic in about 2 weeks for a wound check to make sure no infection has set in. At the wound check, most clinicians will not reevaluate pacing thresholds because the patient is in the midst of the acute-to-chronic threshold transition and thresholds will not have *settled down* to their chronic values. The real first follow-up will occur somewhere around 8–12 weeks postimplant, when the clinician will reevaluate threshold values.

Looking at this process in terms of energy efficiency, it is clear that in the first 8–12 weeks after implant, a lot of energy is wasted in the name of patient safety. The device is programmed to high outputs to be sure capture is maintained during acute-to-chronic threshold change, but most likely, a lot of that energy was unnecessary—and wasted.

Threshold is lowest at implant, then rises upward, and then comes back down partway to about twice what it was at implant. Attaching some round numbers to this example, let's say the patient returns to the clinic at three months after implant with a chronic pacing threshold of 1 V at 0.5 ms. The pacing output pulse should be programmed with a safety margin of two to three times the chronic pacing threshold. In my experience, most physicians would program this device to an output of 2.5 or 3 V at 0.5 ms. The reason is that although pacing experts and the literature allow for a safety margin of two or three times the patient's pacing threshold, most clinicians simply do not feel right at anything lower than 2.5 times.

The purpose of this generous safety margin is simple: patient safety. Pacing thresholds, even chronic pacing thresholds, change all of the time in unpredictable ways. Programming the previously described device to 2.5 V at 0.5 ms is simply a way to help manage these unpredictable deviations in threshold. The problem with this method is that it wastes energy. A pacing output pulse of 2.5 V at 0.5 ms will likely reliably capture the patient's heart every time, but it will also very likely waste a lot of energy most of the time. In fact, programming a safety margin is a way of deliberately wasting energy in the name of patient safety.

Automatic capture algorithms are special features (offered by all manufacturers) aimed at providing reliable and safe capture without wasting energy. They do this by adjusting the pacemaker output frequently so that the patient gets the extra energy only when he or she needs it (see **Table 22.4**).

All of these devices measure the patient's thresholds on an ongoing basis and adjust pacemaker output pulses accordingly. If the threshold increases, the output goes up; if the threshold decreases, the output goes down. When and how

Table 22.4 All pacemaker manufacturers offer at least one feature for automatic capture

Company	Name of features
Biotronik	Active Capture Control™ or ACC™
Boston Scientific	Automatic Capture™
Sorin	V Autothreshold
Medtronic	Atrial/Ventricular Capture Management™ (ACM/VCM)
St. Jude Medical	AutoCapture™ (ventricular) ACap Confirm™ (atrial)

The goal of these features (which work differently) is to assure reliable capture (patient safety) without wasting energy. Note that St. Jude Medical has two distinct features for this function, depending on whether it is used in the atrium or ventricle.

they measure the patient's thresholds vary by algorithm. The main benefit of automatic capture algorithm is to assure patient safety while saving battery energy.

Capture algorithms are so important that they will be discussed in more detail in the next chapter.

Features related to refractory periods

Postventricular atrial refractory periods

The postventricular atrial refractory period (PVARP) is an important timing cycle in dual-chamber pacemakers in that it can affect the point at which a patient will enter 2:1 block in the presence of high intrinsic atrial rates. Automatic PVARP adjustments are available in certain pacemakers (see **Table 22.5**).

These features automatically shorten the PVARP value as the patient's intrinsic atrial rate increases. In fact, the Sorin algorithm—which is unique among these—automatically adjusts the PVARP in all cases such that a clinician never programs any PVARP value but rather allows the device to regulate its length based on the patient's atrial rate. This WARAD feature can be thought of as a dynamic PVARP or a self-adjusting PVARP value.

This feature works well in patients who exhibit a lot of atrial sensed/ventricular paced activity above the base rate; in other words, it works well in patients who have high intrinsic atrial rates and

Table 22.5 Certain pacemaker companies offer features to automatically adjust PVARP in dual-chamber pacemakers

Company	Name of features
Biotronik	AUTO PVARP
Boston Scientific	Dynamic PVARP
Sorin	Window of Atrial Rate Acceleration Detection (WARAD)
Medtronic	Auto PVARP
St. Jude Medical	Rate-responsive PVARP

These features can be useful for upper-rate behaviors. The term used by St. Jude Medical alludes to rate response, but this has nothing to do with sensor-driven pacing—it is a PVARP that responds to the patient's *intrinsic* atrial rate.

experience atrial tracking. Patients who experience nearly constant atrial pacing would not benefit from this feature.

The main concern with automatic PVARP-shortening algorithms is that, in certain patients, a retrograde P-wave could occur and be sensed (outside of the now-shortened PVARP interval). This retrograde P-wave could then launch a pacemaker-mediated tachycardia (PMT). For patients susceptible to PMTs, the PVARP is often carefully programmed to a length sufficient to prevent PMTs. Automatically shortening the PVARP can *undo* that safety net and cause the patient to experience a PMT. Thus, some clinicians will opt not to use this feature for patients with known susceptibility to PMTs and/or known retrograde conduction.

PMT prevention algorithms

All pacemaker manufacturers offer specialty algorithms in dual-chamber pacemakers aimed at preventing PMT by preventing the tracking of retrograde P-waves that might occur following a PVC or premature atrial contraction (PAC) (see **Table 22.6**).

These PMT prevention algorithms work somewhat differently; for example, Sorin's WARAD feature handles this (along with shortening the PVARP). Essentially all PMT detection algorithms will increase the PVARP interval for one cycle after a PVC or PAC is detected. Bear in mind, all pacemakers define a PVC as the second of two consecutive ventricular events without an intervening P-wave

Table 22.6 PMT prevention algorithms are available in dual-chamber devices from all pacemaker manufacturers

Company	Name of features
Biotronik	PVC Response
Boston Scientific	PVARP after a PVC/PAC
Sorin	Window of Atrial Rate Acceleration Detection (WARAD)
Medtronic	PVC Response
St. Jude Medical	A Pace on PVC

Table 22.7 Special features to terminate PMTs are available from all manufacturers

Company	Name of features
Biotronik	PMT Termination
Boston Scientific	PMT Termination
Sorin	PMT Intervention
Medtronic	PMT Intervention
St. Jude Medical	PMT Termination

(this is a sensed ventricular event following either a paced or sensed ventricular event). When a PVC is identified, the PVARP is prolonged for a single cycle to prevent a PMT. The algorithms differ in terms of how long the PVARP is extended.

PMT Termination algorithms

All manufacturers offer special features to stop a PMT once it has gotten started (see **Table 22.7**). All of these algorithms work by identifying a PMT and then extending the PVARP interval for one cycle. This prolonged PVARP period will cause a retrograde P-wave to *fall into the PVARP* and not be tracked, thus breaking the PMT.

These algorithms differ in terms of how they define and identify a PMT and when and how long the PVARP timing cycle is extended. A good example of a PMT Termination algorithm in action appears in Figure 22.2 (Boston Scientific device).

In most patients, the PMT occurs at the programmed maximum tracking rate or MTR (see **Figure 22.2**), but it is possible that the PMT could occur at lower rates as well. In some PMT Termination algorithms, it may be possible to program the PMT rate to a lower-than-MTR value. For example, if MTR is 120 ppm and a PMT rate was

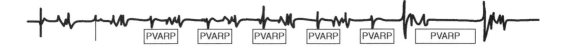

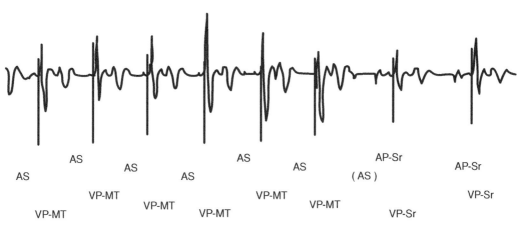

Figure 22.2 A PMT occurs, as evidenced by atrial tracking at the maximum tracking rate (shown on the annotations as MT). After observing this behavior for 16 cycles (not all cycles of PMT are shown on this strip), the device identifies it as a PMT and then prolongs the PVARP for one cycle. This extended PVARP interval allows a retrograde P-wave to *fall into the PVARP* and thus breaks the PMT.

programmed to anything above 110 ppm, the algorithm would identify consistent atrial tracking for a programmable number of cycles at 111 ppm or more as a PMT.

Features related to AT

AT is a broad term that includes all intrinsic high-rate atrial activity, including, but not limited to, atrial fibrillation (AF). AF is a serious arrhythmia that can be challenging to treat and, the fact is, no pacemaker can treat AF or even AT. However, since pacemaker patients may experience AT or AF, pacemakers have to be able to deal with them. This has led to numerous special features that are designed to prevent AT, to avoid tracking AT or AF, or to suppress AF. The goal of these algorithms is to preserve AV synchrony during normal sinus rhythm as much as possible.

Mode switching

All manufacturers offer some form of special feature to help turn off atrial tracking in the presence of an AT (see **Table 22.8**). These features are

Table 22.8 Special features for mode switching are available from all manufacturers

Company	Name of features
Biotronik	Auto Mode Conversion
	Mode Switch
Boston Scientific	Atrial Tachy Response (ATR)
Sorin	Mode Switch
Medtronic	Mode Switch
St. Jude Medical	Auto Mode Switch (AMS)

particularly important because AT can develop in pacemaker patients who did not have it when they were first implanted with a device. The majority of pacemaker patients have some form of sick sinus syndrome and most of them will eventually develop some form of atrial rhythm disorder during their lifetime. This may be relatively mild at first (such as paroxysmal AF, which is intermittent and can be mild), but it can progress to more severe forms (such as chronic AF).

When an AT develops, a dual-chamber pacemaker will try to track the atrium and pace the

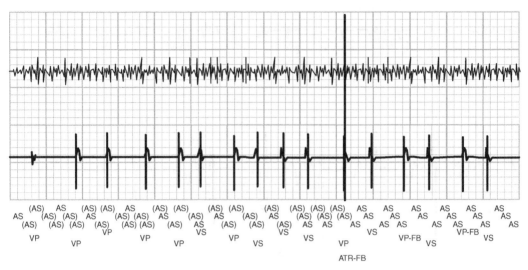

Figure 22.3 This is a stored electrogram showing mode switching in a Boston Scientific device. Notice the atrial fibrillation on the atrial channel (top) and the irregular but rapid ventricular paced response on the ventricular channel (bottom). Mode switching occurred at the vertical line, essentially disabling atrial tracking. The atrial fibrillation continues, but now, ventricular pacing occurs at a slower, more regular rate.

ventricle to try to preserve 1:1 AV synchrony. During AF episodes, where the rate can go far beyond 300 or 400 bpm, the pacemaker is stopped by the MTR. But during AT and *slower* AT, the pacemaker may try to pace the ventricles at very fast ventricular rates in an effort to maintain 1:1 AV synchrony. When the intrinsic atrial rate exceeds a certain programmable limit, the pacemaker can be programmed using any of the features described in Table 22.7 to turn off atrial tracking temporarily. True, this will eliminate any chance of maintaining 1:1 AV synchrony, but it prevents rapid pacing of the ventricle. These features are typically described as mode switching because turning off atrial tracking changes to the mode. Pacemakers switch from DDD or DDDR pacing to DDI or DDIR pacing, which will appear on the ECG as functional VVI or VVIR. Note that some algorithms automatically activate rate response (if it was not on previously) during the mode switch, for instance, if the patient was programmed to DDD pacing and mode switching occurred, the mode switch would be to DDIR pacing (which would look like functional VVIR) pacing.

This mode switch occurs automatically and is temporary; when the patient's intrinsic atrial rate goes back to normal (or slower than normal), the mode switches back to its previously programmed parameter settings. Mode switching is obviously only available in dual-chamber pacemakers. All of these special features to temporarily disable atrial tracking involve several programmable parameters, which may be treated slightly differently by manufacturer:

- The cutoff rate (sometimes called the trigger rate or the atrial tachycardia detection rate or mode switching rate) defining an AT.
- The number of beats and/or duration of time the AT episode must last before the mode switches.
- In some cases, the clinician can specify the mode (e.g., DDDR to VVIR or DDDR to DDIR).

For example, the clinician may say that mode switching should occur whenever intrinsic atrial activity occurs at a rate above 150 bpm for 16 beats or more.

Atrial tracking will be restored when the AT resolves, but different companies handle this in different ways. In some cases, atrial tracking is restored when the AT rate falls below its programmed trigger rate for a specific number of beats; in other algorithms, the atrial rate must be below the MTR or maximum sensor rate (MSR) in order to restore the originally programmed mode. An example of mode switching appears in **Figure 22.3**.

Mode switching is not appropriate for all patients. It is ideal for patients with intermittent episodes of AT or AF and second-degree or higher AV block. Many pacemaker patients are known to have AT or AF; in some cases, it will be evident from electrograms or diagnostic data. While AT and AF can cause symptoms, even severe symptoms, it is important to note that symptoms are not a reliable indicator of AT. Symptoms do not necessarily correlate with the severity of this arrhythmia; in other words, patients with mild AT may have severe and even debilitating symptoms, while patients with more severe forms of AF may have mild symptoms. Some AF patients may even be asymptomatic. Thus, rely on the pacemaker diagnostics and electrograms to assess AF in pacemaker patients rather than their symptoms.

One concern with mode switching is the actual pacemaker behavior during the transition. For example, a patient with a dual-chamber pacemaker set to a base rate of 60 ppm is experiencing high intrinsic atrial rates of about 140 bpm. The pacemaker tried to track this rate as it ramped up, but it bumped into the MTR speed limit (120 ppm) and is now pacing the ventricle at 120 ppm. Once the intrinsic atrial rate hit 150 bpm, the mode switch algorithm was activated and the device turned off atrial tracking. Now, it paces in the non-atrial-tracking mode *at the programmed base rate*! This means that the ventricle would go from being paced at 120 ppm to 60 ppm in a single cycle. This is a very abrupt transition that many patients perceive as quite uncomfortable and unsettling. Some mode switch algorithms offer an interim or mode switch rate that offers a somewhat higher base rate for mode switch episodes. For example, this mode switch base rate might be set to 90 ppm. (Note that if the sensor is controlling the pacing rate in DDDR mode, during a mode switch episode to DDIR, the patient will go to the sensor-indicated rate, which might be higher than the base rate if the patient is active.) This slightly elevated rate helps make the transition less steep and can help to make up for the loss of atrial kick the patient experienced during the AT episode.

Other atrial arrhythmia management features

All of the companies offer some variation of the mode switching algorithm in the presence of AT, but some companies offer additional special features for dealing with AT as well (see **Table 22.9**).

Table 22.9 Some of the manufacturers offer additional special features to help manage atrial tachyarrhythmias

Company	Name of features
Biotronik	None
Boston Scientific	Ventricular Rate Regulation™ (VRR)
Sorin	None
Medtronic	Conducted AF Response
St. Jude Medical	None

Table 22.10 Two manufacturers offer special features with the objective of preventing or suppressing episodes of AF

Company	Name of features
Biotronik	None
Boston Scientific	None
Sorin	None
Medtronic	Atrial Pacing Preference™ or APP™ Post Mode Switch Overdrive™ or PMOP™
St. Jude Medical	AF Suppression™

Ventricular Rate LRegulation™ or VRR from Boston Scientific is designed to regulate the patient's ventricular rate during mode switching episodes. As stated earlier, mode switching episodes can be accompanied by a sharp and abrupt decrease in rate. VRR was designed to control the ventricular rate so that it does not decrease all at once. This is a unique feature to Boston Scientific.

Features to prevent or suppress AF

AF can sometimes be prevented or suppressed, and two manufacturers offer special features aimed at managing AF in this way (see **Table 22.10**). To understand the concept behind these features, it is necessary to understand a little bit about AF. An episode of AF is typically preceded by a multitude of PACs. In the context of these PACs, the patient's intrinsic cardiac cycle length is changing, and with these constant cycle length changes, the patient's physiologic refractory periods are also changing. This condition is sometimes described as the *dispersion of refractoriness*, meaning that the refractoriness of the cardiac tissue is not acting in a coherent, predictable way. One theory about the origin of AF is that it starts with the dispersion of refractoriness. Thus, these algorithms were designed to maintain consistent atrial activity, which, in turn, would eliminate the dispersion of refractoriness. In other words, if the pacemaker could pace the atrium fast enough to avoid these PACs and keep the physiologic refractory periods consistent, this, in turn, would decrease the dispersion of refractoriness and AF would not develop. The algorithms described in Table 22.10 are designed to *overdrive* the atrium by pacing it in such a way to prevent or suppress AF.

Overdrive pacing at a rate of 100 ppm effectively prevents AF, but it has a couple of important drawbacks. Overdrive atrial pacing at 100 ppm paces the patient at 100 ppm as often as AF is likely, which for some patients is all of the time. Even if the patient could tolerate atrial pacing/ventricular pacing at 100 ppm during the day, this is likely to be much too fast for rest at night. Moreover, this kind of rapid pacing drained the battery. Overdrive pacing did indeed work at preventing AF, but its drawbacks limited its applicability in the real world.

The AF Suppression™ algorithm from St. Jude Medical allows atrial overdrive pacing at rates only slightly faster than the patient's own atrial rate. In other words, rather than overdrive atrial pacing at 100 ppm, the algorithm paced only 5–10 ppm above the patient's intrinsic atrial rate. Thus, this algorithm did not overdrive pace all of the time (only in the presence of intrinsic atrial activity), and when it did pace the atrium, it kept the overdrive pacing rates as low as possible. This offered a method of suppressing AF. It should be noted that the AF Suppression™ algorithm works better for dual-chamber pacemaker patients with paroxysmal AF rather than persistent (or chronic) AF.

Features related to rate

One of the challenges in pacing therapy is to accommodate the fact that a healthy heart changes its rate constantly over the course of the day. Besides rate response, pacemakers have added new special features to help pacemakers more closely mimic the behavior of the healthy heart.

Sleep rates
In the early days of pacing, patients had round-the-clock fixed-rate pacing at the programmed base rate. While patients might not

Table 22.11 Hysteresis is available from all manufacturers

Company	Name of features
Biotronik	Hysteresis
Boston Scientific	Rate hysteresis
	Rate search hysteresis
Sorin	Hysteresis
Medtronic	Hysteresis
	Sleep function
St. Jude Medical	Hysteresis
	Rest rate

have minded being paced at 70 ppm during the day, this made sleep very difficult! The healthy heart slows down markedly during sleep, and there are special pacing features aimed at helping paced patients benefit from slower rates during sleep or profound rest (see **Table 22.11**).

An early version of a sleep rate was offered by a company known as Intermedics (since acquired by Guidant, which in turn was acquired by Boston Scientific). This algorithm worked by clock time, so that the clinicians set the patient's bedtime (when the pacemaker decreased its rate) and wake time (when the pacemaker increased its rate). The problems with this algorithm were immediately apparent: patients who did not maintain regular sleep/wake cycles or who traveled to different time zones experienced problems with their pacing rate. St. Jude Medical borrowed from this concept but instead of using clock time, they based rest on accelerometer data. When the accelerometer suggested that the patient was resting or asleep, the device lowers the rate to the programmable rest rate; when the accelerometer found the patient was even slightly active, the rest rate was discontinued. This rest rate could accommodate variations in the sleep/wake cycle.

These features are particularly helpful for patients with intermittent sinus bradycardia and, in particular, those who are aware of their pacemakers when they try to sleep. Some patients report sleep difficulties that they attribute to their pacing.

Rate hysteresis
Rate hysteresis functions can be considered a form of *sleep rate*, but since they work according to a different algorithm, they will be discussed here.

All manufacturers offer some form of rate hysteresis (see **Table 22.11**), which can lower rate during sleep. The goal of hysteresis is to allow the patient's own intrinsic rate to drop below the base rate (or sensor-indicated rate) during rest or sleep. Hysteresis must first be programmed on and then it must be activated, either by the patient's intrinsic activity or following a programmed *search* interval.

Rate hysteresis is available in single- and dual-chamber pacemakers. In a single-chamber pacemaker, rate hysteresis works by prolonging the escape interval following intrinsic activity. For example, in a VVI pacemaker, the pacemaker will automatically prolong the escape interval when it senses intrinsic ventricular activity. If intrinsic activity below the base rate but above the hysteresis rate is detected, it is allowed to prevail (and pacing is inhibited) until the intrinsic activity falls below the programmed hysteresis rate. For example, a VVI or VVIR pacemaker programmed to a base rate of 70 ppm and a hysteresis rate of 50 bpm would allow intrinsic ventricular activity of 60 bpm to inhibit ventricular pacing. However, if intrinsic ventricular activity fell below 50 bpm, then base-rate pacing would resume.

Dual-chamber hysteresis works a little differently. Remember that dual-chamber pacemakers time themselves from the *atrial channel*. Therefore, a DDD or DDDR pacemaker applies the hysteresis rate to the atrial channel. Thus, with a base rate of 60 ppm and a hysteresis rate of 50 bpm, the pacemaker would allow an intrinsic atrial rate of 55 bpm to inhibit atrial pacing, but if the intrinsic atrial rate fell below 50 bpm, then base-rate pacing would resume. The key differentiator between DDD and VVI hysteresis is that the former works on the atrial channel, while the latter works on the ventricular channel. In fact, a good way to think about dual-chamber hysteresis is that it's single-chamber *atrial* hysteresis. This makes sense considering how single- and dual-chamber pacing is timed.

Rate hysteresis is activated by a sensed event; dual-chamber rate hysteresis is thus activated by a sensed atrial event. Hysteresis remains in effect as long as the sensed activity occurs. Should a sensed event fail to occur (i.e., occur below the hysteresis rate), base-rate pacing resumes. Since base-rate pacing may make it difficult for sensed events to occur, rate hysteresis may incorporate a search function, which periodically extends the escape interval (VA interval) for a programmable number of cycles at programmable intervals to *search* for intrinsic activity. For instance, if the patient is being paced in a DDD device at 60 ppm, intrinsic atrial activity at 55 bpm can only emerge during a search. If it is detected, it is allowed to control the device unless and until it falls below the hysteresis rate. Examples of successful and unsuccessful hysteresis searches are illustrated in **Figure 22.4**.

Rate smoothing

Rate-smoothing features are designed to prevent abrupt beat-to-beat rate changes. The healthy heart changes rate frequently over the course of the day, but heart rate changes tend to ramp up gradually and decelerate gradually. Pacemakers are not always so accommodating, so some manufacturers have developed algorithms to address this situation (see **Table 22.12**).

Earlier in the chapter on upper-rate behaviors, the problem of 2:1 block was discussed where the pacemaker might transition from atrial tracking/ventricular pacing at the MTR to 2:1 block and base-rate pacing—in a single cycle. To attach numbers to this situation, imagine that the patient is being paced in the ventricle at around 120 ppm and, then reaching 2:1 block, the pacemaker goes to the 60 ppm base rate, all in one beat (about 1 s). The goal of rate smoothing is to *smooth out* that kind of transition by imposing some interim rates. For example, rate smoothing allows the clinician to program the maximum amount that the ventricular rate can change in a single beat, stated as a percentage. A clinician who programs rate smoothing on and sets a value of 9% is stating that in each beat, the rate can only decelerate 10%, that is, 12 ppm each time (10% of 120 = 12). The pacemaker will still drive the rate down to the base rate, and it will just stairstep each time by 12 ppm (or whatever the programmed value dictates). It is easy to see how this feature got its name: it *smooths* the rate transition.

Rate smoothing also works to *smooth out* rate acceleration. For example, if a DDD patient is being paced at the base rate but suddenly has intrinsic atrial rates of 100 bpm, the rate smooth feature will only allow the rate to accelerate according to its

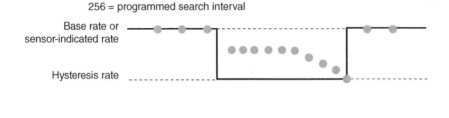

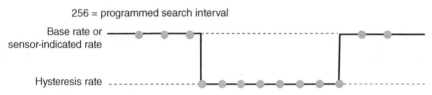

Figure 22.4 This figure was designed based on Boston Scientific's Search Hysteresis for a dual-chamber pacemaker programmed to a base rate of 60 ppm and a hysteresis rate of 50 bpm with 8-cycle search intervals programmed every 256 cycles. In the first example, intrinsic activity occurred in the gap between the lower rate limit (LRL) and the hysteresis rate. It took over the pacemaker until an intrinsic event occurred at the hysteresis rate (50 bpm) and base-rate pacing resumes. This is a *successful search*. In the other example, the search cycle commences at the 256th beat, but no intrinsic activity occurs in the offset between base rate and hysteresis rate. For eight beats, the pacemaker paces at the hysteresis rate (50 ppm) and then resumes normal base-rate pacing. This might be considered an *unsuccessful search* in that no intrinsic activity could be found.

Table 22.12 Most manufacturers offer special features with the objective of preventing abrupt beat-to-beat rate changes

Company	Name of features
Biotronik	Rate fading
Boston Scientific	Rate smoothing
Sorin	Rate smoothing
Medtronic	Rate smoothing
St. Jude Medical	None

programmed intervals. While rate smoothing for rapid rate decelerations is generally a very helpful feature, using rate smoothing for acceleration can delay sharp rate increases. This may be less beneficial for those patients who need rapid rate acceleration. Newer iterations of rate-smoothing special features now allow for independent programming of rate smoothing for acceleration and deceleration (they can be independently programmed on or off and different percentage values used for each).

Another good example of rate smoothing in action can occur during AT (see **Figure 22.5**).

A brief note on pacemaker rates

The bottom line for device clinicians is that pacemakers can have multiple rates: base rate, MTR, MSR, sensor-indicated rate, rest rate, and a hysteresis rate! It is no wonder that clinicians looking at paced ECGs often ask the question: Why is this pacemaker not pacing at the base rate?

While active patients can benefit from these rate-modifying special features, when the patient is in the hospital for device implantation, the clinician really ought to only program two rates: the base rate and the MTR. Those are the two most important rates and they are all that the patient needs right after implant. The other rates are useful once the patient is up and about, because they serve to fine-tune pacing therapy. Base rate and MTR *define dual-chamber pacing therapy*; the other rates help fine-tune and improve it.

Features related to neurocardiogenic syncope

Neurocardiogenic syncope, also known as vasovagal syncope or neutrally mediate syncope, is characterized by an abrupt drop in heart rate. Special pacemaker features to address this will

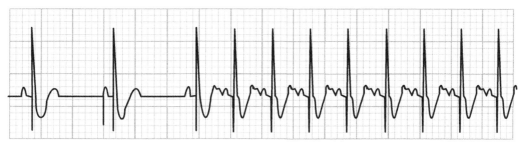

Atrial flutter without rate smoothing

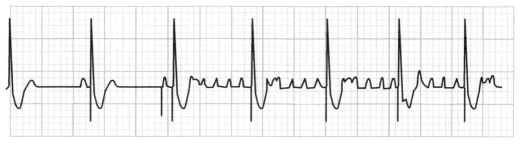

Atrial flutter with rate smoothing

Figure 22.5 Rate smoothing in a patient with atrial flutter. Note that as the rate transitions from normal sinus rhythm to atrial flutter, the patient without rate smoothing experiences atrial tracking at the maximum tracking rate, while the patient with rate smoothing experiences a more gradual transition to the maximum tracking rate.

Table 22.13 All manufacturers also offer special features to help address the sudden decrease in rate associated with neurocardiogenic syncope

Company	Name of features
Biotronik	Closed-Loop Stimulation (CLS)
Boston Scientific	Sudden Brady Response (SBR)
Sorin	DDD/AMC with acceleration
Medtronic	Rate drop response
St. Jude Medical	Advanced Hysteresis

Note that in common clinical parlance, this feature is often called *rate drop response*.

increase the pacing rate in the presence of this abrupt decrease in heart rate in order to preserve cardiac output (see **Table 22.13**). These algorithms rely on the device sensor to help guide the feature. Note that the St. Jude Medical name for this feature is Advanced Hysteresis.

Rate drop response works in that when the device detects a sudden drop in heart rate, it will pace the patient at a rate above the programmed base rate. For example, if a rate drop is determined by the pacemaker, it will start to pace

the patient at a programmable rate, typically around 90–110 ppm, for a programmable duration of time. After that duration expires, the rate goes back down to sinus rate, sensor-indicated rate, or the base rate (whichever one is in control). This feature is recommended for patients with known or suspected neurocardiogenic syncope and it may benefit those with hypersensitive carotid sinus syndrome as well.

The goal of rate drop response is that the suddenly increased pacing rate will sufficiently increase cardiac output to the point that the patient may not experience syncope.

Conclusion

Even after this admittedly *brief* overview of pacemaker special features, it is easy to see why so many pacemakers are never reprogrammed from their *out-of-the-box* settings. These features—which can really help fine-tune pacing for specific patients—can increase device complexity exponentially. A top-of-the-line dual-chamber pacemaker today offers clinicians over a million programmable combinations if you consider all of the programming choices for all of the parameters. While this can be overwhelming, there are a few key take-away messages. First, clinicians should have a good overview of the available features not because they will always be programmed but because clinicians need to know what is available for individual patients. Rate smoothing, for instance, may not be necessary for every patient, but if you have a patient who is having problems with rate *bumps* during mode switching and 2:1 block, it is helpful to know that there is a feature that can address this. Second, pacing clinicians must also be prepared to see the results of these features on paced ECGs and electrograms. There are so many special features that can potentially alter the pacing rate; it is good for clinicians to know that they may see a dual-chamber pacemaker pacing above the base rate and below the base rate and be functioning appropriately! In fact, every now and then, a clinician may find a dual-chamber pacemaker pacing at the base rate! These are important features to know about. Third, these special features can be important but do not use them if they create more problems than they solve. Not every patient needs or can even benefit from these features.

The nuts and bolts of special features

- All manufacturers offer special features in their pacemakers to help better manage particular types of patients, to streamline function, or to make the device operation more automatic. Sometimes, all or many manufacturers offer a similar feature but call it by different names; the algorithm may work slightly differently by device. In other cases, special features (such as rate smoothing) may only be available from a couple of manufacturers.
- Clinicians should not go overboard programming all special features for every patient. In many cases, special features are intended to help a subset of the pacing population, not all patients. Furthermore, every special feature added increases the complexity of the device. Thus, it is important to know about all of the special features but to program only those that are actually helpful for the patient.
- Some special features automatically shorten the AV delay when the pacemaker is pacing at rates above the base rate. This mimics what the healthy heart does when rates accelerate. These may decrease the AV delay by a specific number of ms for each 1 ppm the rate increases or it may shorten the AV delay only after the rate reaches a certain level. This feature works well in patients with heart block, but should probably not be used in patients with good intrinsic conduction except in unusual cases. (That's because this feature may pace the right ventricle when it can be avoided.)
- Note that any feature that affects the AV delay also, in turn, affects TARP, which resets the point at which 2:1 block sets in. Shortening the AV delay means that 2:1 block would occur at a higher rate (provided that the PVARP stays the same). Here's an example. Imagine a patient with a PVARP set to 300 ms and a paced AV delay of 200 ms; TARP is 500 (300 + 200), which means that 2:1 block occurs at 120 ppm (500 ms = 120 ppm). Leaving the PVARP alone, if the paced AV delay shortens to 100 ms, TARP is now 400 and 2:1 block would occur at 150 ppm (400 ms = 150 ppm).
- Sometimes, it is useful to prolong the AV delay in an effort to encourage intrinsic ventricular activity and reduce right ventricular pacing. The best candidates for this special feature are those with first- or second-degree AV block. It should not be used in patients with complete heart block, since they do not have intrinsic conduction.
- The SafeR™ feature from Sorin and the MVP™ feature from Medtronic both work to prolong the AV delay by operating as functional AAI or AAIR devices, which switch to DDD or DDDR when no intrinsic ventricular activity is present. This could be thought of as function atrial single-chamber pacing with ventricular backup

pacing. Do not be confused when these algorithms describe what they do as *mode switching*. Classic mode switching is something else (it involves turning off atrial tracking in the presence of high-rate intrinsic atrial activity).

- In other AV delay-lengthening algorithms, the device periodically extends the AV delay to *search* for intrinsic ventricular activity.

- Be aware that when special features are activated, they can cause potential confusion when the clinician reviews tracings. For instance, just as it is possible to have multiple rates on a rhythm strip (base rate, sensor-indicated rate, maximum tracking rate (MTR), and so on), it is also possible to see variations in the AV delay!

- All manufacturers today offer a type of automatic sensing such that the pacemaker monitors intrinsic activity and self-adjusts its sensitivity settings appropriately. Automatic sensing can be a time-saving feature that promotes patient safety.

- Pacemakers also offer automatic capture algorithms to assure reliable capture with the most efficient use of energy.

- Just as AV delays can shorten automatically as rate increases, many manufacturers offer a dynamically shortening PVARP value. In Sorin devices, PVARP is not programmable as an absolute number but constantly adjusts itself to the paced rate. The potential pitfall with shortening PVARP is that it can lead to a pacemaker-mediated tachycardia (PMT) in patients with retrograde conduction. This is not a good feature to use with patients who are known to be susceptible to PMTs.

- All manufacturers offer algorithms to prevent PMTs and to terminate PMTs once they start. PMT prevention is a matter of extending the PVARP for one cycle when the device detects a PVC. Pacemakers define PVCs as two ventricular events (the second one sensed) without an intervening atrial event. Automatically prolonging the PVARP when a PVC is sensed will allow any retrograde P-waves to *fall into the PVARP* and not be sensed, thus preventing the onset of a PMT.

- The same concept works to terminate a PMT. When the device detects a PMT, usually as a programmable number of cycles at the MTR, the pacemaker automatically prolongs the PVARP for one cycle, allowing a retrograde P-wave to fall into the PVARP and be missed. Note that most PMTs occur at the MTR, but it is possible for a PMT to occur at a rate slightly below that. In some special features, the PMT definition may allow for a number of cycles at the MTR or another rate.

- Mode switching—in the classic sense—refers to temporarily disabling atrial tracking in the presence of high-rate intrinsic atrial activity. To program mode switching, the clinician must define what high-rate atrial activity is (usually, this is an atrial tachyarrhythmia, say, at 120 or 150 bpm), how many cycles this high-rate activity must last, and how the mode switch is to be made (some devices allow some programming choices as to the mode and mode switch rate). When the atrial tachycardia ceases, the mode is returned to the originally programmed settings.

- Atrial overdrive pacing refers to the technique of pacing the atrium slightly faster than the intrinsic rate in an effort to *control* it and suppress potential atrial fibrillation. While this technique can be very effective, it requires the patient to be paced at rates which may be uncomfortable, for instance, 80 or 90 ppm.

- The rest rate or sleep rate is a programmable base-rate option that allows the pacemaker to pace at slower rates when the patient is asleep. In the early days, pacemakers tried to use clock time to define sleep and wake cycles; today, the accelerometer is used such that the patient's rest rate is activated when the accelerometer shows the patient is very still.

- Rate hysteresis is a feature that is beneficial for many patients and somewhat confusing for clinicians encountering it for the first time. The goal of rate hysteresis is to allow the patient to conduct intrinsically as much as possible. Rate hysteresis imposes a second rate—a so-called hysteresis rate—that is below the base rate. A typical hysteresis rate is 50 bpm (but any

Continued

Continued

number of rates is programmable). Periodically, the pacemaker will *search* for intrinsic activity at or above the hysteresis rate in *search cycles*. If the pacemaker finds such intrinsic activity, it allows that intrinsic activity to control the pacemaker and inhibit pacing. For example, assume a VVI device is programmed to a base rate of 60 ppm and a hysteresis rate of 50 bpm. During a hysteresis search, the pacemaker prolongs the V-to-V or pacing interval long enough that intrinsic ventricular activity at 52 bpm emerged. Since that is above the hysteresis rate, the pacemaker will now inhibit pacing for this 52 bpm rate. As long as the intrinsic activity is above the hysteresis rate, the pacemaker stays inhibited. Should intrinsic activity fall below the hysteresis rate, the pacemaker resumes base-rate pacing (at 60 ppm).

- The goal of hysteresis is to give intrinsic rates maximum opportunity to prevail.
- Hysteresis is available in single-chamber devices, where it operates on the channel of the devices (ventricular single-chamber pacemakers have ventricular channel hysteresis, while atrial single-chamber pacemakers have atrial channel hysteresis). Dual-chamber pacemakers also offer hysteresis, but it is on the atrial chamber, since dual-chamber systems time themselves based on the atrial channel.

- Rate smoothing is an interesting and important feature offered only by Medtronic, Biotronik, Sorin, and Boston Scientific. Rate smoothing will only allow the pacing rate to change (increasing or decreasing) by a programmable percentage for each cycle. For instance, let's say a DDDR pacemaker at a base rate of 60 ppm reached atrial tracking at the MTR of 120 ppm, which happened in this device to be the 2:1 block rate; this means ventricular pacing would go from 120 to 60 ppm in one beat. With rate smoothing programmed to 10%, the rate change could only be 10% in each step, that is, when 2:1 block was reached, the ventricles would be paced at 108 ppm (120 minus 10% of 120 or 120 minus 12) and then 97 ppm (108 minus 10% of 108 or 108 minus 11) and then 87 ppm (97 minus 10% of 97 or 97 minus 10) and then 79 ppm (87 minus 10% of 87 or 87 minus 8) and so on until the desired rate was achieved.
- Neurocardiogenic syncope is also called vasovagal syncope or neurally mediated syncope and it is characterized by an abrupt drop in heart rate. Pacemakers with a rate drop response feature will accelerate the pacing above the base rate during such episodes in an effort to boost cardiac output.

Test your knowledge

1 Mrs. Broussard has a DDDR pacemaker programmed to a base rate of 60 ppm, an MTR of 120 ms, an MSR of 130 ppm, and a sensed AV delay of 175 ms. A special feature to adjust the sensed AV delay in response to higher atrial tracked rates has been activated. At what point would her sensed AV delay be *the shortest*?
    A At 60 ppm.
    B At 120 ppm.
    C At 130 ppm.
    D The sensed AV delay would not change.

2 What is the main purpose of dynamic or rate-adaptive AV delays?
    A Better rate response to exercise
    B Reduced battery drain on the pacemaker

    C Less right ventricular pacing
    D Better upper-rate behavior

3 Which of the following features is associated with the *dispersion of refractoriness*?
    A Atrial overdrive pacing and AF suppression
    B Rate hysteresis and rest rates
    C Rate-responsive AV delays and rate-responsive PVARPS
    D PMT prevention and termination algorithms

4 In a DDDR pacemaker, the hysteresis interval is applied to which channel?
    A Atrial.
    B Ventricular.

C It can be programmed to either atrial or ventricular channels.

D It can be programmed to atrial, ventricular, or a blended channel (both atrial and ventricular).

5 During a period of high intrinsic atrial activity, a pacemaker that mode switches is actually doing what?

A Overdrive pacing the atrium

B Changing from single-chamber to dual-chamber sensing

C Temporarily disabling atrial tracking

D Shortening the AV delay

6 Mr. Williams was just implanted with a new single-chamber pacemaker. Which of the following special features would definitely *not* be available in his new device?

A Rate hysteresis

B Automatic sensing

C Automatic capture

D Mode switching

7 Rate drop response is intended to help patients with neurocardiogenic syncope by doing which of the following?

A Smoothing out rate drops that might occur at 2:1 block

B Allowing a temporarily decreased hysteresis rate

C Increasing pacing rate when a sudden rate decrease is detected

D Turning on the sensor when a sudden rate decrease is detected

8 As a rule of thumb, about 25% of pacemaker patients will experience atrial fibrillation. Which of these features would benefit this subset of patients?

A Autosensing

B Mode switching

C Rest rate/rate hysteresis

D PMT Termination

9 How does a PMT Termination algorithm work?

A When it detects a PMT, it prolongs the PVARP for one cycle.

B When it detects a PMT, it shortens the PVARP for one cycle.

C When it detects a PMT, it turns off atrial tracking.

D When it detects a PMT, it increases base-rate pacing by a programmable percentage.

10 What is one of the main goals of automatic capture algorithms?

A To reduce battery drain

B To assure reliable sensing

C To generate good diagnostic reports

D All of the above

CHAPTER 23

Automatic capture algorithms

Learning objectives

- Give a very brief history of automatic capture algorithms and their general goals.
- Name the main benefit of automatic capture algorithms and two secondary benefits.
- Explain the role of the initial pulse and backup safety pacing.
- Briefly name the key parameters or features in the St. Jude Medical AutoCapture algorithm.
- Define *evoked response* and explain how it is assessed automatically by the pacemaker.
- Explain why polarization presented a challenge to engineers working on automatic capture algorithms and one way this problem was solved.
- State briefly the programming considerations and a recommended value for evoked response sensitivity, using the example of a 20 mV evoked response signal.
- Name the times that AutoCapture is typically turned on for a new pacemaker patient and state a reason to support the timing you favor.

Introduction

The automatic capture algorithm has done much to reshape the world of cardiac pacing, and it is important that we review it in detail. This chapter becomes a bit complex in that each manufacturer offers its own special version of automatic capture. To some extent, specific manufacturers and

algorithms will be presented, but when possible, the chapter will try to offer *generic* information. Basically, all capture algorithms attempt to automatically regulate and adjust pacemaker output in response to fluctuations in capture threshold. The goal of these algorithms is to provide safe, reliable capture at the most energy-efficient settings possible. All manufacturers offer some version of this algorithm in their devices, and clinicians can expect to routinely encounter automatic capture features.

So why is automatic capture so important? To be sure, automatic capture algorithms have done many important things for the pacing industry. These algorithms have allowed engineers to design and develop radically downsized devices—and that is a good thing, because small devices enhance patient comfort. And these algorithms have given pacemakers a big boost in terms of longevity—modern pacemakers can sometimes last a decade or more. In today's cost-conscious healthcare market, the importance of this cannot be overstated. But that is not the reason that this feature was developed or why it was so aggressively promoted and why it is so common today. The reason for that is simple. It's about patient safety.

A pacemaker is only effective as long as it captures. Loss of capture is the same as *not pacing*. A pacemaker patient could have a world-class brand-new dual-chamber pacemaker but if it failed to capture, the patient could still have syncope. Thus, the development of automatic capture was a drive for patient safety that netted the industry and its patients many other benefits.

The Nuts and Bolts of Implantable Device Therapy Pacemakers, First Edition. Tom Kenny.
© 2015 John Wiley & Sons, Ltd. Published 2015 by John Wiley & Sons, Ltd.

A short history of automatic capture

The history of automatic capture algorithms begins in 1995 when St. Jude Medical introduced its unique Microny™ pacemaker with AutoCapture™ to the market. Microny was unique because, at the time, it was the world's smallest pacemaker. This single-chamber device was about the size of a quarter! Part of the reason that a VVIR pacemaker could be so radically downsized is owed to the fact that it used a proprietary new algorithm that automatically adjusted device output to match the patient's pacing threshold. This meant that the old-fashioned 2:1 or 3:1 safety margins were no longer necessary, which, in turn, led to minimal energy demands on the system. This allowed the Microny pacemaker to provide reliable single-chamber pacing with a relatively small pacemaker battery.

Today, all St. Jude Medical pacemakers offer AutoCapture. This is an interesting decision on the part of the company. Most pacemaker clinicians recognize that there are *tiers* of pacing devices with top-tier pacemakers offering all special features, lower-tier pacemakers offering few if any special features, and midtier products offering a subset of advanced features. This marketing strategy is used to some degree by all pacemaker manufacturers and, indeed, manufacturers of other medical and consumer devices. However, St. Jude Medical decided that its AutoCapture algorithm would be included in every device, even low-tier products, probably because the company recognized the tremendous value of this particular feature. Remember that the main goal of automatic capture is to improve patient safety by assuring reliable capture.

In the 1990s, the pacing industry was under pressure from two different camps to achieve two apparently mutually exclusive goals. On the one hand, doctors and their patients wanted smaller and smaller devices. Not so long ago, pacemakers could be very large and thick. They sometimes protruded through the chest. Patients, especially women and smaller-framed individuals, wanted smaller devices. The clinical community thought these might also be easier to implant and handle. So there was pressure to downsize the pulse generator. At the same time, the healthcare industry was eager to reduce device replacements so it is advocated for longer-lasting devices. Early in pacing history, a pacemaker might be expected to last only 2 or 3 years; this meant frequent replacements, particularly for younger patients. So while engineers were trying to make pulse generators smaller, they were also trying to make them last longer. That did not seem possible, since most of the real estate inside the pulse generator is taken up by the battery. How could engineers downsize the pulse generator and upsize the battery at the same time?

The goal was first achieved by St. Jude Medical that found a way to use less battery energy to capture the heart, which allowed a device to have a small battery, which, in turn, allowed the pulse generator to be much smaller. But the real goal of automatic capture was actually to protect the patient from loss of capture.

The problem of noncapture

Noncapture refers to the condition when a pacemaker delivers an output pulse but fails to capture the heart. Noncapture can have serious consequences and can even be a potentially life-threatening situation for pacemaker-dependent patients. While noncapture is relatively rare, it is not rare enough. Roughly, clinicians estimate noncapture incidence at around 1–5%.

Noncapture can occur for any number of reasons. First, thresholds change. There is the well-known acute-to-chronic threshold change and then there are daily fluctuations in capture threshold. Capture threshold can also change with disease progression or with certain medications. In short, programming the pacemaker outputs is like trying to hit a moving target! Threshold changes are not predictable, so the best way to solve the problem of noncapture had previously been to program very generous safety margins. A good way to think of this is that the 5-fold safety margin in the acute-to-chronic phase and the 2:1 or 3:1 safety margin for chronic pacing are appropriate for most patients, but it is not going to be sufficient for all patients, and since threshold changes are not predictable, clinicians do not know who will need extra safety margin and when.

Thresholds change with everything from sleep, eating meals, exercise, illness, metabolic imbalances, posture, and medications. There are probably even more things that can influence threshold. The problem is that even knowing that certain things affect threshold, we still do not know how much they will impact thresholds in which patients.

The optimal safety margin

Clinicians routinely program safety margins and prevailing wisdom has long held that a 2:1 safety margin was sufficient for chronic implants. That may not be the case for all patients. Some clinicians err on the side of caution and select 3:1 safety margins for chronic use. This may be safer, but it uses up a great deal of energy—in fact, it likely will waste much energy in most patients. The optimal device output is whatever will reliably capture the heart at the most energy-efficient settings.

How these algorithms work

Automatic capture algorithms have some important features that had never been seen in devices before. Previously, pacemakers delivered an output pulse and that was that—the pacemaker *thought* that every output pulse captured the heart. Automatic capture algorithms incorporate features in them that help the pacemaker to recognize capture and confirm it. These algorithms do something new, namely, they verify appropriate capture and they can do it for any and every beat.

Second, these devices are able to assess the patient's threshold regularly and to adjust the output pulse to an energy-efficient setting that will capture the heart. This assures that energy is used efficiently and does not go to waste. Automatic capture algorithms allow devices to consistently capture the heart using only a fraction of the energy they used to use. And even though they use far less energy than they used to, capture verification assures that the patient is benefiting from consistent capture.

Historical advances

The automatic capture algorithms in use today are a far cry from the original features that hit the market in the mid-1990s. Originally, automatic capture had some limitations. It would only work with unipolar pacing (but it required bipolar sensing). Sometimes, as in the case of the original St. Jude Medical AutoCapture, it was available for ventricular use but not in the atrium. It was incompatible with ICDs. Today, all of those limitations have been overcome. As is typical in pacing, innovation occurs in a series of incremental improvements!

Capture confirmation

Up to now, I have encouraged clinicians to learn to think like a pacemaker. When it comes to capture, clinicians and pacemakers think very differently. If a clinician is asked to confirm capture in a pacemaker patient, he or she is going to look at the surface ECG. It is often easy to confirm capture—there is a pacemaker spike and an immediate depolarization. Pacemakers do things a little differently and it is hard for us to do it as they do it; pacemakers confirm capture on the electrogram.

A capture confirmation system was developed by St. Jude Medical for its AutoCapture algorithm. The information that follows is specific to St. Jude Medical—we will go over the other algorithms in later sections.

AutoCapture Pacing Systems™ from St. Jude Medical

As St. Jude Medical developed the world's first automatic capture algorithm, it seems appropriate to start by describing their proprietary algorithm. Many of the concepts presented here will apply to the algorithms of the other manufacturers.

Every time a pacemaker spike is delivered, the automatic capture algorithm is going to use the electrogram and go back and confirm that capture indeed occurred. To a pacemaker, capture is the *evoked response*, that is, the depolarization (response) caused (evoked) by the spike. To accomplish this, pacemakers have now built in a separate sensing circuit that looks for only evoked responses. Thus, each time the pacemaker delivers an output pulse, this separate sensing circuit uses the electrogram to examine the myocardium to see if there was a resulting event. In the St. Jude Medical system, AutoCapture works on the ventricular channel only.

If capture is lost, the St. Jude Medical algorithm is programmed to automatically deliver a backup pacing pulse intended to capture the heart. This backup safety pulse is a high-output pulse (see **Figure 23.1**). The purpose of backup safety pacing

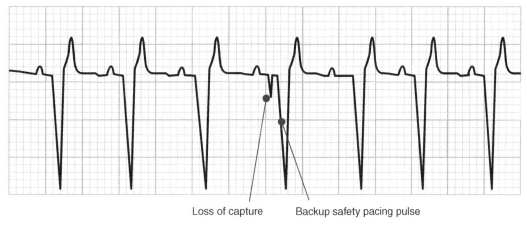

Loss of capture   Backup safety pacing pulse

Figure 23.1 St. Jude Medical's AutoCapture algorithm. Note that capture is lost and a backup safety pulse is delivered that captures the heart.

is to make sure the pacemaker does not lose ventricular capture.

Therefore, on an AutoCapture pacing strip, there may occasionally be two ventricular pacing spikes next to each other (80–100 ms apart). If the first fails to capture, the backup safety pulse is delivered. Whenever the pacemaker experiences loss of capture followed by a backup safety pulse, on the next cycle, the pacemaker automatically prolongs the sensed AV delay interval to encourage intrinsic conduction. At issue is fusion. Just as a clinician can be tricked when a pacemaker spike and intrinsic beat collide (fusion), the capture algorithm is concerned that perhaps fusion had caused it to see loss of capture. Recall from earlier sections that fusion occurs when a pacemaker spike and intrinsic beat occur at the same time, such that the pacemaker spike makes no contribution at all to the intrinsic depolarization. Fusion is not a capture problem at all; it's a timing issue. Thus, the pacemaker *is concerned* that what it saw as loss of capture might actually have been fusion and the patient has some degree of intrinsic conduction. For that reason, on the very next beat, it extends the AV delay interval by 100 ms to provide maximum opportunity for intrinsic conduction and intrinsic ventricular activity. If fusion occurred earlier, this extended AV delay interval would encourage an intrinsic ventricular event. If fusion did not occur (as is the case in Figure 23.1), this prolonged AV delay interval lasts for only one cycle and does not interfere with device operation.

In the St. Jude Medical device, the backup safety pulse is 5.0 V at 0.5 ms in newer devices and 4.5 V at 0.5 ms in older devices. (Note that pulse duration of the backup pulse will always be at least 0.5 ms; if the device is programmed to a longer pulse width value, say 0.75 ms, then that longer value will be used. On the other hand, if the pulse width of the device is set to 0.4 ms, the backup safety pulse will be 0.5 ms. In all cases, the backup safety pulse minimum pulse duration is 0.5 ms.) The backup pulse comes in about 80–100 ms after a primary pulse (or first output pulse) fails to capture the heart.

Much of what clinicians first learn about capture and pacing involves safety margins; clinicians are urged to use safety margins at least 2.5 times the patient's capture threshold. Yet AutoCapture pacing can successfully capture the heart at outputs of 1.0 V or even lower. So what happens to the safety margin? Actually, these algorithms maintain a very generous safety margin. Imagine an AutoCapture pacing system pacing the ventricles consistently at 1.0 V. Now, imagine that for one beat the ventricular spike fails to capture, so in 80–100 ms, a backup safety pulse of 5.0 V is delivered. A 5.0 V pulse at 0.5 ms is literally a 5:1 safety margin—a huge safety margin! However, the device uses a fivefold safety margin *only when it is needed*. Most of the time, pacing at 1.0 V is perfectly adequate and results in reliable capture. If and when more energy is needed, the pacemaker delivers it—but only if and when it is needed. This is how the

AutoCapture algorithm can save energy while still preserving patient safety.

This scenario raises one question. What if loss of capture occurred in a patient and the 5.0 V at 0.5 ms backup safety pulse was insufficient to capture the heart? That is possible, although it is unlikely. Right now, these algorithms do not allow the backup safety pulse to be programmed. One of the innovations that we may expect in the future is programmable backup safety pulses, such that clinicians could set a maximum-output pulse (typically 7.5 V at 0.5 ms). Returning to the original scenario, what happens if the pacemaker observes two consecutive losses of capture? If that should happen, the device carries out what St. Jude Medical calls the *loss of capture recovery*. If two consecutive capture losses occur, the pacemaker will increase its pulse amplitude by 0.25 V (one-quarter of a volt) for one beat. Should that capture the heart, the pacemaker will deliver the same amplitude again for another beat just to reconfirm capture. If that does not capture the heart, the pulse amplitude will continue to increase by one-eighth of a volt (0.125 V) increments until two consecutive captures occur.

Once capture is confirmed twice, the pacemaker launches a *threshold search,* which is another term for an automatic threshold test. The goal is that the pacemaker will base its future output on this new pacing threshold. If capture cannot be confirmed by a 3.875 V output at 0.5 ms, then the pacemaker automatically switches to the backup safety pulse value for pacing (5.0 V in newer St. Jude Medical devices, 4.5 V in older ones). After 128 cycles at this output, a new threshold search is initiated (see **Figure 23.2**).

As Figure 23.2 shows, AutoCapture allows for pacing with reliable capture at very low outputs—down to as low as 0.5 V! The backup safety pulse was needed a few times, but when capture was restored at 0.875 V, capture could still be reliably maintained at output amplitudes of less than 1 V. This is remarkable, and it shows the potential these algorithms have to save battery energy. In fact, in St. Jude Medical systems with AutoCapture™ turned on, it is very common to see pacing at outputs under 1 V.

After a threshold search, the pulse amplitude will then decrease by a quarter-volt (0.25 V) two beats a

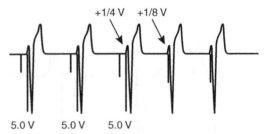

Figure 23.2 AutoCapture from St. Jude Medical. In the first complex, the pacemaker spike is delivered at 0.5 V and fails to capture, so a backup safety pulse is delivered at 5.0 V. This backup pulse captures the heart. The scenario repeats itself in the second complex: loss of capture at 0.5 V occurs with a 5.0 V backup safety pulse capturing the heart. The pacemaker has now recorded two consecutive losses of capture, so it increases the output of the primary pacing pulse by one-quarter volt in the third complex. The primary pulse is delivered at 0.75 V (0.5 + 0.25 V = 0.75 V), and it, too, fails to capture the heart, so the backup pulse comes in at 5.0 V. In the fourth complex, the primary output pulse is increased by an eighth of a volt to 0.875 V. Note that in this case, this new output captures the heart for this and the subsequent beat.

time until loss of capture occurs for two consecutive beats. Now the pacemaker has homed in on a threshold. It then increases voltage of an eighth of a volt (0.125 V) until two consecutive captures occur. When these two consecutive captured events appear, the device calls this the new *capture threshold*. The new primary output pulse is adjusted to be 0.25 V above the new capture threshold. This 0.25 V increment is the working safety margin of the AutoCapture pacing system. As an example, if the device determined that the patient's new capture threshold was 0.875 V, then the new working primary output pulse would be 1.125 V (0.875 + 0.25 V = 1.125 V) (see **Figure 23.3**).

Since capture thresholds fluctuate frequently and can change many times over the course of an ordinary day, the AutoCapture pacing system was designed to monitor capture on a beat-by-beat basis and to conduct a threshold search whenever two consecutive losses of capture occur. This means that a patient's primary output pulse setting may change several times over the course of the day.

One advantage of the St. Jude Medical AutoCapture algorithm is its track record. It has been around for almost 20 years. And combined with other automatic capture algorithms, there are

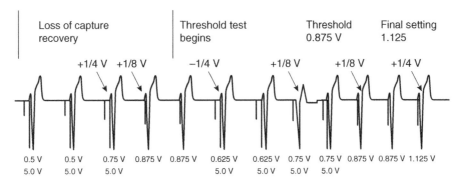

Figure 23.3 This strip continues Figure 23.2. Following the loss of capture recovery (described in detail in Figure 23.2), the pacemaker begins a threshold test by decreasing the output voltage 0.25 V each time. This results in two consecutive losses of capture, so the voltage is incremented by 0.125 V. Two captures at this output setting confirm the threshold of 0.875 V. Adding the working safety margin of 0.25 to the threshold, the new primary output pulse setting is 1.125 V.

over a million pacemakers using such algorithms. The take-away message is that –to some degree— we clinicians have come to trust these algorithms (from all manufacturers) to reliably capture the heart at very low outputs. Clinicians can expect to encounter these various algorithms in their many forms in real-world clinical practice. However, there are still physicians who resist the use of these algorithms and prefer instead to program fixed output settings based on the old 2:1 or 3:1 safety margins. In my experience, physicians who do not use these algorithms mainly do so out of habit. Once these algorithms are understood and implemented, they usually become a routine part of practice.

St. Jude Medical pioneered ventricular AutoCapture. It was originally available in single-chamber pacemakers and also in dual-chamber devices but only on the ventricular channel. More recently, an atrial version of AutoCapture has been introduced (called ACap Confirm) and even an LV version for the left ventricular channel of a cardiac resynchronization therapy (CRT) device.

Threshold search

Threshold search in St. Jude Medical's AutoCapture algorithm occurs whenever there are two consecutive losses of capture occur, but it also occurs on other occasions:

- Automatically every 8 h or every 24 h (depending on the device)
- Upon magnet removal (if the magnet has been in place for at least 5 s)

- When the telemetry wand is removed
- When the AutoCapture threshold test is initiated from the programmer
- When the device resumes its originally programmed parameters after a mode switch episode (mode switch exit) in some devices

Thus, AutoCapture provides automatic threshold testing on a regular basis as well as during specific instances, such as when capture is lost for two consecutive beats. A very handy feature for follow-up is the programmer-based threshold search. A clinician conducting a conventional capture threshold test must—by definition—lose capture. That's how the test is done! But now, if the patient comes to the clinic, the threshold search can be initiated right from the programmer, and it can complete a threshold test without ever losing capture. This feature saves time and offers clinical convenience, but it is particularly important for threshold testing in pacemaker-dependent patients.

Backup pulses

In the first generation of St. Jude Medical AutoCapture pacing systems, the backup pacing pulse was always unipolar. Unipolar signals are those that make their *antenna* from the lead electrode back to the pulse generator. At 5 V, this very large unipolar signal was powerful enough for patients to perceive—and many did not like the sensation! A patient who perceives this signal will often state that they *feel their pacemaker* or are *aware of their pacemaker*. Since these older devices provide for routine automatic threshold searches every 8 h, patients got backup pulses three times a day, and a few were bothered enough by it to discuss it with their physicians. For patients with those older systems, sometimes, patient education sufficed to allow the algorithm to stay on. Patients were told that the sensations they perceived occurred when the pacemaker was *testing itself* to be sure it was providing enough energy to the heart. Patients who understood this feature and its purpose often could live with it.

In the next generation of St. Jude Medical AutoCapture pacing systems, the unipolar backup pulse was changed to a bipolar pulse. Bipolar pulses form an antenna between the tip and ring electrodes on the pacing lead—a very small, concentrated area. Such pulses are almost impossible for patients to perceive.

But there was another issue that came about as a result of the threshold search. During a threshold search, the pacemaker automatically shortened the paced AV delay and sensed AV delay to 50 and 25 ms, respectively. Threshold search requires pacing in order to assess capture, and shortened AV delay intervals would cause ventricular pacing. These abbreviated AV delays were very helpful in forcing pacing and allowing for capture testing, but they did not allow much time for ventricular filling. As a result, some patients experienced Cannon A waves in their neck region. So even with bipolar backup pacing pulses, some patients still have unusual sensations during threshold search. Again, patient education helped but some patients still disliked these periodic tests.

In the next generation of devices, St. Jude Medical allowed for some programmability in the AV delays for the threshold search (the options were 120 and 100 ms, 100 and 70 ms, or 50 and 25 ms for paced and sensed AV delays, respectively). This gives clinician more flexibility in programming the threshold search and decreases the chances that patients will have uncomfortable or unpleasant sensations. In addition, clinicians may be able to choose every 8 h or every 24 h for the threshold search.

Evoked response test

The AutoCapture algorithm is based on the pacemaker being able to recognize capture, which it does by sensing the so-called evoked response. The evoked response is the depolarization (response) caused (evoked) by the pacemaker spike. A more thorough definition is that evoked response is depolarization of the heart at the myocardial level. Evoked response is measured at the lead tip. Every time the pacemaker delivers an output pulse, it checks to see if that pulse generated a depolarization at the myocardial level (evoked response) or not (loss of capture).

In order for the pacemaker to be able to identify an evoked response, a test has to be conducted when AutoCapture is first programmed to help *show* the pacemaker what the evoked response is going to look like. While this section relates to the St. Jude Medical algorithm for AutoCapture, algorithms from all manufacturers rely on the *evoked response* to confirm capture. This term will come up again in discussions of other algorithms.

Capture verification

If the pacemaker's ventricular output pulse captures the ventricle, it will produce an evoked response. The evoked response is measured from the ventricular lead's tip electrode using a unique sensing circuit. The sensing circuit is unique in that it is used only to sense the evoked response (in other words, it is not involved in sensing intrinsic cardiac depolarizations). The algorithm measures the amplitude of the evoked response in mV. Note that the algorithm looks for an evoked response when a *normal* pacing output is delivered; it does not verify evoked response when a backup safety pulse is delivered.

In the St. Jude Medical algorithm, there is an evoked response detection window of 60 ms. In the first 14 ms of the window, no evoked response can be detected, but in the next 46 ms, the device looks for an evoked response.

Every pacing output pulse causes an electrical phenomenon in the heart known as polarization or *afterpotential*. Polarization refers to the fact that there is some residual electrical charge present at the pacing electrode after any output pulse, which leads to a buildup of ions around the lead electrode. For example, when energy is sent out with one charge, it tends to attract energy of the opposite charge. Polarization occurs because of the output pulse; it is present to equal degrees whether the output pulse captures or does not capture. The

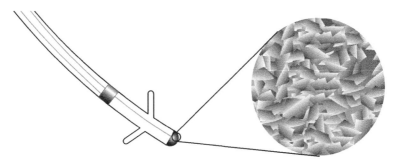

Figure 23.4 A fractal surface on a pacing electrode adds surface area to the electrode without increasing its size.

great challenge to pacing engineers in developing automatic capture algorithms was overcoming the problem of polarization, because the pacemaker's tip electrode could easily *confuse* the electrical charge buildup due to polarization with an evoked response. The problem was solved by recognizing that polarization dissipates very quickly, in just a few milliseconds. With that knowledge, the evoked response detection window was given a brief *blind spot* of 14 ms to allow polarization to dissipate before the pacemaker looked for the evoked response.

Polarization can be reduced by increasing the surface area of the electrode. The larger the surface area of the electrode, the less polarization occurs. While this sounds like an easy solution, pacemaker leads must be kept small for optimal lead design. These seemingly contradictory design goals were solved by creating a fractal surface on the lead; think of this as a highly textured surface. The *texture* expands the surface area of the lead without necessarily increasing its overall size (see **Figure 23.4**). The goals of achieving the optimal low-polarization lead have also led to adding titanium nitride coating to the electrode (reducing polarization). The so-called high-impedance leads do not diminish polarization; they do the opposite. Although high-impedance leads were heavily marketed some years ago, their popularity is decreasing because they are associated with high polarization. (High-impedance leads offer the benefit of reducing current drain, which, in turn, might extend battery life.) High-impedance leads cannot be used with automatic capture algorithms because they encourage rather than reduce polarization. And since automatic capture prolongs device longevity, the move away from high-impedance leads

toward low-polarization leads with automatic capture makes sense in that clinicians are not giving up increased device service life.

When the automatic capture algorithm in a St. Jude Medical pacemaker is activated, a test must be conducted to make sure that the evoked response can be appropriately sensed. This E/R sensitivity test, as it is called (renamed AutoCapture Setup in newer devices from St. Jude Medical), can only be performed with the programmer. In simple terms, the E/R sensitivity test measures the amplitude of the evoked response signal and the amplitude of the polarization signal and determines if there is sufficient difference between them for AutoCapture to work reliably. During the test, the pacemaker delivers 10–20 *double pulses* (at backup parameters, typically 5.0 V at 0.5 ms) about 100 ms apart at the various evoked response sensitivity settings. For each output pulse, the pacemaker takes two measurements: polarization signal and evoked response signal. This is then reported back on the programmer (see **Figure 23.5**). A typical evoked response signal often falls in the range of 15–20 mV, while a typical polarization signal is around 1 or 2 mV. The actual value of the signal amplitude is less important to the algorithm than whether there is sufficient difference between the two values to allow the algorithm to reliably differentiate the signals based on amplitude size. Based on the sensitivity measurements, the algorithm sets up its own *sensitivity wall* so that low-amplitude polarization signals are blocked out, while higher-amplitude evoked response signals can be seen *over the wall*. Using the example in Figure 23.5, the sensitivity could be set at 10 mV, meaning that the AutoCapture algorithm would only respond to signals of at least 10 mV amplitude, effectively *blinding* the algorithm

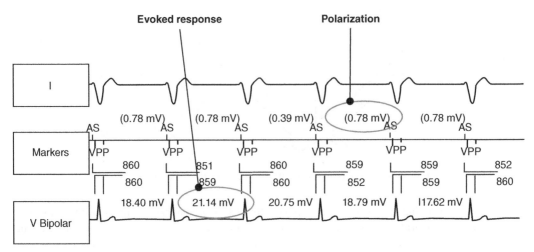

Figure 23.5 Programmer report from St. Jude Medical Identity ADx device for AutoCapture Setup.

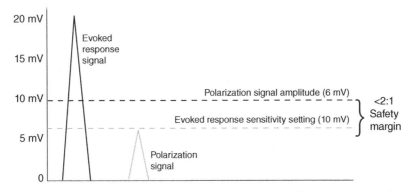

Figure 23.6 In the AutoCapture Setup on the programmer, this patient had an evoked response signal of 10.0 mV and a polarization signal amplitude of 6.0 mV. AutoCapture would not be recommended because the polarization signal is too large (>4 mV) and a 2:1 safety margin between polarization and evoked response signals is not possible (6.0 mV and 10.0 mV = 6:10 or 3:5).

to the lower-amplitude polarization signals. The evoked response sensitivity is set automatically by the programmer; a 2:1 safety margin is recommended such that a 20 mV evoked response signal would merit a 10 mV sensitivity setting.

In some instances, the St. Jude Medical programmer may alert the clinician that AutoCapture is not recommended for a particular patient. AutoCapture may not be recommended in these cases:

• The patient has a polarization signal amplitude greater than 4.0 mV.
• There is no way to program a safety margin for the evoked response sensitivity signal that is at least 1.8–1 (2:1 is recommended).

• There is no way to program a safety margin for the polarization signal that is at least 1.7–1 (2:1 is recommended).

Figure 23.6 shows an example where the patient's signals would not allow for AutoCapture. In the event that AutoCapture is not recommended, the clinician would program output settings the conventional way (capture threshold test and adjustment of output parameters pulse amplitude and pulse width). This *not-recommended* verdict will occur in about 10% of patients trying to use St. Jude Medical's AutoCapture algorithm. It is possible to turn on AutoCapture when it is not recommended—but this is not recommended! If AutoCapture is desired but not recommended, a good strategy is to keep trying, that is, retest the evoked response sensitivity periodically (perhaps every 8 weeks or so). In some cases, signal amplitudes will change sufficiently over time to the point that AutoCapture is recommended. In my experience, about half of the patients who get a *not-recommended* report can eventually use AutoCapture once the system matures (after several weeks or months).

AutoCapture is not activated in the device as shipped; it must be activated by a clinician. There continues to be some debate among pacing experts as to when AutoCapture should be turned on. Providing AutoCapture is recommended for a patient; here are the prevailing points of view:

- It is not a good idea to activate the AutoCapture algorithm while the patient is in the hospital as the AutoCapture algorithm can cause nonpacing experts to suspect a device malfunction, in particular if backup safety pulses are delivered. This can generate worried calls about pseudomalfunction and waste a lot of time.
- Some advocate that AutoCapture be turned on at predischarge, right before the patient leaves the hospital. This reduces the change of potential confusion about the patient's paced ECG but allows him or her to get the benefits of AutoCapture right away.
- Others state that AutoCapture ought to be turned on only at the first follow-up at around 8 weeks. This allows the clinician to use the 5:1 safety margin during the acute-to-chronic threshold transition and then activate AutoCapture as thresholds stabilize.

While both methods (turning AutoCapture on at predischarge and first follow-up) make sense, I recommend that AutoCapture be turned on at predischarge because there is no waste of energy at all. Pacing clinicians will see both methods used in real-world practice.

One question that comes up with clinicians who regularly use AutoCapture involves changes in the signals. Since it is well known that thresholds change, studies have been done to see if evoked response and polarization signals might change as well. It appears that polarization signals are stable but the evoked response signal can change over 6 months, but that this change may go either way, that is, the evoked response signal may increase or decrease in size. Fortunately, there is a very easy way to manage these potential fluctuations. Every 6 months, the evoked response sensitivity test should be done again. The test requires the programmer but it is largely automatic and takes only a couple of minutes. This test automatically resets the algorithm's sensitivity, so it is an easy way to manage potential changes in the evoked response and polarization signals. In many cases, no change has occurred but it reassures the clinician that the sensitivity is appropriate.

Long-term threshold record

When St. Jude Medical first marketed AutoCapture pacing systems, it promoted long-term threshold trends to help clinicians get a better picture of how often noncapture occurred in a given patient. Most physicians assume that noncapture occurs at about 1–5% of the time in their pacemaker patients, but this was not based on data from individual patients of theirs for the simple reason that it was too hard to get that kind of data. The long-term threshold trends offered that kind of insight for the first time. While most patients had stable thresholds, occasionally, this diagnostic report revealed episodes of noncapture that might occur with an illness, electrolyte imbalance, or other conditions. These threshold trends show the value of AutoCapture in the real-world setting in that AutoCapture can adjust to sudden changes in threshold.

ACap™ Confirm (Automatic Atrial Capture)

ACap™ Confirm is the proprietary St. Jude Medical algorithm for automatic capture in the atrium; it was first made available in the Zephyr® pacemaker and has been available for a few years. The goal of ACap Confirm is exactly the same as ventricular AutoCapture, namely, to make sure that the output pulse delivers only the amount of energy needed to capture the heart. The main difference, of course, is that ACap Confirm™ works on the atrial channel of the dual-chamber pacemaker.

Clinicians can use a *Monitor* setting for ACap™ Confirm that allows them to measure capture automatically and plot the values on a trend graph without actually adjusting the output signal. This might be compared to the *Passive* setting for sensors—it allows the clinicians to test ACap™ Confirm before implementing it or to use it as a handy way to monitor atrial threshold values over time. Whether ACap™ Confirm is turned on (and adjusts the output pulse) or is set to *Monitor* (graphs threshold trends but does not adjust output pulse), a setup test is needed.

ACap™ Confirm requires that the primary pacing lead in the right atrium is bipolar; this feature will not work with unipolar leads. Just like with the ventricular algorithm, the backup pacing pulse and the sensing configuration can be programmed to unipolar or bipolar.

One of the main distinctions between ventricular AutoCapture™ pacing systems and ACap™ Confirm involves the timing of the backup safety pulse. If the pacemaker's atrial output pulse fails to capture the atrium, the backup safety atrial pulse is delivered 40 ms later rather than the 80–100 ms on the ventricular side. Otherwise, features are similar: the backup safety pulse output is fixed at 5.0 V with a minimum pulse width value of 0.5 ms. While primary pacing must be bipolar for atrial automatic capture, the backup safety pulse can be programmed to be either bipolar or unipolar.

Atrial automatic capture works in three phases:
1 Capture verification
2 Atrial rate overdrive
3 Atrial threshold search

Unlike ventricular automatic capture, ACap Confirm is not a beat-by-beat algorithm, that is, it does not verify capture every single output. Capture verification can be programmed to occur every eight or every 24 h. Unlike ventricular AutoCapture, ACap Confirm will not automatically conduct a threshold search if two losses of capture occur. In order to verify capture, the device must obviously pace the atrium. If it is not pacing the atrium at the time the test is to be conducted, it may overdrive the atrial rate. Rate overdrive begins with the pacemaker pacing the atrium for 16 cycles and calculating the average atrial rate and the average variance. The overdrive interval is based on the average rate and triple the variance. Capture is tested by decreasing the atrial output amplitude by 0.25 V until three consecutive pulses at the same amplitude setting confirm loss of capture. (During these three losses of capture, a backup safety pulse is delivered.) For the atrial capture test, the AV delay is set to 120 ms. Once the capture is lost, the

amplitude is then increased in 0.125 V increments until two consecutive pulses at the same amplitude value confirm capture. This confirmed value becomes the capture threshold.

There can be some limitations on the atrial threshold search. First, the atrium has to be paced for the test to be run, and while the pacemaker will overdrive the atrium if need be, it will not go above the *speed limit* of 120 ppm. The test will only be run when programmed, that is, every eight or every 24 h; it is not a beat-by-beat algorithm.

Once the threshold is established, the safety margin is automatically applied according to a formula. For thresholds of 0.125–1.5 V, it takes the measured threshold and adds 1.0 V. For thresholds measuring 1.625–2.25 V, it adds 1.5 V to the measured threshold. For 2.375–3.0 V measured thresholds, it adds a 2.0 V safety margin to the measured threshold. Anything above 3.0 V will result in the output pulse being set to 5 V. Thus, if the patient's measured atrial threshold during the threshold search is 1.0 V, the output will be set to 2.0 V (1.0 + 1.0 V); if the patient's measured threshold is 2.0 V, the output will be set to 3.5 V (2.0 + 1.5 V); and if the patient's measured threshold is 3.0 V, the output will be set to 5.0 V (3.0 + 2.0 = 5.0). The output is 5.0 V for any measured threshold over 3.0 V as well. These safety margins are markedly larger than those on the ventricular channel, but there is a good reason for this. Being able to sense evoked response on the atrial channel is more difficult than on the ventricular channel, and the larger safety margin promotes more reliable capture.

Review of St. Jude Medical AutoCapture pacing systems

St. Jude Medical first introduced the AutoCapture algorithm in 1995 in Europe (and in 1999 in the USA) and continues to offer newer-generation versions of this algorithm in all of its pacemakers today. Some key take-away messages about AutoCapture:
• It looks for capture on every single beat.
• If loss of capture is determined, a backup safety pulse is delivered to assure capture.
• It conducts an automatic capture threshold test (called *threshold search*) every 8 or 24 h (depending on the device model and/or how it is programmed).

- It adjusts voltage in the pacing pulse output automatically to pulse at energy-efficient parameter settings.
- The evoked response sensitivity test measures the evoked response and polarization signals and determines if AutoCapture is recommended.
- The difference between the polarization signal and the evoked potential signal must be large enough for the pacemaker's sensing circuits to reliably distinguish them. The polarization signal occurs immediately after an output pulse for a few milliseconds and is a result of a gathering of charged ions around the tip electrode.
- If AutoCapture is recommended, turn it on at predischarge or first follow-up. Do not activate it in the hospital because AutoCapture ECGs can be confusing and generate reports of pseudomalfunction.
- AutoCapture is an algorithm for the ventricular channel; ACap Confirm is a similar feature for the atrial channel.
- The main difference between ventricular and atrial automatic capture is that the ventricular algorithm works on every beat, while the atrial algorithm checks capture every 8–24 h, depending on how it is programmed.
- First and foremost, AutoCapture promotes patient safety, although its added benefits are reduced device size and extended device longevity.

Automatic Capture from Boston Scientific

The proprietary algorithm from Boston Scientific provides automatic capture in the ventricle only, and it relies on the same concepts presented earlier. Automatic threshold measurements are taken and used to adjust the ventricular output pulse so that it captures the ventricle without wasting energy. It does this by optimizing the output voltage to 0.5 V above the capture threshold at a pulse width of 0.4 ms. Ventricular capture is confirmed with every beat using an evoked response test. If an output pulse fails to capture the ventricle, the algorithm provides for a backup safety pulse.

The Boston Scientific threshold test is called the Ambulatory Ventricular Automatic Threshold Test, and it is performed every 21 h and whenever

a confirmed loss of capture (C-LOC) occurs. Based on this measurement, the device programs the output (threshold + 0.5 V at 0.4 ms). On those rare occasions when the Ambulatory Ventricular Automatic Threshold Test cannot measure the threshold successfully, the algorithm allows for a *Retry* mode.

The clinician programs automatic capture on the programmer by selecting *AUTO* for the pulse amplitude setting (see **Figure 23.7**). Automatic capture will work with any lead and can be set up to work in unipolar and bipolar modes, but the bipolar mode is probably the better choice for most patients.

When automatic capture is programmed on, it starts out with a ventricular output pulse of 3.5 V and 0.4 ms. The device then uses the Ambulatory Ventricular Automatic Threshold Test to ascertain the patient's capture threshold by working down in increments to the minimum ventricular output that will effectively capture the ventricle. Once the threshold test determines the threshold, the ventricular output is set using the formula: threshold + 0.5 V at 0.4 ms.

If two consecutive losses of capture occur, a backup safety pulse is delivered 100 ms after the primary pulse. If there is no capture in two out of four consecutive cardiac cycles, the pacemaker declares this C-LOC and the automatic threshold test is conducted (see **Figure 23.9**). Note that whenever this automatic threshold test is conducted, loss of capture will be observed. Since this test is run automatically every 21 h, this means clinicians can expect to see one loss of capture each time, that is, about once a day. This should not be a cause for alarm. After all, if a clinician were conducting a threshold test in the clinic, there would also be a loss of capture for one beat! If C-LOC is declared and the automatic threshold test can be run successfully—which is typically the case—then the pacemaker returns to normal operation and beat-by-beat automatic capture resumes (see **Figure 23.8**).

On the other hand, if the automatic threshold test is unsuccessful after a C-LOC has occurred, then the output pulse will be set to an amplitude value twice that of the measured threshold (minimum 3.5 V and maximum 5.0 V settings). For example, if the patient's threshold had previously been determined to be 1.0 V but the automatic

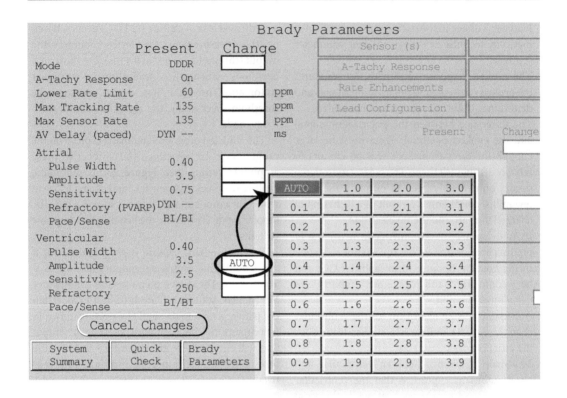

Figure 23.7 To program automatic capture in a Boston Scientific pacemaker, the clinician selects the AUTO setting for the ventricular pulse amplitude. Automatic capture can work with any lead (both unipolar and bipolar); lead configurations are programmable.

threshold test failed after a C-LOC, the pacemaker will automatically program the ventricular amplitude to 3.5 V (1.0 V × 2 = 2.0 V, which is lower than the 3.5 V minimum). This behavior is known as the Retry mode. If the pacemaker is in Retry mode, ventricular output pulses are going to be between 3.5 and 5.0 V. The device can come out of the Retry mode with a successful automatic capture Test. It will try the automatic threshold test again in 1 h. If this test can be completed successfully, the device resumes automatic capture and the next automatic threshold test occurs on schedule (the 21 h schedule is not affected by the Retry mode; this clock is never reset).

The automatic threshold test can also be initiated by the clinician from the programmer; the test runs essentially in the same way (3.5 V, stepping down in small increments until capture is lost).

Automatic capture provides a graphic depiction of the evoked response signal, which is how the pacemaker *sees* capture. In the event that the evoked response signal is not larger enough or is unclear, the programmer will report *V-ER?* or *Inadequate Evoked Response Signal*. If this occurs with some regularity, automatic capture may not be a good feature for that particular patient; in such cases, ventricular output should be set manually to the customary 2:1 to 3:1 safety margin.

The backup pulse is delivered 100 ms following the primary ventricular output pulse that failed to capture. The backup pulse interval has a 10 ms blanking period immediately after the ventricular output pulse to prevent the inappropriate sensing of polarization at the right ventricular lead tip. There is also a so-called noise window within this interval to prevent sensing of noise or fusion detection. The backup pulse will be 1.5 V greater than the last-measured threshold at 0.4 ms with a minimum setting of 3.5 V at 0.4 ms and a maximum value of 4.5 V at 0.4 ms. For example, if the

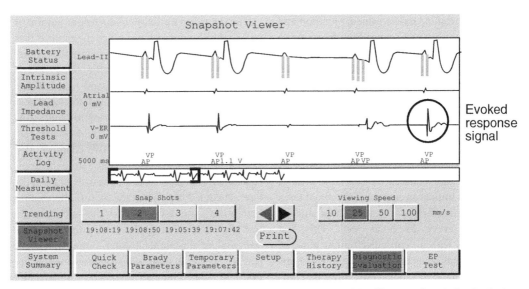

Figure 23.8 The Ventricular Automatic Threshold Test in a dual-chamber Boston Scientific pacemaker. Notice that in the first two complexes, there are two spikes for an atrial and ventricular output pulse, respectively. Capture is evident on the ECG. On the third complex, atrial and ventricular outputs occur but there is a loss of capture on the ventricular channel. The fourth complex shows atrial output (capture), ventricular output (loss of capture), and a backup safety pulse. Note that the evoked response signal appears on the V-ER line. Where loss of capture occurs, there is a corresponding lack of an evoked response signal.

previously measured threshold value was 1.0 V at 0.4 ms, the backup safety pulse will be 2.5 V at 0.4 ms (1.0 + 1.5 V = 2.5 V).

The System Summary screen on the Boston Scientific programmer offers an automatic capture Threshold trend graph to allow for rapid evaluation of the patient's threshold values. You should expect to see steady values at an appropriate voltage setting (see **Figure 23.9**).

According to the manufacturer, automatic capture can extend device longevity 10–15% at 100% pacing. This difference can be substantial, adding up to an added year of device life in some cases.

The automatic capture algorithm can be programmed on while the patient is in the hospital (predischarge) or at the first follow-up. It is not advised to program it on sooner since automatic capture algorithms can produce confusing ECGs that may result in calls about *pacemaker malfunctions* that turn out to be the normal and expected behavior of the device. If the automatic capture algorithm reports an unsuccessful threshold test the first time, it is recommended that the clinician program the automatic threshold OFF and perform a conventional threshold test. If that threshold

Automatic capture threshold

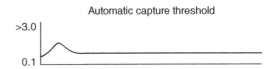

Figure 23.9 The automatic capture Threshold trend appears on the programmer in Boston Scientific devices. Note that this trend shows an initial upward trend that came down and then plateaued. The higher area initially corresponds to the acute-to-chronic threshold transition. Trend graphs give clinicians a good *high-altitude* view of how the device and patient are interacting. Thresholds should be consistent after about 6–8 weeks and at an appropriate voltage value; substantial changes in threshold may warrant investigation.

test is unsuccessful, the pacemaker and its leads must be evaluated. There is clearly a problem with the system. On the other hand, if a manual threshold test is successful, it is recommended that the automatic threshold test be attempted again in an hour or at some later point.

Boston Scientific automatic capture summary

- This is a beat-by-beat capture algorithm and is available for the ventricle only.

- When the threshold is determined, the automatic capture output is 0.5 V above that threshold at 0.4 ms.
- The algorithm evaluates evoked response to confirmed capture.
- The backup safety pulse is delivered 100 ms after the primary pulse and is 1.5 V above the previously measured threshold with a maximum setting of 4.5 V.
- C-LOC occurs when there is loss of capture in two out of four consecutive cardiac cycles. A C-LOC will initiate an automatic threshold test.
- An automatic threshold test is automatically conducted every 21 h as well. This test commences with a ventricular output pulse of 3.5 V and steps down until loss of capture occurs.
- If the automatic threshold test cannot be completed successfully, the device enters the Retry mode. The automatic threshold test is tried again in an hour; this pattern will repeat until the test can be completed successfully.
- The 21 h automatic threshold test clock is never reset, even if the device has been in Retry mode and has run other threshold tests in the past few hours.
- The clinician can *command* an automatic threshold test from the programmer. It runs the same way as the automatic version.

Capture management from Medtronic

While the St. Jude Medical and Boston Scientific algorithms share similar concepts, Capture Management from Medtronic is quite different. Capture Management is not a beat-by-beat algorithm. Instead, it automatically monitors pacing thresholds in both the atrium and the ventricle at periodic intervals. Once the threshold is determined, the pacemaker determines a target output value based on the minimum pulse amplitude plus a programmable safety margin. Capture Management as an algorithm can be programmed to *Adaptive* (which means it is on), *Monitor Only* (which provides data to the clinician on how the algorithm would have worked had it been on), or Off. Only the Adaptive setting will result in reprogramming of the pulse amplitude of the output pulse.

The algorithm works by conducting an automatic pacing threshold search test called the capture Test. The clinician programs how frequently the capture Test should be performed with fixed-interval values of every 15 min, 30 min, and 1, 2, 4, 8, and 12 h. It can also be programmed to occur at a certain time during the day. Prior to conducting the Capture Test, the pacemaker seeks stable pacing in the chamber the respective chamber. If it cannot confirm stable pacing at the time the test is scheduled, it cancels the test; it retries again at the next scheduled test. When the capture threshold is determined, the device applies the safety margin that the clinician programs (called the *amplitude margin*) and minimum allowable output amplitude (called the *minimum adapted amplitude*). For example, the clinician can set up Capture Management to threshold test every 15 min, to never let the output pulse get lower than 1.5 V, and, when the capture threshold is determined, to apply a 2:1 safety margin. In many instances, Capture Management more or less automates the values that would occur in conventional programming, that is, the 2:1 safety margin.

Capture Management does not confirm loss of capture and has no backup pulses to pace in the event of noncapture. It is available on both atrial and ventricular channels but works somewhat differently in each. They are also independently programmable; the clinician can set up ventricular Capture Management but not atrial Capture Management.

Medtronic capture management summary

Capture Management from Medtronic is a fundamentally different algorithm than the automatic capture algorithm from Boston Scientific and the AutoCapture algorithm from St. Jude Medical, in particular because it is not a beat-by-beat algorithm. Capture Management assesses the patient's pacing threshold automatically at programmable intervals and then adjusts the output pulse amplitude based on a safety margin that the clinician can adjust (such as 1.5:1 or 2:1, and so on). For many clinicians, these programmable options are intuitively understandable and closely mirror conventional output pulse programming. Capture Management does not confirm capture with an evoked response test or deliver a backup safety pulse.

Table 23.1 A very short overview of some of the key characteristics of automatic capture algorithms from the three largest manufacturers of pacemakers

Features	Boston Scientific	Medtronic	St. Jude Medical
Name	Automatic capture	Capture Management	AutoCapture
Available in A and V	No	Yes, but works differently	Yes, but works differently
Threshold search	Every 21 h, not programmable	Programmable from every 15 min to every 12 h	Programmable every 8 to 24 h
Beat-by-beat capture assessment	Yes	No	Yes
Detects loss of capture	Yes	No	Yes
Backup safety pulse in the event of loss of capture	Yes	No	Yes
Safety margin of output pulse	0.5 V above threshold	Programmed by clinician	0.25 V above threshold

A look at all three algorithms

This chapter reviewed briefly only three capture algorithms; Sorin and Biotronik also have automatic capture algorithms. Furthermore, each new generation of devices can bring enhancements and changes to these algorithms—so please take this chapter with a grain of salt. The best advice to clinicians is to keep up-to-date with the latest products from all manufacturers. All manufacturers offer excellent instructions about these and other algorithms in their physician manuals, which may be available online and are certainly available upon clinician request to the company.

St. Jude Medical pioneered the algorithm and has worked to continually refine it, advancing from a ventricular-only system to an atrial version. Boston Scientific has an algorithm that works on the same principles (beat-by-beat evaluation, measurement of evoked response, capture confirmation, and backup safety pulses) but, at the time of this printing, has only ventricular automatic capture. The Medtronic algorithm is substantially different but offers some distinctive characteristics that clinicians may like: it can be programmed to test capture thresholds frequently and it imposes a clinician-defined safety margin. A short overview of these algorithms appears in **Table 23.1**.

Conclusion

Automatic capture algorithms have absolutely changed cardiac pacing and, in my opinion, for the better. These algorithms automate the once tedious function of threshold testing, allowing it to be conducted more frequently. The information from these capture tests can then be effectively applied to the output pulse of the pacemaker, with the result that the pacemaker saves energy. This energy efficiency has contributed to device downsizing. But more than that, algorithms that evaluate capture can enhance patient safety.

Despite these good things, clinicians routinely will encounter physicians and other colleagues who do not use automatic capture algorithms. Sometimes, these are *old-school physicians* who over the years got used to programming pacemaker output settings a certain way and dislike changing their routines. More often, they are physicians who just do not trust automatic algorithms. The best way to win over a skeptic is to ask them to manually conduct a threshold test—the way they *have always done it*—and then launch the same automatic threshold test from the programmer to compare results. When the clinician sees that the automatic threshold test can get the same value, it can often relieve anxiety that the automatic algorithm is somehow less reliable than the conventional method.

While this chapter attempted to briefly go over the main concepts behind the algorithms offered by three of the five pacemaker manufacturers, consider this chapter more theoretical than a *how-to* guide. Most manufacturers offer excellent *how-to* programming guides, brochures, and manuals to explain their features, and these are going to be far more specific—and up-to-date—than what appears here.

The nuts and bolts of automatic capture algorithms

- Automatic capture algorithms have changed pacing. They are available from all manufacturers and they are in widespread use today. Their main advantage is that they promote patient safety while also being energy efficient.
- St. Jude Medical first introduced AutoCapture pacing systems in 1995 (Europe) and in 1999 in the USA. This original algorithm worked only on the ventricular channel and it was debuted in a tiny device called the Microny® pacemaker.
- Noncapture is a serious problem because the whole point of cardiac pacing is capture. Most clinicians would estimate that noncapture occurs in about 1–5% of patients.
- Noncapture can be caused by any number of conditions. First, it may be that the device was improperly programmed and the output is too low. Second and more likely, the patient's threshold may have changed such that the output is no longer sufficient for capture.
- Threshold changes occur every day in patients. They are known to occur with changes in posture, with meals, with certain medications, and with certain activities. Thresholds can also change with disease progression. The big problem with threshold fluctuations is that they are unpredictable.
- For most patients, the capture threshold is lowest at implant, then it rises upward at peaks at about 2 weeks. At 4–6 weeks, it goes back down and plateaus at a low level that is somewhat above the implant value. In a normal patient, the threshold plateaus at that level for the rest of the device's service life. Since the initial threshold is measured at implant (when it is lowest) but must work when the threshold rises (when it reaches it maximum value ever), clinicians program a 5:1 safety margin at implant. For example, if the capture threshold at implant is 0.5 V, then the pacemaker should be programmed to no less than 2.5 V. After the acute-to-chronic transition when the threshold decreases and plateaus, it is measured again and a 2:1 or 3:1 safety margin is used; for instance, the threshold may be 1.0 V and the physician programs 2.5:1. (Physicians tend to say that they use a 2:1 or 3:1 safety margin, but very few are comfortable actually programming a 2:1 margin—they tend to round up a little to 2.5:1.)
- The problem with 5:1 or 3:1 or 2.5:1 safety margins is that they routinely waste battery energy. Automatic capture algorithms allow the clinician to shrink the safety margin to the point that much less energy is wasted.
- Automatic capture algorithms must confirm that they have captured the heart. A pacemaker on its own will deliver an output pulse and then assume it captures; there is no verification. The algorithms for automatic capture added a feature that allowed the pacemaker to verify capture.
- Capture verification uses something called the *evoked potential* or ER. This is engineer-ese for the captured (evoked) beat (potential) as seen on an intracardiac electrogram. After a pacemaker output pulse is delivered, the pacemaker checks that an ER occurred. The presence of an ER of sufficient size to be a cardiac depolarization means the spike captured the heart.
- If an output pulse is delivered and does not capture the heart, the device delivers a backup safety pulse. The exact specifications of this pulse (voltage, pulse duration) vary by manufacturer, but it tends to be a high output (such as 5.0 V at 0.4 ms). It may be delivered 80–100 ms following the spike that did not capture. There is often a short blanking period right after the spike of about 10 ms to prevent the pacemaker from sensing polarization at the lead tip.
- If a loss of capture occurs, the algorithm is able to automatically measure the threshold and adjust its output settings again. This threshold test or threshold search occurs with loss of capture or at regular intervals (which may or may not be programmable, depending on the manufacturer).
- The threshold test is automatic but it works on the same premise as a conventional, manual threshold test. A value is selected that captures the heart and then it is reduced step by step in small increments until capture is lost; when capture is lost, the output is increased by a small increment to regain capture. This arrives at the threshold.

- With some algorithms, the pacing output is just slightly above the threshold (0.25 V for St. Jude Medical and 0.5 V for Boston Scientific). This may sound very low—these algorithms often work at output values of 1.0 V! But remember that there is a backup safety pulse in place.
- Some automatic capture algorithms work beat by beat (St. Jude Medical and Boston Scientific), while Capture Management (Medtronic) uses a different approach by automatically testing thresholds at programmable intervals and adjusting device output to the physician-programmed safety margin. Capture Management does not offer a backup safety pulse.
- Polarization refers to the collection of charged ions that gather around the pacing lead electrode tip immediately after an output pulse; polarization is very short-lived (about 10 ms) but it can create a signal that can obscure the evoked potential.
- Do not activate an automatic capture algorithm while the patient is in the hospital. Turn on this feature either immediately before the patient is discharged or at the first follow-up. The reason for this is that automatic capture may create pseudomalfunctions on the ECG that can confuse hospital staff and even result in calls to the pacing physician.

- All manufacturers offer an automatic capture algorithm for the ventricle, and some companies also have a corresponding function for the atrial channel. Atrial automatic capture is more challenging for engineers to develop because of the relatively small difference in size between an evoked signal potential and the polarization signal.
- St. Jude Medical's atrial AutoCapture algorithm is called ACap Confirm™ and it is not a beat-by-beat algorithm. It verifies capture, periodically overdrives the atrium, and conducts an atrial threshold search. Once it has established the atrial threshold, it then adds a safety margin value to it, for example, for thresholds between 0.125 and 1.5 V, the system adds a safety margin of 1.0 V.
- Boston Scientific has a beat-by-beat automatic capture algorithm called automatic capture, and it is available only for the ventricle. It has a backup safety pulse delivered 100 ms after the primary pulse in the event of loss of capture. Confirmed loss of capture is defined by the device as two losses of capture in four consecutive events; this initiates the automatic threshold test. If the automatic threshold test fails to find a threshold, it enters Retry mode and retries the test every hour.

Test your knowledge

1 Which manufacturer brought to market the first pacemaker with an automatic capture algorithm?
  A Medtronic
  B St. Jude Medical
  C Boston Scientific
  D Biotronik

2 Which of the following was *not* accomplished with automatic capture algorithms?
  A Enhanced patient safety
  B Longer service life of the pulse generator
  C Reduced device prices
  D Smaller devices

3 Which manufacturer's system is known as Capture Management?

  A Medtronic
  B St. Jude Medical
  C Boston Scientific
  D Biotronik

4 When is a backup safety pulse delivered?
  A After a failure to capture
  B After an evoked potential
  C After a polarization signal
  D After a threshold search

5 Mr. Garcia has a DDDR pacemaker from St. Jude Medical with the AutoCapture algorithm. He is in for follow-up and has just had a magnet placed over the pacemaker for about 30 s. When the magnet is removed, how does the AutoCapture system respond?

A AutoCapture automatically disables itself upon magnet application.

B AutoCapture continues operating normally.

C AutoCapture automatically runs an E/R sensitivity test.

D AutoCapture automatically runs a threshold search.

6 What is the best reason of those listed below to *not activate* an automatic capture algorithm while the patient is in the hospital right after device implantation?

A The acute-to-chronic threshold transition.

B Lead/tissue interface issues.

C The paced ECGs can be confusing to the hospital staff.

D The algorithm must gather at least 48 h of data before it can start.

7 Studies have shown that a patient's polarization signal amplitude remains stable but that the evoked response signal can change over the course of about 6 months. What is a good way to manage this?

A Measure the evoked response signal at least every 6 months.

B Measure the polarization signal at least every 6 months.

C Increase the evoked response sensitivity every 6 months.

D Monitor the patient and discontinue automatic capture if the evoked response signal changes more than 10%.

8 Which of the following statements *does not apply* to Boston Scientific's automatic capture algorithm?

A It works beat by beat.

B It is available for the atrium and ventricle.

C It is activated by programming pulse amplitude to AUTO.

D It runs an automatic capture test every 21 h and this is not programmable.

9 Which company has an algorithm that delivers a backup safety pulse after the second loss of capture (not the first)?

A Capture Management for the atrium

B ACap Confirm

C Automatic capture

D AutoCapture

10 In the AutoCapture algorithm from St. Jude Medical, once the capture threshold is determined, how is the output pulse set?

A It is 0.25 V above the threshold.

B It is 0.5 V above the threshold.

C It is 10% above the threshold.

D It relies on a programmable safety margin (2:1, 2.5:1, 3:1).

CHAPTER 24

Pacemaker follow-up

Learning objectives

- Compare the three main *types* of pacemaker follow-up.
- Briefly describe what the guidelines allow in terms of frequency of pacemaker follow-up.
- Name at least one drawback to transtelephonic monitoring (TTM).
- Explain how information is conveyed using TTM and RM.
- Using the acronym PUBL-STOP, name the key steps in systematic pacemaker follow-up.
- Define the recognized boundaries of the role of the industry-employed associated professional in the pacemaker clinic.

Introduction

There are roughly one million new cardiovascular implantable electronic devices (CIEDs) implanted every year, many of which are pacemakers. Remembering that a pacemaker can last a dozen years or more, this means there are millions of CIED patients all over the world. Follow-up for these patients is the lion's share of work done at the average device clinic. Whether you are a doctor, nurse, other healthcare professional, or industry representative, if you work at a device clinic, you will be involved in follow-up.

Getting to know and understand follow-up is crucial to success in the device clinic. In many ways, follow-up seems deceptively simple. Most clinics have systematized the process to streamline the workflow and programmers today have automated

many tests. Sometimes, follow-up work is routine; the device is functioning appropriately and the patient is doing well. In many cases, no device adjustments are required. On the other hand, sometimes, follow-up involves troubleshooting, which we will cover in the next chapter.

Types of follow-up

There are three main types of follow-up: transtelephonic monitoring (TTM), remote monitoring (RM), and the in-clinic visit. All three are widely used today and you may even use all three types for one single patient. The trend in follow-up is to move to the increasing use of RM, but RM will never completely replace the in-clinic visit.

Transtelephonic Monitoring (TTM)

Pioneered in the early days of cardiac pacing, TTM can make a strong claim to be the first widespread form of telemedicine, in that it enabled a pacemaker clinic to follow their remote patients. TTM is still used today, although for reasons we will see shortly, it is not as popular today as it once was.

Patients using TTM receive a kit from the clinic with equipment to attach to a landline and electrodes to be used on their body. The patient would then call the clinic on the landline and establish a connection between his or her transmitter and the clinic's receiver. The pacemaker then sent a paced ECG via the phone line to the clinic's receiver. This paced ECG could be used to assess appropriate capture and sensing. In some cases, the paced ECG might show other issues as well. After this transmission, the patient would place a magnet

The Nuts and Bolts of Implantable Device Therapy Pacemakers, First Edition. Tom Kenny.
© 2015 John Wiley & Sons, Ltd. Published 2015 by John Wiley & Sons, Ltd.

(provided in the TTM kit) over the implanted device. This caused the pacemaker to go into magnet mode. A magnet mode ECG would be transmitted to the clinic, from which the clinic could estimate battery status. (Battery mode changes as the battery nears its elective replacement indicator.)

There are a lot of things that TTM cannot do: it cannot download diagnostic data or reports from the pacemaker, it cannot make adjustments to the pacemaker, and it cannot provide the clinic with alerts or messages about unusual conditions. The average TTM session is brief and fairly simple for the patient: only two ECGs are transmitted (one paced, one magnet mode). The great advantage to TTM is that it provided patients with a fast, convenient way to have routine device checks from the convenience of their home. Today, one of the biggest *threats* to TTM is the fact that landlines are rapidly becoming a thing of the past and TTM does not work with cell phones. Also, new technologies like RM may displace TTM. Nevertheless, it is still in widespread use.

Remote Monitoring (RM)

RM, sometimes called home monitoring, is the latest generation of long-distance follow-up equipment available for pacemakers. The two main distinctions between TTM and RM are that RM relies on the Internet for high-speed data transmission and RM offers downloaded reports and stored electrograms rather than paced and magnet ECGs. Except for Sorin, all of the major companies have their own RM systems but they have different names, unique features, and programming nuances.

With RM, the patient also receives a transmitter kit. The transmitter is designed so that when the device is in the vicinity, it can wirelessly communicate with the implanted pacemaker. For that reason, doctors often tell patients to keep the transmitter on the night stand near their bed, and then the doctor sets up the system to automatically communicate with the pacemaker every night at, say, 2 a.m., when the patient is asleep near the transmitter. Patients are unaware of the transmission, which is completely painless and requires no action on their part. The transmitter communicates with the pacemaker and is able to *pull* from the pacemaker diagnostic data, reports, trends,

histograms, stored electrograms, and other information. This information travels via the Internet to a secure website, which is usually not at the clinic at all. Special centers exist to receive and store these downloaded reports, which clinicians can then retrieve at their convenience. Think of RM as the ability to conduct a full device interrogation. However, RM does not allow for transmission of paced or magnet ECGs (like TTM) and it cannot make adjustments to the device.

RM has the unique ability to allow for special programmable *alerts*. An alert is a message that is sent automatically to the doctor (or nurse, clinician, technician, or other specified individual) by text, email, or fax that is triggered by a programmable event or condition. For example, the clinician may program an alert that if the RM ever sees out-of-range lead impedance values, it should trigger an alert. He may even be able to specify exactly what lead impedance values should generate the alert message. Alerts may be programmed for arrhythmic activity (atrial fibrillation, ventricular tachycardia), system status (elective replacement), or device-related conditions (mode switching episodes). Clinicians can also prioritize alerts individually for patients, making some *red alerts* or emergencies and others more like notifications.

The value of the system is better illustrated with an example. Let's say a dual-chamber pacemaker patient has a device with a lead that is under surveillance because of potential malfunction. The doctor has decided not to replace the lead in the patient because the patient is too frail to withstand another surgery, but he is concerned about lead function. He may program that any marked fluctuation in lead impedance generates a top-priority alert. In this way, if there is a lead problem, it will be caught at the very latest point by the next RM follow-up at 2 a.m.

The terminology for RM is a little fuzzy. RM refers to the regular monitoring of the pacemaker using the remote system. Sometimes, clinicians talk about remote follow-up, which is a way of initiating an RM session from the clinic. For instance, the clinic may contact a patient and ask them to sit near their transmitter as a data download takes place. The clinician can then review the reports; in some cases, the clinician will even call the patient with the results, which is often just the reassurance that everything is working fine. Thus, RM works automatically, but it can also be used as a specific follow-up tool as well.

RM is used as a tool to consistently monitor the pacemaker and generate alerts about unusual or remarkable events. It can also be used for follow-up. Even though RM works on a daily basis, clinicians do not conduct a full-blown follow-up every day—alerts serve to bridge the gap between follow-ups. For this reason, RM is considered a system that enhances patient safety. Take this example: Mr. Smith and Mr. Jones both have dual-chamber pacemakers but only Mr. Smith has RM. Both of them experience a long episode of AF. Mr. Smith's RM generated an alert message, which was received by the clinic, which called him in for an exam and some device adjustments plus a prescription. Mr. Jones waited several more months until his next in-clinic visit when the clinic discovered he had been experiencing prolonged episodes of AF. Similar case reports of the value of RM in finding problems early (often before the patient developed symptoms) appear in the medical literature.

In-clinic follow-up

The traditional in-clinic follow-up visit may be the most *old-school* version of follow-up of all, but nothing will ever totally replace this form of checkup. An in-clinic visit allows the clinical team to meet with the patient face-to-face, to interact, to observe the patient for signs of potential cardiac disease or other comorbid conditions, and to adjust

the pacemaker. No other form of follow-up allows for the clinician to make changes to how the device's parameters are set. During an in-clinic visit, the patient is typically interviewed about possible changes in his or her condition and medications and the programmer is used to download reports and diagnostics. An in-clinic visit allows for the recording of a paced ECG as well as retrieval of information stored in the pacemaker. In many ways, the in-clinic follow-up is the *ideal scenario* for follow-up, but it can be a hardship for the patient to come to the clinic several times a year (particularly when the report is usually that everything is functioning normally) and it places a huge burden on the clinics and healthcare system to see so many patients.

Benefits of follow-up

Follow-up is more than what most of us think. Whenever you follow a pacemaker, you are going to check the device, but you are also checking the patient, assessing how the patient and the device are interacting, and monitoring the patient's underlying and possible comorbid disease states. Clinicians should remember they are evaluating the patient, the device, and how the two are interacting, and they must also be mindful of the patient's underlying disease (see **Table 24.1**). It is not unusual for pacemaker patients to be geriatric and have comorbid conditions prevalent in that population, including hypertension, diabetes, heart failure, and arthritis. Furthermore, cardiovascular

Table 24.1 No matter how follow-up is conducted, the clinician must evaluate the patient, the device, how they interact, and the patient's underlying and possible comorbid conditions

Patient	Device	Interactions	Disease
Does device meet patient's current needs?	Is this device working appropriately? Is there good capture and sensing?	Would the patient benefit from any special features that are not currently on?	What arrhythmia(s) does the patient have and how severe and frequent are they?
Is the patient at risk for arrhythmias or other conditions, such as heart failure?	Has the device reached end of life?	Is there evidence of fusion, pauses, frequent PVCs, and frequent mode switches? Can these be addressed or minimized?	Is the patient suffering hemodynamic compromise?
Does the patient need a referral to any kind of specialist?	Are there abnormal or suboptimal device behaviors that can be fixed?	Is rate response adjusted appropriately? If it is not on, should it be turned on?	What is transthoracic impedance? Is the patient having pulmonary problems?

disease tends to get progressively worse, so the patient's cardiac condition will likely worsen over time and require pacemaker adjustments.

Communication

Not so long ago, the average pacemaker clinician was buried in paper, having to print out histograms and trends and ECGs and to handwrite follow-up results in the patient's folder. Sometimes, the print-outs from the old programmers used long, skinny thermal paper that never folded up right and would stick out of the folders. Today, that is changing. In fact, many clinicians today work in paperless clinics where all of these reports are digitized and retained. Electronic medical records (EMR), sometimes called electronic health records, represent a major advance in how clinicians document care. With EMR, the patient's entire record (in theory at least) is available digitally and travels with the patient. This means that the pacing clinic or the diabetes clinic or the emergency room will all have access to the same complete record. EMR could mean more thorough records and more complete records. The potential of EMR is that records could travel securely around the hospital, from clinic to clinic, or even around the world.

There is one important danger in the transition to EMR and that is that clinicians will assume that *electronic* means *automatic*. The fact is whether we use the old paper files or EMR, the system relies on clinical personnel to document and communicate. At the time this book was written, it was rare for a pacemaker to be able to download records directly into an EMR; but that may change in the future. As a result, clinicians still have to retrieve information and assure that it gets recorded.

Good communication also means sharing information with colleagues inside and outside of our own clinic.

Frequency of follow-up

Guidelines are considered important roadmaps to clinical care; they are written by experts who get a consensus among the leaders in the field. For cardiac pacing, we look to the Heart Rhythm Society (HRS), the American College of Cardiology (ACC), and the American Heart Association (AHA) for clinical guidelines relating to the care of pacemaker patients. Another type of guideline—and perhaps one of greater interest to the business side of the clinic—is issued by the Centers for Medicare and Medicaid Services (CMS). CMS controls Medicare reimbursements and most pacemakers are covered by Medicare. Now, the last time CMS updated its guidelines with respect to frequency of pacemaker follow-up was 1984! That's over 30 years ago and a lot has changed, but reimbursement guidance for pacemaker follow-up has not.

Speaking as a clinician, the main thing that should influence the frequency and type of pacemaker follow-up is the patient. For instance, a stable patient may require less frequent follow-up than an unstable one. A patient who is dependent on the device requires more rigorous follow-up than one who is not. A patient who cannot reliably report his or her own symptoms may require closer monitoring than one who knows and reports symptoms clearly. Patients and their families may have their own preferences that should be taken into account. For instance, some patients dislike the RM system, typically for one of two reasons. The first is technical—it's too complicated, and the patient gets frustrated trying to work the equipment. The second is because of concerns about privacy; some people are distrustful of personal or medical information traveling on the Internet. Clinicians will encounter patients who could benefit from RM but will refuse it. There may also be social factors that come into play, for instance, some patients may want to see the doctor face-to-face at regular intervals, while others may find travel to the clinic a hardship (this can be particularly true for patients who are in wheelchairs or have limited mobility).

Planned procedures may be a reason for a device check. In some cases, patients may be able to undergo certain types of interventions when precautionary steps are taken. It may be necessary to check the device both before and after the procedure. For instance, a patient who requires therapeutic radiation may have to undergo the procedure with caution (radiation may damage the device) and require a postprocedural device check to verify proper device function. (Note that diagnostic radiation doses are much lower than therapeutic radiation; diagnostic radiation is unlikely to be a source of problem.) Therapeutic radiation can damage the complementary metal-oxide semiconductors (CMOS) within the pacemaker. The great challenge in managing this situation is that CMOS damage has unpredictable consequences; therapeutic radiation may cause no damage or it may lead to no output or conditions in between. Since the device damage may be cumulative (it builds up over time), the pacing clinic should work together with the radiology team to develop a plan for the pacemaker patient. Pacemaker patients who require therapeutic radiation typically have the device shielded with lead, but radiation within the body scatters so that even if the radiation does not hit the pacemaker directly, it can still *ricochet* and hit the pacemaker. Shielding the device is a good strategy, but it is not 100% guaranteed. A better strategy (but one that is rarely used) is to move the device to an implant site more distant to the site of radiation and shield it there. In actual clinical practice, the most effective solution to therapeutic radiation in a pacemaker patient is to conduct a follow-up after each and every radiation session. In each of these follow-ups, the clinician checks to assure that the device is functioning properly.

Follow-up frequency may also be affected by the age of the device; it is good practice to follow an older device more closely than a newer device. As the device nears battery depletion, it may be useful to accelerate follow-up to be sure that the patient continues to receive therapy.

Other factors can also influence how often follow-up should occur: changes in medication or condition, frequency or severity of arrhythmic episodes, and changes in cardiovascular therapy. For instance, if the patient's disease state is intensifying and their condition is worsening, their follow-up frequency should probably intensify as well.

The guidelines

The HRS together with the European Heart Rhythm Association has issued a consensus statement from experts for the minimum recommended follow-up for pacemaker and other CIED patients [1]. A short summary appears in **Table 24.2**. These follow-ups stated in the following are reimbursable by CMS.

Thus, a pacemaker patient can have a follow-up visit every 3 months, which would be reimbursable

Table 24.2 A summary of minimum recommended pacemaker follow-ups

Timing	Type
Within 72 hours after implant	In person
Two to 12 weeks after implant	In person
Every 3–12 months (at least annually until battery depletion)	In person or remote
Every 1–3 months at signs of battery depletion	In person or remote

Note that *remote* could be a remote follow-up using RM equipment or it could be TTM. Pacemakers are recommended to be monitored at least annually until battery depletion.

by CMS in the USA. However, many pacemaker patients are stable enough that their follow-up visit is more of a routine check confirming everything is fine. In the USA, some doctors manage this by having their stable pacemaker patients come to the clinic for an in-person visit once a year and then doing the other three follow-ups remotely.

Lost to follow-up

Despite the clinic's best efforts, some patients will simply not show up for their scheduled follow-up visits. Such patients are described as *lost to follow-up*, meaning that the clinic lost touch with them during the follow-up phase of their treatment. At the highest level, it is the patient's responsibility to come to follow-up, but physicians bear a secondary responsibility. As a result, many clinics spend time calling, writing letters, and making all reasonable efforts to get these *lost* patients in for a device check. Anecdotally, I have heard of clinics contacting the police to find *lost* patients. Police cannot arrest a person for missing a follow-up; ultimately, the patient has the right to refuse follow-up. However, physicians bear a responsibility as well and will make efforts to find *lost* patients. Note that the police in this anecdote were contacted to be sure nothing had happened to the patient, not to coerce the patient to come to the clinic. Patients have the full legal right to refuse follow-up, although that is obviously not a very wise decision.

Patients can be lost to follow-up for many reasons, not just refusal of services. Patients may move away and fail to tell their doctor. A patient may have found another physician or device clinic that he or she prefers and does not tell the doctor. Sometimes, patients become very sick or incapacitated and the clinic is not informed, such as an elderly, frail patient who is taken to a nursing home. Such patients may be followed at the residential facility. And, last but not least, it must be mentioned that some patients die and their families do not necessarily think to notify the pacemaker clinic.

Thus, patients who are *lost to follow-up* may be haphazard about their care or there may be valid reasons that they no longer come to the clinic. *Lost* patients represent a major problem for most clinics in that physicians need to make reasonable efforts to track them down.

The complete pacemaker follow-up

Although there are three main types of follow-up, a complete pacemaker follow-up can only be obtained by an in-clinic visit. Below are the things that must take place in a complete follow-up:

- Patient interview
- Interrogation of the device
- Review of device data (diagnostic data, stored electrograms, histograms, and so on) and currently programmed parameters
- Temporary programming so that the following tests can be conducted:
  - Capture threshold test
  - Sensing threshold test
- Evaluate impedance values
- Changes to programmable parameter settings, if necessary
- Assessment of rate response and special features, if necessary (including programming them on or off or making programming adjustments)

TTM and RM are useful follow-up alternatives, but they do not offer complete pacemaker follow-up, which should be conducted in person at least once a year. The follow-up visit may be conducted by a physician, a nurse, clinician, or even a properly trained industry representative, but permanent programming changes should only be made or at least approved by the physician. Setting pacemaker parameters is essentially the same as writing a prescription—and the physician should be involved even if he or she does not do the actual programming.

Interrogation evaluation

The pacemaker patient can be interrogated at an in-clinic visit or using RM. A so-called interrogation evaluation is a review of the pacemaker's data and programmable parameter settings. It is appropriate for a physician or an allied healthcare professional to conduct this kind of follow-up. This kind of follow-up is appropriate for:

- Checking the patient's response to an arrhythmia or other cardiovascular drug, particularly if the prescription is new or has changed
- Monitoring battery voltage to estimate device longevity as the device nears end of service
- Monitoring a pacemaker that is subject to a *field notification* (recall)

If device parameter changes are indicated, these must be programmed by or approved by a physician.

Periprocedural evaluation

If the pacemaker patient is scheduled to undergo some sort of procedure, an interrogation of the pacemaker is appropriate. Depending on the type of procedure, it may be necessary to temporarily reprogram certain pacemaker parameters or even to turn the device off. The patient should also be educated as to the potential risks (if any) to the device during the procedure. If the device must be reprogrammed or turned off, the patient should be told this clearly and instructed as to when the device would be turned back to previously programmed parameters. In many cases, it is good practice to interrogate and check the device following the procedure, even if the chance of damage to the device is slim.

Patient-initiated RM

Previously, we discussed RM as an automatic function with alerts to notify clinicians about important changes in the patient's condition. The patient can also initiate an RM transmission from home. For example, if a pacemaker patient is home and experiences sudden palpitations or shortness of breath, he or she might call the clinic and be asked to initiate an RM transmission. Not all patients will be prepared or able to do this, but it can be an important way to get immediate information about a symptomatic spell.

Follow-up steps

When a pacemaker patient is to undergo a routine follow-up (every 3 or 6 months) whether this is conducted in clinic or by RM, it should include:
- Battery voltage
- Magnet rate
- Pacing and sensing thresholds
- Lead impedance
- Percentage paced and percentage sensed (in each chamber)
- Review of programmed parameter settings
- Review of diagnostic data
- Review of stored electrograms, if any
- Review of any device alerts

In the real-world clinical practice, one of the biggest challenges in follow-up is remembering to do all of the right steps. It is very easy to get distracted in the hectic day-to-day world of a device clinic, and because many tests are routine and produce routine results, even experienced clinicians can forget to do all of the necessary tests. For that reason, device clinicians need a system for follow-up. It is not nearly as important which system you select as that you find and regularly use a follow-up system. A systematic approach to follow-up does many things:
- It assures you do not accidentally overlook or forget important tests or downloads.
- It prevents you from *jumping ahead* and making rash assessments instead of carefully reviewing all of the information.
- It keeps you honest—so that you are not tempted to skip a step in the heat of the moment.

There are many systems out there and many device clinicians have come up with their own methods over the years. Several years ago, Medtronic created a great systematic approach to follow-up, which they call PBL-STOP. I modified this a bit to PUBL-STOP, but I have to give most of the credit for this to the folks at Medtronic (see **Table 24.3**).

Roles in follow-up

Even a relatively healthy patient meets a lot of different people along the *continuum of care*.

Pacemaker clinics are staffed with doctors and nurses but also administrators, technicians, and other healthcare professionals. One nuance in the pacemaker clinic that is perhaps less evident in other fields is that pacemaker clinics also include industry-employed allied professionals (IEAP) who are usually called industry reps. The main role of the IEAP is to provide technical expertise on the implant, use, and operation of the company's products (pacemakers), but there are some important limitations:
- The physician must request the services of the IEAP; IEAPs may not appear at implants or in clinics uninvited or stay on if the physician asks them to leave.
- An IEAP may attend the implant procedure. This is actually not unusual, and the presence of an IEAP can be very helpful to the surgical team as the IEAP is the *product expert*. However, the IEAP should stay out of the sterile field unless he or she has privileges at that institution.
- The IEAP should only perform technical support functions when the physician is nearby (either in the same room or close enough that the physician could be there in a matter of minutes).

IEAPs play a crucial role in modern device clinics; they bring knowledge of their company's products to the team and can assist the team whether they are handling routine device-related tasks or troubleshooting challenging cases. Note that IEAPs must always be invited by the physician, work in close proximity to the physician, and work only with or using equipment from their own company. An IEAP from one company should not be conducting an interrogation on a device from another company. Never should an IEAP provide technical support at the clinic when they are unsupervised or alone. An IEAP should not provide technical assistance in the home of a patient unless the responsible physician is present or nearby. Under very rare emergency circumstances, an IEAP can assist a patient without supervision if the responsible physician has issued direct written orders to this effect and even then, the IEAP must restrict his or her work to only the extent specified in writing by the doctor. This might happen if the IEAP is called in remotely to help assist in a particular case.

Although IEAPs must be invited by the physician, they often find themselves working closely

Table 24.3 The PUBL-STOP method, taken from Medtronic's PBL-STOP system for follow-up

Letter	Stands for	What to do
P	Presenting rhythm	Greet the patient, apply the surface ECG electrodes, and record the presenting rhythm
		As much as the tracing allows, determine the pacing mode, rate, and if capture and sensing are appropriate
		At this point, briefly review the interrogation screen to identify what sort of pacing behavior has occurred since the last follow-up (percentage paced/sensed by chamber) (see **Figure 24.1**)
U	Underlying rhythm	If the patient is not pacemaker dependent, it is a good idea to assess the underlying or native rhythm. You may have to make some temporary adjustments to the pacemaker to expose the underlying rhythm. For example, you may be able to temporarily lower the base rate. Some manufacturers offer a button on the program to temporarily inhibit pacing in both chambers; as long as the button is depressed, the pacemaker will not pace. Releasing the button restores pacing at the previously programmed parameters
		Knowing the underlying rhythm, verify that the presenting rhythm and the percentages paced are appropriate. For instance, if the patient is paced mainly in the AP/VP state but appears to have good intrinsic conduction across the AV node, the pacemaker should be adjusted to allow for intrinsic conduction (AP/VS), typically by extending the AV delay interval
B	Battery status	Use the programmer to get a report on the battery (you may have to navigate from the interrogation main screen to a screen or subscreen on battery status or battery measurements) (see **Figure 24.2**). The main goal is to estimate when the device will require replacement
L	Lead impedance	Check the lead impedance for all leads in the system (see **Figure 24.2**) (look for *measured impedance*). Normal impedance falls in the range of 300–1800 ohms. Large changes in lead impedance (which can be set up as an alert) suggest a lead problem (lead fracture, insulation damage)
S	Sensing	Sensing verifies that the pacemaker can see intrinsic cardiac signals. This can be done automatically; the programmer will report P-wave and R-wave amplitudes. The test can also be done semiautomatically where the sensitivity setting is increased in small steps until sensing is lost
T	Threshold	This is absolutely the most crucial step in the whole sequence!
		There may be automatic or semiautomatic methods of assessing capture, but in order to run the test, you must have consistent pacing. If the patient does not have consistent pacing, you may have to change some settings for the test. Using temporary programming, decrease the base rate (for single-chamber systems or the atrial channel of a dual-chamber pacemaker) or shorten the AV delay (for the ventricular channel of dual-chamber pacemakers)
		Be cautious about this test as some patients do not tolerate even a brief loss of capture well
		Note that capture is not the point at which you lose capture but the lowest value at which you consistently show capture
O	Observations	From the interrogation screen, review the observations or alerts that have been reported since the last follow-up (see **Figure 24.1**). Download reports or stored electrograms associated with these observations. At this point, you may also want to download other counters, histograms, or trends
P	Programming	At this point, all of the necessary tests are done and the relevant diagnostic data have been downloaded and assessed. For most patients, the follow-up confirms that all is well. For a subset of patients, changes are appropriate, such as adjustments to the pacing output pulse (pulse amplitude and pulse width) for capture issues and sensitivity for sensing issues or adjustments to rate, AV delays, refractory periods, lead polarity, or special features (see **Figure 24.3**). Once these adjustments are made on the programmer, then these should be saved; they go into effect when the *program* button is pressed. Only a physician should make or supervise permanent changes to pacing parameter settings

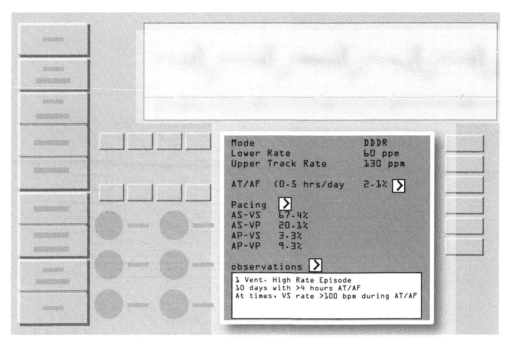

Figure 24.1 In the first step of follow-up, briefly compare the patient's presenting rhythm to the pacing states recorded since the last follow-up. Verify that the mode and rate are appropriate and reflected in the tracing. In this case, the patient is paced only about one-third of the time. Note if the screen calls attention to any unusual events (called observations or alerts) that should be reviewed in detail in the observation step of the systematic follow-up.

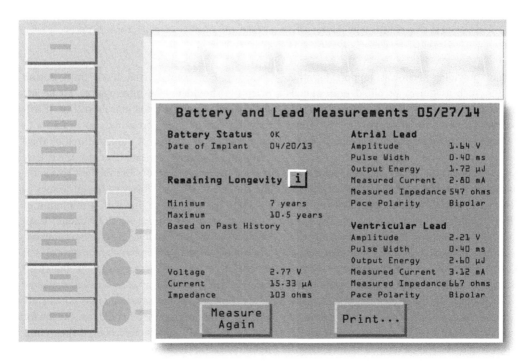

Figure 24.2 Battery status is available from the programmer and, fortunately, will estimate battery service life. The challenge in predicting battery longevity is that it changes based on how frequently the pacemaker paces and at what outputs—things that change over time. Thus, this programmer provides service life in a range, basing its calculations on how the patient has been paced to date.

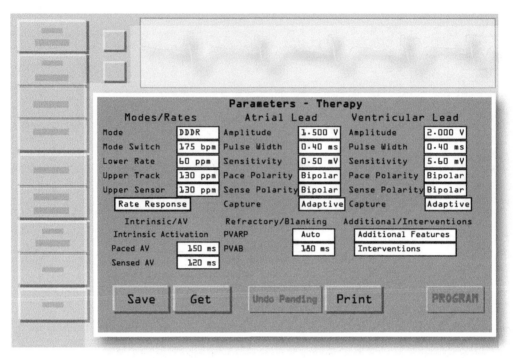

Figure 24.3 Permanent changes to parameter settings is the final step in systematic follow-up and should be done by a physician or under a physician's supervision. The main parameter changes are conveniently grouped together on one programmer screen. Values can be scrolled up or down. Note that the programmer will not allow the programming of incompatible features (such as rates that conflict with each other). Many features are automated, for example, this device is programmed to an automatic algorithm for adjusting PVARP. While clinicians can program such values manually, automatic features save time and, for the right patients, may enhance safety.

with and providing technical support to other clinicians, such as nurses or allied professionals who practice *incident to* the responsible party (the physician). However, the presence of an IEAP does not change requirements of this allied professional to work under physician supervision.

An IEAP is—as the name tells you—employed by industry. If an IEAP provides services to the patient, for example, conducting a follow-up visit, the IEAP cannot bill for those services. The IEAP cannot bill the patient or the clinic or anyone else; the IEAP is employed by industry. The physician or clinic may bill for the services they provide with the assistance of an IEAP, so in the case of the IEAP-conducted follow-up, the doctor may bill Medicare. Note that if the clinic bills Medicare for a follow-up, the physician must have been involved in that follow-up (even if he or she did not actually touch the programmer).

One last word of caution: an IEAP should work only on the equipment manufactured by his or her company. For example, the IEAP from Boston Scientific should not be interrogating Medtronic pacemakers. In real-world clinical practice, IEAPs may be asked, even pressured, to work with equipment other than that manufactured by their company. It cannot be said that no IEAP ever crossed the line—some do. But the best advice for the IEAP is to stick as closely to the guidelines as possible. In order to do this with a minimum of problems from the clinic, the IEAP should learn the specific rules and policies of his or her company. Then, when asked by the physician or clinical staff to operate a competitive programmer, the IEAP can say, "I'm sorry, but my company will not allow it. My company's policy says that I may not operate a competitive programmer. I could lose my job for that." If all IEAPs consistently obeyed their company's rules, no clinic would expect IEAPs to bend the rules. Following this rule, even if the clinic is disappointed, will help you maintain the highest standards of clinical care, preserve your professional integrity, and keep you on the right side of any legal issues that could come up—plus they also show a respect for your employer.

Naturally, there is one exception in the guidelines to the rule that an IEAP can only operate equipment from his or her own company. Let's say an IEAP is called into an implantation procedure for a patient who is having a competitive device replaced. It is important for the implant procedure that the physician know how the indwelling competitive device is programmed. In such a case, the IEAP—under physician supervision—can interrogate the device and retrieve the programmed parameter settings. This specific and limited scenario is considered acceptable under the guidelines.

Conclusion

Follow-up is one of the *constants* of any pacemaker clinic and clinicians need to be aware of how important this seemingly routine chore can be. Follow-up may be conducted by TTM, by RM, or in clinic. There are pros and cons to all three methods, but nothing can replace the in-clinic visit, which should be conducted at least annually. Pacemaker guidelines allow physicians to reimburse for one follow-up every 3 months; these may be done remotely or in clinic but one face-to-face visit should be conducted every year. It is the patient's responsibility to come for follow-up, but the physician bears a secondary responsibility so clinics try to avoid having patients *lost to follow-up* although this inevitably happens to a subset of patients for any number of reasons. Of course, patients also have the right to refuse follow-up. The IEAP often assists during follow-up and implantation but his or her presence is outlined in the guidelines and is likely also governed by company-specific rules. An IEAP should only come to the clinic by invitation of the physician and work under the physician's supervision and in his or her close proximity. The IEAP plays a crucial role in today's device clinic.

The nuts and bolts of pacemaker follow-up

- With millions of pacemaker patients around the world and follow-up recommended at least annually (but as much as four times a year), pacemaker follow-up is a major activity at the pacemaker clinic.
- There are three main types of follow-up: transtelephonic monitoring (TTM), remote monitoring (RM), and the old-fashioned in-clinic face-to-face checkup. The in-clinic visit should be done at least once a year, but the other follow-ups may be replaced with TTM or RM.
- TTM may be thought of as one of the first forms of telemedicine. It is still used today, although with RM and fewer and fewer land-line phones, it is becoming less popular. TTM transmits a paced and magnet mode ECG via a landline phone to a receiver station at the clinic.
- RM transmits diagnostic data and parameter settings (a complete device interrogation) over the Internet to a secure website. RM can be set up to obtain and transmit daily. The clinician then accesses a secure server to download the information. RM offers programmable *alerts* that can notify clinicians about important events.
- The wireless RM system from Biotronik is called CardioMessenger. It operates a little differently in that it transmits signals using the cell phone network.
- An in-clinic visit allows the follow-up to also examine the patient. Follow-up should ideally be about more than the device. It should also be about the patient, the underlying disease, and how the device and patient are interacting.
- Electronic medical records are making more and more pacemaker clinics paperless. Clinicians should still be careful to document their findings. Most pacemakers cannot download diagnostic data directly into patient records, at least at the time this book was written; diagnostic data must be downloaded from

Continued

Continued

the pacemaker and then uploaded to medical records.

- Follow-up frequency is governed by guidelines and, in the USA, by what CMS will reimburse through Medicare. Reimbursement for pacemaker follow-up is available within 72 hours of implant and 2–12 weeks postimplant (in clinic), every 3–12 months (in clinic or RM), and every 1–3 months at signs of battery depletion (in clinic or RM).
- Many factors govern how often the device should be followed, including the patient's condition and health, the age of the device (older devices should be followed more closely), changes in the patient's medicines, upcoming or recent procedures, and even psychosocial factors.
- When considering whether to use TTM, RM, or in-clinic visits, there are many factors to consider: the guidelines and reimbursements, the patient's preferences, the clinic's preferences and capabilities, and the patient's condition.
- A good rule of thumb is that a pacemaker patient can be followed every 3 months with three RM visits and one in-clinic visit a year.
- For some patients, in-clinic visits represent a hardship either because they live far from the clinic, they have limited mobility, it is hard for them to get a ride, or they are frail. RM has been a great boon to such patients.
- Some patients will refuse RM even though it is a convenient and efficient way to monitor their devices. They typically either dislike technological *gadgets* or they suspect it will somehow compromise their privacy.

- A patient is *lost to follow-up* when a patient fails to return for scheduled follow-ups. The patient is ultimately responsible for his or her own care, but the physician and clinic are secondarily responsible. Clinics will try to find these patients, but some will never come in for follow-up. There may be many reasons for this. Some reasons are legitimate: patients may move, find a new doctor, or enter a long-term care facility, and simply not bother notifying the doctor. Some patients are haphazard about keeping follow-up appointments. The patient has the legal right to refuse follow-up, but this is not a wise decision.
- Many programmers automate or semiautomate follow-up. The main steps include downloading programmed parameter settings, estimating battery voltage, evaluating magnet rate, testing pacing and sensing thresholds, measuring lead impedance, and checking diagnostics, including percentage of pacing/sensing in each chamber, stored electrograms, histograms and trends, and a review of device alerts.
- The industry-employed allied professional (IEAP) may help clinics with follow-up but there are rules that govern and define what they can do. IEAPs must be invited by the physician and work under physician supervision; they can only work on products or programmers from the company that employs them. The IEAP may attend implant but should not enter the sterile field (unless the IEAP happens to have privileges at that hospital). IEAPs play a large and growing role in the management of device patients.

Test your knowledge

1 TTM uses a telephone landline to transmit what two things?

A A paced ECG and programmed parameters

B A paced ECG and a magnet mode ECG

C Programmed parameters and stored electrograms

D Diagnostic data and impedance values

2 RM uses the Internet to transmit what kind of information?

A Real-time ECGs and electrograms

B Programmed parameters, diagnostic data, stored electrograms

C A paced ECG and impedance values

D A list of alerts with time codes

3 Which of the following would be a good
example for an *alert* for RM?

  A Episode of atrial fibrillation.

  B Activation of rest rate.

  C Lead impedance values are unchanged and in
normal range.

  D Rate response is on.

4 Alerts can be programmed by priority (triage)
and sent to the physician and other clinicians.
How are they sent?

  A Someone from a call center telephones the
doctor.

  B A letter is sent to the clinic and the patient.

  C The clinic can select text, email, or fax.

  D They are not sent out; the clinic must log in to
the server to pick them up.

5 Mrs. Houghton is a stable patient with a DDDR
pacemaker that is 3 years old. What is the
maximum number of pacemaker follow-ups a
year that would be reimbursed for her in the
USA?

  A 1

  B 2

  C 3

  D 4

6 Mrs. Houghton (above) hates coming to the
clinic. What is the minimum recommended
number of in-clinic follow-ups that she must
have in a year to stay within the guidelines?

  A 1

  B 2

  C 3

  D 4

7 Which items below would *not* be a
consideration to alter the frequency of
follow-up?

  A The patient has become demented and
cannot reliably report symptoms.

  B The patient is 72 years old.

  C The patient was just diagnosed with cancer
and may be undergoing therapeutic radiation treatments.

  D The device is 9 years old.

8 Which two people are most responsible in a
situation where the patient is *lost to
follow-up*?

  A The patient and the nurse

  B The patient and his or her spouse

  C The patient and the doctor

  D The patient and the IEAP

9 An IEAP may assist and perform valuable
services at a pacemaker clinic. What one
condition must be met for the IEAP to assist
at a clinic or hospital?

  A The IEAP must be a PA or MD.

  B The IEAP must hold a state license.

  C The IEAP must be invited by the physician
and work under the physician's supervision.

  D The IEAP must be bonded.

10 An IEAP has conducted a follow-up for a
dual-chamber pacemaker patient under the
supervision of the patient's physician. This
follow-up is reimbursable by Medicare. Who
can charge Medicare for the follow-up?

  A The physician

  B The IEAP

  C The IEAP's employer

  D None of the above

Reference

1 Wilkoff, B.L., Auricchio, A., Brugada, J. *et al.* (2008) HRS/
EHRA Expert Consensus on the Monitoring of
Cardiovascular Implantable Electronic Devices (CIEDs):
description of techniques, indications, personnel, frequency, and ethical considerations. *Europace*, **10**, 707–725.

CHAPTER 25

Follow-up and troubleshooting

Learning objectives

- Name the three principles behind pacemaker troubleshooting.
- List the invasive and noninvasive ways of identifying the cause of an issue.
- Define magnet mode and how it might be helpful in troubleshooting.
- Name three noninvasive *tools* for troubleshooting pacemakers.
- State several corrective actions and how they might be applied.

is human nature to overreact to things you do not understand. Thus, when a clinician on the night shift notices a pacemaker pacing at a rate other than the programmed base rate, there can be an urgent call to the physician. These calls usually get delegated to other clinicians. In some cases, you may be able to ask that the rhythm strip be faxed or emailed to you—since many of these *unusual behaviors* are actually perfectly appropriate. In some cases, the clinician may be able to troubleshoot by phone (reassuring the hospital that the pacemaker is behaving appropriately) or know definitively if there is a real problem that must be addressed in person.

Introduction

Unlike the previous chapter, this chapter is going to focus on what clinicians actually do during follow-up. Today's follow-up routine has been automated and streamlined to the point that clinicians may only need to press a few buttons to conduct a full follow-up. Remote follow-up may just involve reviewing some reports. But the crucial aspect of follow-up is managing problems. When everything is working fine, follow-up is simply a verification that all is well. Most of the time, follow-up is routine. I call it the *well-baby check*. But there are times—important times—when follow-up uncovers a problem that the clinician must address. Follow-up and troubleshooting go hand in hand, so they are presented together in this chapter.

Clinicians are also called to the telemetry unit or the hospital when pacemakers exhibit unusual behavior. This usually happens in the middle of the night when the monitor technicians and clinical staff seem to have more time to watch monitors! It

Principles of troubleshooting

Troubleshooting is simply the term that is often used in pacemaker clinics to refer to addressing a device problem. Although troubleshooting can seem like a daunting task, breaking it down into its three main principles will make it easier:

1 Identify the issue.
2 Determine the cause.
3 Take corrective action.

Identify the issue

The routine steps in follow-up are actually designed to reveal any potential device problems, such as pacing problems (loss of capture, no output), sensing problems (undersensing, oversensing), and other abnormalities. The troubleshooter also has to look for what can be called a pseudomalfunction, that is, something that *looks wrong* but in reality is appropriate device behavior. Pseudomalfunctions

The Nuts and Bolts of Implantable Device Therapy Pacemakers, First Edition. Tom Kenny.
© 2015 John Wiley & Sons, Ltd. Published 2015 by John Wiley & Sons, Ltd.

are more common than you think! Of course, sometimes, a pseudomalfunction indicates that the device could be programmed more optimally for that patient.

Determine the cause

Many pacemaker issues have multiple causes. Take the fairly common problem of oversensing. This might be due to having a sensitivity setting that is too sensitive; it could be a lead problem or even a problem with the device; it might be caused by myopotentials or interference. Thus, once a problem can be identified, the troubleshooter has to figure out what is causing it.

The troubleshooter's tool box includes a variety of tools; the noninvasive tools are the ones that are used first and foremost. They include the surface ECG, pacemaker diagnostic data, stored electrograms, magnet mode behavior, and a chest X-ray. In evaluating the surface ECG, determine the patient's pacemaker mode and programmed rate. Measure out intervals; look for pacing spikes, capture, sensing, and the patient's underlying rhythm. It is best to develop a systematic approach to tackling an ECG, but the exact sequence of the steps is not as important as that the clinician evaluates all aspects (mode, rates, intervals, timing, capture, sensing, underlying rhythm) thoroughly. In some cases, it may be helpful to use a multilead ECG.

If the clinician has access to the intracardiac electrograms, these should be reviewed as well along with annotations or markers. Remember that the electrogram is what the pacemaker *sees* and the annotations are what the pacemaker *thinks*. This should match up with the surface ECG. If there is a discrepancy, the ECG wins in terms of *what actually happened*. Thus, if you see a surface ECG with a lot of pauses but an intracardiac ECG showing sensed ventricular events at the same time, the *pauses* are the reality, but the ventricular sensed events are what the pacemaker *thought* was going on (oversensing).

Magnet mode is an important tool in pacemaker follow-up and troubleshooting. Just as a review, when a magnet is applied over a device, the pacemaker enters *magnet mode*. This causes the device to change over to asynchronous pacing, that is, it

temporarily disables the sensing function. For a VVI pacemaker, magnet mode is VOO; for a DDD pacemaker, magnet mode is DOO. Because magnet mode causes asynchronous pacing, magnet mode confirms device output and will allow the clinician to evaluate capture. The rate of magnet mode asynchronous pacing can be used to estimate device longevity; many devices will pace asynchronously at faster or slower rates as the device nears its end of service. The specifics of magnet mode can also identify the device manufacturer. For example, magnet mode in a Medtronic pacemaker at the beginning of life involves asynchronous pacing at 85 ppm. St. Jude Medical's magnet mode rate at the beginning of life is 98.6 ppm.

A potential lead problem is suggested by large and sudden changes (up or down) in lead impedance values and/or inappropriate pacing and sensing behavior (intermittent or continuous). To verify appropriate lead position and lead connection, a chest X-ray can be helpful. Chest X-rays are another useful noninvasive tool for troubleshooting lead problems. However, most clinicians and IEAPs would not be the ones to order or interpret the X-rays; that is the doctor's role. Lead position and lead connection are fairly easy to evaluate on an X-ray, but lead integrity can be extremely difficult if not downright impossible to see on an X-ray. Lead integrity issues might be nicks or cuts to the insulation or damage to the conductor coil. An X-ray can also reveal false-positives in lead integrity; the suture sleeve or other abnormalities may look like insulation breaches. This does not mean that an X-ray should not be ordered if a lead integrity problem is suspected—they may help. Overall, X-rays are good at indicating what might be the problem: lead fracture, lead dislodgement, and loose lead connections. But an X-ray is not helpful in ruling those same problems out; just because the lead connection looks fine on X-ray does not mean that there is no problem there. Likewise, the lead may not look fractured, but there may be a fracture present.

The pacemaker contains a wealth of diagnostic data that can be used to help troubleshoot pacing problems. These include everything from intracardiac electrograms with annotations to event markers, histograms, event counters, and trends. The clinician can also access real-time telemetry. Whenever possible, activate the intracardiac electrogram with markers along with the ECG. Do not hesitate to use all of the tools and shortcuts at your disposal!

One item in the troubleshooter's toolkit is often overlooked—the patient. When troubleshooting pacemaker problems, ask the patient about:
- Changes in status
- Changes in how they feel
- Limitations in their everyday activity
- New medications and discontinued medications
- New over-the-counter drugs or supplements
- Procedures and surgeries
- Hospitalizations
- MRI scans

Changes in the patient's condition and routine can be reflected in unusual or possibly abnormal pacemaker behavior. For example, a new drug may elevate the patient's capture threshold and cause intermittent loss of capture. That is technically not a *device problem*; it's the result of a changed threshold. Some procedures or an MRI can damage the device. (The exception to this is Medtronic, which offers an *MRI-safe* pacemaker. Other companies are developing or have developed *MRI-conditional* pacemakers, which may undergo MRIs under certain conditions.)

The skillful pacemaker troubleshooter knows a lot about probability. The fact is that there are certain pacemaker problems that occur more commonly than others and clinicians should try to explore these *probable* causes before digging into very unusual scenarios. One of these *usual suspects* is myopotential oversensing. Myopotential oversensing shows up on an ECG as a pause—the pacemaker stops pacing. The cause is that noise from the muscles of the body is being sensed by the pacemaker and inappropriately interpreted as sensed ventricular events, causing the pacemaker to inhibit the ventricular output pulse. Myopotential oversensing is fairly common and it typically occurs with muscle movement, like big gestures or arm movements. If a clinician sees pauses, his or her first thought should be that it is oversensing and it may very well be related to myopotentials. Sharp and abrupt changes in lead impedance suggest a lead problem. *Overpacing* (a term I made up) suggests that the device is not sensing all of the cardiac signals it should and sensitivity should be adjusted. Fusion and pseudofusion are not really serious

problems at all but can be resolved by adjusting timing; these are timing problems rather than capture problems. Frequent mode switch episodes suggest that the patient has prolonged periods of atrial fibrillation or AF; the pacemaker cannot actually address that but the physician may wish to treat the AF pharmacologically or with an intervention.

Sometimes, the troubleshooter must play the role of a detective. Take the patient who experiences dizziness when he uses his electric shaver. It happens every time he tries to shave. The troubleshooter has identified the problem (oversensing) but not its cause. Is the pacemaker sensing the electric shaver or is it myopotential oversensing from the patient's arm movements? To get to the bottom of the problem, the clinician can have the patient simulate the arm movements of shaving and monitor the device to see if myopotentials are to blame. It may be useful to have the patient bring in the shaver and see if holding the shaver near the patient (without arm movements) causes the problem.

Take corrective action

The first step in troubleshooting is to identify the problem. There may be several options on how to go about correcting the problem:

Reprogram the pacemaker   Some pacemaker problems can be addressed by changing output settings (loss of capture), adjusting sensitivity settings (oversensing, undersensing), or changing special features (such as turning off rate response in the patient with rate-related angina).

Replace the hardware   Problems to the pulse generator itself (such as damage to the CMOS during therapeutic radiation treatments) or to the lead (such as lead fracture or insulation breaks) may require replacement. This necessitates a surgical procedure to replace the lead(s) and/or pulse generator.

Reposition the lead.   If the lead is malpositioned, a surgical procedure may be able to properly position it. No lead replacement is required.

Reconnect the lead   If there is a loose connection between the lead(s) and the pulse generator, it may be possible to tighten that connection without replacing any hardware. This must be done surgically.

Repair the lead   Although in rare instances, physicians may seek to repair an indwelling lead, it is generally better just to remove a damaged lead and replace it with a new one.

Counsel the patient   Myopotential noise can be a difficult problem to address because making the device too insensitive (which fixes the myopotential noise problem) may cause the pacemaker to undersense (and introduces a new problem). If a patient only has myopotential noise in very specific, very limited situations (such as reaching overhead), the patient can be counseled to avoid that movement. By the same token, other problems, such electromagnetic interference, may be most effectively solved by avoidance.

Conclusion

Pacemaker troubleshooting involves dealing with problems that are either raised by the patient (symptoms, signs) or revealed during follow-up or both. The pacemaker clinician must first identify and define the problem, determine its cause, and then select a corrective action. Not all pacemaker problems are easy to solve. Some problems—such as myopotential oversensing—may be treated by asking the patient to avoid certain movements. Other problems may require surgical revision to tighten a loose lead connection or replace a damaged pulse generator. Many programs can be handled by programming fixes, which is a fast, easy, noninvasive solution. Most pacemaker follow-ups simply confirm that the device is working well, but when troubleshooting is necessary, the pacing clinician will benefit greatly from this systematic three-step approach (identify problem, determine cause, correct).

The nuts and bolts of pacemaker follow-up and troubleshooting

- The best approach to pacemaker troubleshooting involves these three principles: identify the issue, determine the cause, and take corrective action. When tackling difficult pacing challenges, clinicians can stay on course by remembering effective troubleshooting is simply answering three questions: What is the issue? What is the cause? How can this be corrected?

- Clinicians have many noninvasive tools for troubleshooting: the surface ECG, pacemaker diagnostic data, stored electrograms, and magnet mode behavior are at the top of the list. A chest X-ray may be a useful and noninvasive device for checking on potential lead issues (lead connection problems, lead position, and lead integrity—although it can be difficult to verify lead integrity on an X-ray).

- Magnet mode ECGs are an old-fashioned but useful tool. Magnet mode converts the device to asynchronous pacing (no sensing), so that VVI becomes VOO mode and DDD becomes DOO mode. The forced pacing allows for the evaluation of appropriate output and capture. The rate of the magnet mode indicates battery status and for experienced clinicians can even tip them off as to the device manufacturer (for

instance, magnet mode at 98.6 ppm is St. Jude Medical while magnet mode at 85 ppm is Medtronic).

- Rapid and substantial changes in lead impedance values (up or down, in or out of specification) suggest potential lead problems. These should be checked by chest X-ray. Lead problems may require surgical intervention to correct.

- Troubleshooters at a programmer should always access the paced ECG and the intra-cardiac electrogram with markers. The markers reveal what the pacemaker is *thinking* and the intracardiac electrogram shows what the pacemaker is *seeing*. This should align with the surface ECG—but there may be a *disconnect* that can lead to pacing problems. Typical for this kind of problem is oversensing or undersensing.

- Sometimes, a device develops issues after the patient has done something that may have damaged the device, such as undergone therapeutic radiation, had an MRI, or undergone some other types of procedure. A great troubleshooter tool is the detailed patient interview. Many patients are unaware that other medical procedures can affect their pacemakers

Continued

Continued

and may not think to report them unless specifically asked.

- Changes in the patient's condition, health, activities of everyday life, and pharmacological regimen can affect how the patient and device interact. For instance, a new medication might raise the patient's capture threshold and result in intermittent loss of capture. This is not the device's fault—it is the result of programmed output values that are no longer sufficient.
- Sometimes, a troubleshooter is called to address what might best be called a pseudomalfunction. This is something unusual on the paced ECG that is actually the normal and expected behavior of the device. For instance, when pacemaker Wenckebach occurs, some clinicians may report this to the pacemaker clinic, feeling that it is a device malfunction when,

actually, it is the expected behavior of the device in a given situation. Pseudomalfunctions are also reported for fused beats and pacing at rates other than the base rate.

- Troubleshooting also involves knowing probabilities. There are many common pacemaker problems and it is a good idea to explore them as first potential causes rather than try to track down some obscure cause.
- Corrective actions basically fall into six main categories: reprogram the pacemaker, replace the hardware (lead and/or pacemaker), reposition the lead, reconnect the lead, repair the lead, and counsel the patient. Repair the lead is not usually an effective solution. Patient counseling refers to situations where it is most effective if the patient simply avoids certain activities or environments.

Test your knowledge

1 Mr. Sanders has a DDDR pacemaker and is hospitalized for a knee replacement. While in the hospital, the orthopedic unit notices that he experiences periodic PMTs that go away. The orthopedic nurse calls the pacemaker clinic to report this activity as a device malfunction. What is the issue?
   A Inappropriate high-rate activity.
   B Oversensing.
   C Mode switching is not working.
   D This is a pseudomalfunction.

2 Mr. Bowman is a symptomatic VVIR pacemaker patient; his ECG shows lots of pauses with the device not delivering output pulses. Identify the issue.
   A Oversensing
   B Undersensing
   C Loss of capture
   D Lead problem

3 Mr. Elliott has a DDDR patient and is experiencing intermittent loss of capture. Lead impedance values are in the normal range and have not changed significantly in the past year. His lifestyle is the same but he has recently added some new

medications. What is the most probable cause of this issue?
   A Ventricular sensitivity is too sensitive (mV setting is too low).
   B The output parameters are too low.
   C Myopotential interference.
   D The lead is not securely connected to the device header.

4 Mrs. Garrison has a DDD pacemaker. She has had trouble-free device operation for almost a decade but suddenly reports frequent and unpleasant symptoms. Evaluation shows that her device has intermittently stopped delivering output pulses. From the ECG, it is clear that this is not oversensing; it is failure to output. Battery life shows the device is not at the elective replacement indicator and could last another year or two. What information do you need from Mrs. Garrison?
   A Ask if she has been to a region where certain fungal infections are common.
   B Ask if she has recently had an MRI or surgical procedure.
   C Ask if she takes beta-blockers.
   D Ask if she has changed her everyday routine activities.

5 The identified issue is undersensing, caused by inappropriate device programming. What is the corrective action?

A Reprogram the device.

B Replace the device.

C Counsel the patient.

D All of the above.

6 The doctor received an alert that impedance values suddenly increased by over 300 ohms, strongly suggesting a lead problem. The patient was quickly brought into the clinic and reported no symptoms. Downloading the diagnostics showed a recent spell of intermittent loss of capture and intermittent undersensing. What is the logical next step for the doctor?

A Replace the device.

B Call the manufacturer's technical support line.

C Order a chest X-ray.

D Reprogram the device settings.

7 If a patient is known to have a damaged lead, what can be done?

A The damaged lead can be left in place (but abandoned) and a new lead added.

B The damaged lead can be repaired.

C The damaged lead can be removed and a new lead added.

D Any of the above.

8 A new DDDR pacemaker patient has intermittent loss of capture and alternating oversensing and undersensing. A chest X-ray determined that her lead is intact but it is not properly positioned in the ventricle. What is the corrective action?

A Surgery to reposition the lead.

B The device can be reprogrammed to compensate for this problem.

C Surgery to replace the lead.

D No corrective action is required.

9 Which of the following is *the most difficult* to verify on a chest X-ray?

A Lead connection to the pacemaker header

B Lead position in the ventricle or atrium

C Pulse generator position

D Lead integrity (no insulation breaches or conductor fracture)

10 What should be considered if a pacemaker patient must undergo therapeutic radiation?

A The high doses of radiation may damage the pulse generator.

B The radiation therapy may reprogram the pacemaker to odd settings.

C The radiation therapy can overheat the lead tip.

D Radiation can erase the pulse generator's diagnostic counters.

Answer key

Chapter 01

1 B
2 B
3 A
4 D
5 D
6 C
7 D
8 A
9 C
10 A

Chapter 02

1 D
2 A
3 B
4 A
5 D
6 C
7 C
8 C
9 A
10 D

Chapters 03

1 B
2 C
3 A
4 C
5 D

6 A
7 C
8 C
9 D
10 C

Chapters 04

1 B
2 D
3 A
4 C
5 A
6 C
7 D
8 A
9 C
10 B

Chapter 05

1 B
2 A
3 C
4 D
5 A
6 C
7 C
8 A
9 D
10 B

The Nuts and Bolts of Implantable Device Therapy Pacemakers, First Edition. Tom Kenny.
© 2015 John Wiley & Sons, Ltd. Published 2015 by John Wiley & Sons, Ltd.

Chapter 06

1 A
2 D
3 B
4 B
5 A
6 A
7 C
8 B
9 D
10 B

Chapter 07

1 B
2 C
3 C
4 A
5 B
6 C
7 C
8 A
9 C
10 A

Chapter 08

1 A
2 B
3 D
4 B
5 B
6 D
7 A
8 C
9 B
10 A

Chapter 09

1 B
2 B
3 A
4 D
5 C
6 C
7 C
8 B
9 D
10 B

Chapter 10

1 D
2 A
3 B
4 A
5 D
6 C
7 D
8 A
9 B
10 B

Chapter 11

1 C
2 C
3 A
4 B
5 C
6 C
7 B
8 A
9 D
10 A

Chapter 12

1 A
2 C
3 A
4 D
5 B
6 B
7 A
8 C
9 B
10 D

Chapter 13

1 C
2 D
3 A
4 A
5 D
6 A
7 C
8 B
9 D
10 A

Chapter 14

1 D
2 C
3 B
4 B
5 B
6 A
7 C
8 D
9 D
10 A

Chapter 15

1 B
2 C
3 D
4 A
5 B
6 C
7 B
8 C
9 A
10 A

Chapter 16

1 B
2 D
3 A
4 D
5 C
6 B
7 A
8 C
9 B
10 D

Chapter 17

1 A
2 D
3 C
4 A
5 C
6 C
7 D

8 A
9 B
10 A

Chapter 18

1 B
2 C
3 B
4 D
5 C
6 A
7 C
8 D
9 D
10 B

Chapter 19

1 A
2 A
3 D
4 B
5 C
6 B
7 C
8 B
9 C
10 B

Chapter 20

1 C
2 A
3 B
4 C
5 C
6 A
7 B
8 D
9 B
10 C

Chapter 21

1 B
2 C
3 C
4 D

5 A
6 D
7 B
8 D
9 B
10 A

Chapter 22

1 B
2 D
3 A
4 A
5 C
6 D
7 C
8 B
9 A
10 A

Chapter 23

1 B
2 C
3 A
4 A
5 C
6 A
7 B

8 B
9 C
10 A

Chapter 24

1 B
2 B
3 A
4 C
5 D
6 A
7 B
8 C
9 C
10 A

Chapter 25

1 D
2 A
3 B
4 B
5 A
6 C
7 D
8 A
9 D
10 A

Index

The Nuts and Bolts of Implantable Device Therapy Pacemakers, First Edition. Tom Kenny.
© 2015 John Wiley & Sons, Ltd. Published 2015 by John Wiley & Sons, Ltd.

Printed and bound by CPI Group (UK) Ltd, Croydon, CR0 4YY

09/06/2025

14686004-0001

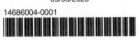